Sensor Networks and Systems for Healthcare Applications

Sensor Networks and Systems for Healthcare Applications

Editor: Karly Lundberg

FOSTER ACADEMICS

www.fosteracademics.com

www.fosteracademics.com

FOSTER ACADEMICS

Cataloging-in-Publication Data

Sensor networks and systems for healthcare applications / edited by Karly Lundberg.
p. cm.
Includes bibliographical references and index.
ISBN 978-1-64646-599-6
1. Biosensors. 2. Medical informatics. 3. Medical care--Data processing. 4. Medical care--Technological innovations. 5. Biomedical engineering. 6. Medical innovations. 7. Wireless communication systems in medical care. 8. Telecommunication in medicine. I. Lundberg, Karly.
R857.B54 S46 2023
610.28--dc23

Foster Academics,
118-35 Queens Blvd., Suite 400,
Forest Hills, NY 11375, USA

ISBN 978-1-64646-599-6 (Hardback)

Contents

Preface

Every book is initially just a concept; it takes months of research and hard work to give it the final shape in which the readers receive it. In its early stages, this book also went through rigorous reviewing. The notable contributions made by experts from across the globe were first molded into patterned chapters and then arranged in a sensibly sequential manner to bring out the best results.

Sensor networks and systems provide smart and efficient solutions for healthcare systems. Sensor networks are vital tools to understand the health of human beings. Some of the different types of sensors are ECG patches, wearable spirometers, and hemodynamic/pressure monitoring devices. A network of connected devices is created when a person wears two or more sensors at one time, which is known as body area network. These networks can gather physiological signals through many sites, calculate vital health metrics, and transfer data on the cloud. Wearable sensors consist of a wide range of applications that help in health monitoring and fitness tracking. They play a major role in developing a connected personal healthcare system. These sensor networks and systems are also helpful in preparing disease management plans for healthcare organizations monitoring patient health. This book strives to provide a fair idea about sensor networks and systems to help develop a better understanding of their healthcare applications. It will serve as a reference to a broad spectrum of readers.

It has been my immense pleasure to be a part of this project and to contribute my years of learning in such a meaningful form. I would like to take this opportunity to thank all the people who have been associated with the completion of this book at any step.

Editor

1

Double-Diamond Model-Based Orientation Guidance in Wearable Human–Machine Navigation Systems for Blind and Visually Impaired People

Xiaochen Zhang [1], Hui Zhang [1], Linyue Zhang [2], Yi Zhu [1,3] and Fei Hu [1,*]

[1] Department of Industrial Design, Guangdong University of Technology, Guangzhou 510006, China; xzhang@gdut.edu.cn (X.Z.); zhanghui2018@mail2.gdut.edu.cn (H.Z.); zhuyi@gdut.edu.cn or zhuyi@gatech.edu (Y.Z.)

[2] School of Communication and Design, Sun Yat-Sen University, Guangzhou 510275, China; zhlyue@mail3.sysu.edu.cn

[3] School of Industrial Design, Georgia Institute of Technology, Atlanta, GA 30332, USA

* Correspondence: hufei@gdut.edu.cn

Abstract: This paper presents the analysis and design of a new, wearable orientation guidance device in modern travel aid systems for blind and visually impaired people. The four-stage double-diamond design model was applied in the design process to achieve human-centric innovation and to ensure technical feasibility and economic viability. Consequently, a sliding tactile feedback wristband was designed and prototyped. Furthermore, a Bezier curve-based adaptive path planner is proposed to guarantee collision-free planned motion. Proof-of-concept experiments on both virtual and real-world scenarios are conducted. The evaluation results confirmed the efficiency and feasibility of the design and imply the design's remarkable potential in spatial perception rehabilitation.

Keywords: tactile feedback; navigation aids; user-centric design; double diamond; blind and visually impaired people

1. Introduction

The World Health Organization factsheet stated that there are approximately 217 million people suffering from moderate to severe visual impairment, with 36 million blind people worldwide [1,2]. Compared to normally sighted people, they have difficulties in accessing visual cues in daily surroundings.

Obviously, blind and visually impaired (BVI) people have a strong dependency on travel aids, tools, and advanced systems [3]. Fortunately, advances in robotics, computer vision, geographic information systems (GISs), and multimodal sensory technology allow for modern smart systems to perform mapping, positioning, and decision-making while users navigate through urban areas [4].

Conventional travel aids for BVI, including white canes, guide dogs, and volunteers, have their intrinsic restrictions [5]. Modern assistive solutions borrow power from mobile computing, robotics, and autonomous technology to overcome these restrictions, as well as to empower new capabilities such as representing the external world digitally in hybrid human–machine systems [5,6].

According to References [7–9], numerous systems are capable of understanding the features of surroundings efficiently and effectively by taking advantage of various onboard sensors and intelligence decision-making advances, especially for travel scenarios. However, most of the studies treated the human–machine system as a conventional mobile robotics system, e.g., using waypoint-based path planning and discrete instructions [5]. The lack of focus on human-centric issues in innovations brings about an insurmountable gap between human and machine cognition [6].

Specifically, BVI people prefer continuous guidance to discrete guidance, so that they retain the tracking of steering instructions at will. They prefer smooth guidance to interruptive coded instructions, so that they do not have to pause to understand the guidance before proceeding. To enhance the readability of this paper, we use the term "continuous" to indicate that the instructions are continuously readable, with clear one-to-one correspondence with the corresponding physical meaning at any time, the term "smooth" to indicate that the reading and perception of guidance instructions are not interruptive and are burden-less, so that people do not have to suspend their current action to understand the guidance instructions.

Moreover, the capability of guidance following is also a part of human spatial cognition. A series of studies by Mosers, winner of the 2014 Nobel Prize in medicine, found that the ability of a moving person to roam in space depends on how much they know about the scene [10]. By consciously imagining and perceiving spatial position and orientation, BVI people may obtain a certain degree of situation awareness and spatial cognition in navigation [11]. Successful design and application of an orientation guidance system may potentially aid training programs for spatial perception rehabilitation.

In this work, we propose a new design of a sliding tactile feedback wristband that guides orientation for BVI navigation systems. The design process is based on the double-diamond design model, with a clear, comprehensive, and visual description of the design thinking process. After the four-phase design process, a design aiming to resolve the numerous limitations of current state-of-the-art solutions is proposed. A Bezier curve-based path planning is proposed to guarantee collision-free path planning. The proof-of-concept prototype is evaluated with blindfolded and BVI volunteers. Proof-of-concept experiments on both virtual and real-world scenarios are conducted. The evaluation results confirm the efficiency and feasibility of the design and imply its potential in applications of spatial perception rehabilitation.

The contributions of this work are manifold. Firstly, it is the first hand-free tool that provides "smooth" and "continuous" sliding tactile orientation guidance for BVI pedestrians. Secondly, it successfully applies the double-diamond design model to address the numerous limitations of existing acoustic and vibration orientation guidance solutions. Thirdly, the experiments in a virtual test field and real test field imply the potential of the designed wristband and testbed in spatial perception rehabilitation applications. Fourthly, a proof-of-concept prototype was produced, which was demonstrated to be functionally capable, portable, and affordable.

The rest of the paper is organized as follows: Section 2 reviews relevant related works. Section 3 presents the details of the design using a double-diamond design model. Section 4 presents the experiments and results. Section 5 presents the discussion regarding the design and experiment. Section 6 summarizes the work.

2. Related Works

2.1. Smart Travel Aids for BVI People

Recent advances in sensor technology and artificial intelligence supported the design and development of smart travel aids for BVI people. Katz [12] designed an assistive device that aids BVI people in multi-scale object identification and route planning. Zhang [13] proposed a hybrid-assistive system using both stereo sensors and a web camera to localize BVI users on pre-built maps. Ahmetovic [14] designed a waypoint-based BVI navigation system that takes advantage of previously deployed wireless beacons in positioning. Remarkably, Bing [15] used a sparse-mapping-based Project Tango Tablet with no extra sensor to guide BVI users. Zhu [16] proposed and implemented the ASSIST (Assistive Sensor Solution for Independent and Safe Travel) system on a Project Tango smartphone that helps BVI users navigate indoors. To date, many researchers and scientists made efforts to deliver affordable high-tech travel aids for BVI users [17]. Benefiting from the rapid development of artificial intelligence and autonomous driving [18], the localization, mapping, and navigation technology for smart travel aids are developing rapidly and promisingly day by day.

Nevertheless, most of the existing devices were only tested in laboratory scenarios [19–22]. One of the core reasons is that the current human–machine interaction-based cooperative perceptions are asynchronized and insufficient. In other words, humans and machines each have their own perception in tasks. If humans and machines could simultaneously share and understand their perceptions, the difficulty in applying human–machine system in the real world would be limited. However, the fact is that humans take time and effort to understand real-time machine perception, while machines can only feed a limited portion of their perceptions to humans.

Enlighted by the hierarchy of decision-making processes in self-driving urban vehicles [23], we considered planning-related decision-making of BVI navigation systems in three layers, as shown in Figure 1. The top layer plans the waypoint-based raw path for BVI pedestrian, a procedure similar to autonomous mobile robots. The middle layer generates behavior and motion plans assuming that the reference trajectory can be carried out by BVI users. The bottom layer aims to guarantee that the reference trajectory can be followed or an equivalent goal can be reached via human–machine interactions. Our work contributes to the bottom action control layer.

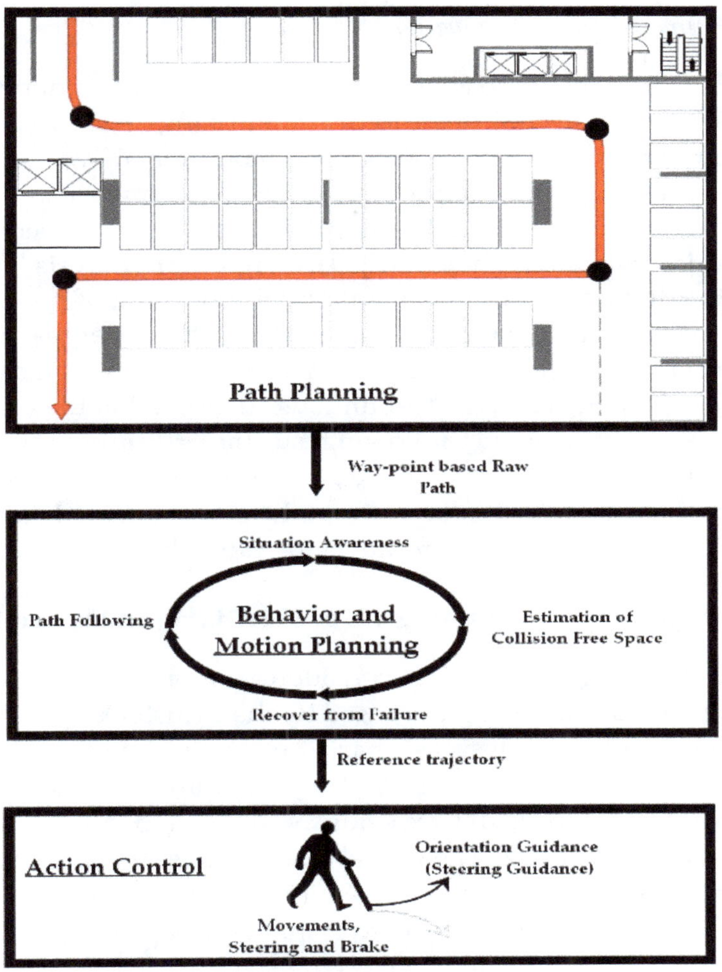

Figure 1. A three-layer planning-related decision-making structure for blind and visually impaired (BVI) navigation systems.

2.2. Human–Machine Interaction and Multimodal Feedback for Orientation Guidance

Most BVI travel aids use auditory and tactile interactions in human–machine systems [22]. Shah [24] used a handheld array of actuators to convey complex meaning via various vibrations. Rizvi [25] presented a simple navigation aid for BVI people using a buzzer and haptic feedback to deliver obstacle alerts. Sohl-Dickstein [26] used stereo sound to provide spatial information. Meanwhile,

Bai [27] proposed a lightweight glasses-mountable device to aid BVI people using guiding sounds. Patil [28] designed NavGuide, an electronic aid using vibration and audio to provide simplified high-priority surrounding information. Amemiya [29] proposed a pseudo-attraction haptic direction indicator, but the device was handheld and bulky. Kaushalya developed "AKSHI" system [30], which verbally guides the BVI user to avoid obstacles. Cardillo [31] used vibration and acoustic signals to indicate the objects of interest in navigation. Although significant progress took place, there is still a nonnegligible deficiency in feedback mechanisms in the action control layer. There are two major issues. Firstly, the capabilities of fulfilling descriptive guidance instructions differ from BVI user to user. In practice, they cannot acquire sufficient guidance from discrete instructions to adjust their actions in each action period, e.g., steering and movements. Secondly, it is unsatisfactory for BVI users to spend much time and effort on perceiving the instructions, especially for coded guidance instructions. Most state-of-art works are insufficient in one of the above two issues in the action layer, while they pay more attention to the path-planning, behavior, and motion-planning layers. Therefore, a continuous and smooth action control layer guidance mechanism is highly worthwhile.

2.3. Design Thinking in Human-Centric Innovations

Design thinking is a methodology to achieve human-centric innovation while ensuring technical feasibility and economic viability [32,33]. Instead of emphasizing objective technic-centric evaluation criteria, design thinking treats the innovative design as a comprehensive and iterative human-centric problem-solving process. Throughout the process, several different design science approaches are proposed and applied to explore and fill the gap between human needs and implementations. In addition to conventional stakeholder analysis [34], competitor analysis [35,36], the British Design Council [37] proposed the double-diamond design model consisting of problem and solution spaces. This model allows for a systematic design analysis with double diverge–converge phases to find a feasible solution. The attempted "continuous" and "smooth" solutions of this work are coincident with Nielsen usability heuristics [38]. Specifically, "continuous" denotes that the system should always keep users informed about the status of guidance following, i.e., the principle of "visibility of system status". It also allows a timely adjustment of orientation, i.e., the principle of "error prevention". On the other hand, "smooth" denotes that the instructions do not take much time to learn, read, and understand, i.e., the principle of "recognition rather than recall" and "flexibility and efficiency of use".

3. Design of BVI Orientation Guidance Using a Double-Diamond Design Model

The double-diamond design model [37] is considered among the most efficient and convincing design thinking process models since being proposed by the British Design Organization in 2005. The model entails emphasis on problem analysis as a basis for creating solutions for clients, and it presents four main stages across two adjacent diamonds. The two diamonds are the problem and solution spaces. In each space, a diverging phase that expends the space is followed by a converging phase that narrows the space, as shown in Figure 2. The model distinguishes itself from others by systematically splitting the human-centric design into two successive diverging–converging phases. To synthesize the design opportunity and contact points gathered from the need-finding stage, insights and primary design goals are formulated in the following converging stage. Then, the collection of user and expert feedback after ideating and modeling in the idea implementation stage allows converging to a final solution in the finalization stage [33]. The process is highly couplable with user-centric usability design principles such as visibility of system status, match between system and the real world, user control and freedom, flexibility, and efficiency of use [39]. Moreover, the four stages are termed discovery, define, develop, and deliver [37].

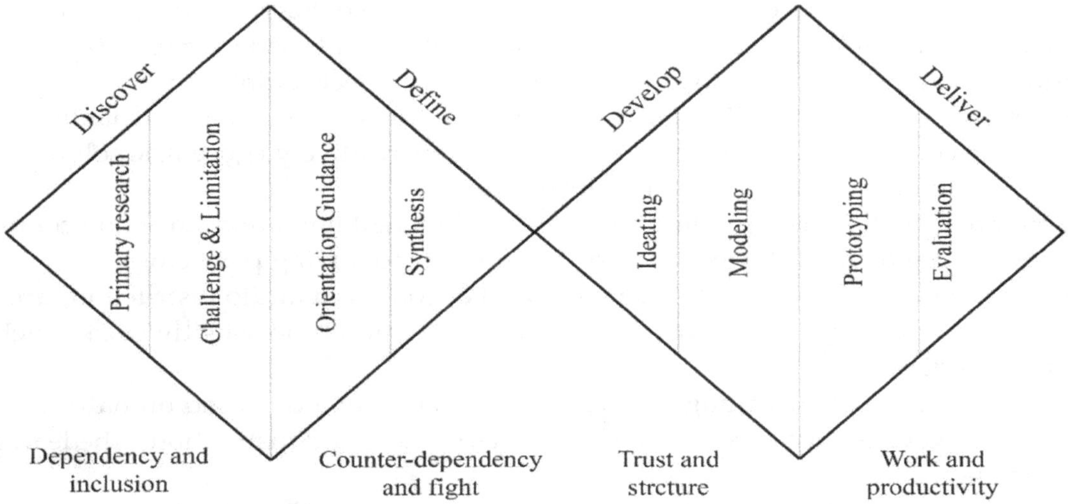

Figure 2. The four-stage double-diamond design model.

3.1. *Discover Stage*

3.1.1. Primary Research Goal

There is a consensus that BVI users' quality of life would be significantly improved by smart travel aids that take advantage of scientific advances and service innovations [4]. In this work, we consider human–machine navigation systems which are capable of performing localization, path and motion planning, and motion action guidance. Currently, technology for localization and planning is significantly improved due to the rapid development of automatous robots and self-driving vehicles [40]; however, the progress of autonomous systems is by no means an equivalent bonus for BVI human–machine systems since there is a lack of adequate human–machine cooperative perception support. Among the numerous human–machine cooperative perception issues in BVI travel aids, orientation guidance is one of the most important since it determines whether the motions planned by the machine can be properly carried out by humans in real time.

Researchers [15,41,42] reported the significance of acquiring augmented localization information by perceiving and processing the surrounding spatial information via multimodal perception in BVI navigation. Joseph [43] stated that the acquired augmented localization information significantly supports the motion planning and navigation of autonomous robots and commercial self-driving vehicles. However, these achievements are still in the machine perception stage instead of synchronized human–machine cognition. Consequently, BVI human–machine systems are theoretically useful but only partially meet the requirements of application; they lack a suitable bridge to convey the knowledge and decisions of machines to BVI people especially in the action controls. A better bridging tool or service that conveys navigation-related knowledge and guidance from the machine to the BVI user needs to be designed [3].

3.1.2. Challenges and Limitations of Existing Work

According to Bujacz and Balan [44,45], acoustics is the most suitable channel to deliver long-term path-planning knowledge since the other candidate interaction channels may not be able to deliver much knowledge of rich data in a timely manner with a certain degree of ambiguity. However, when it comes to the planning details in the action control layer, there are different designs.

Most existing designs rely on acoustic feedback [27,46–48]. Well-formulated verbal instructions of motion cues are the most popular, while other studies either used frequency modulation-based three-dimensional (3D) acoustic signals or composed a mixed symphony (or noise) to guide BVI people.

Another widely accepted opinion is that tactile-based feedback is qualified to dominate the motion-related feedback in BVI navigation. For instance, vibration-based interactions are used to imply further motion actions and alerts for upcoming obstacles or objects of interests.

Moreover, lots of recent studies provided combinations of acoustic and tactile feedback for guidance in action control [15,22]. Their integration delivers relatively egocentric solutions that seek a balance between cognition loads and explicit instructions.

As a matter of fact, the existing solutions have their inherent limitations in action control planning. Firstly, designs relying on acoustic feedback suffer from the following problems:

Inevitable information delivery latency. The delivery and decoding of audio instructions are not instant. In most cases, the verbal commands are not suitable for reaction time-sensitive tasks such as motion and orientation guidance.

Excessive learning burden. The learning burden for verbal commands based on natural languages is not significant. However, when it comes to frequency-based sound instructions, the learning burden becomes immense.

Difference between descriptive instructions and executive actions. Acoustic instructions deliver descriptive instructions with a certain degree of ambiguity. This limitation results from the inherent low capacity of the linear acoustic transmission channel; complete semantics are composed only after a certain period of communication.

None-multiplexing channel. In most cases, it is not recommended that the channel is shared by more than one communication task. The interference between independent signals is serious and inevitable. Moreover, the length of communication time is proportional to the information capacity. Since hearing is the most important sensory receiver for BVI people in daily life, the non-multiplexing property makes the hearing channel more precious.

Results-oriented instructions. The instructions aim to accomplish short-term and medium-term goals, i.e., they are results-oriented, which makes guidance during a detailed action insufficient.

Meanwhile, the existing tactile feedback-based designs have the following limitations:

Discrete guidance on continuous motion tasks. Most of the solutions use three to five vibration units to indicate the approximate orientation. Combinations of vibrations allow the BVI user to find clues of motion guidance. Nonetheless, this is contradictory to the continuous nature of dynamics and motion in navigation.

Instructions are prone to be misperceived. Firstly, depending on the tactile perception of the specified user, the combination of vibrations might be perceived quite differently. Secondly, the partial misbehaviors of vibration units are difficult to be self-diagnosed during operation.

Raw ergonomic user experience. The frequent vibration makes navigation annoying. Moreover, it tends to shorten the device's life span.

Despite fusing the merits of the acoustic and tactile mechanisms, the existing integrated designs have the following flaws:

Waypoint finding-based routing and motion planning are not human-friendly. The waypoint finding-based planning is perfect for autonomous robots, but it is not reasonable to expect that BVI users could follow the planned track as well as robots.

Discrete guidance on continuous motion tasks. Existing designs combining acoustic and tactile feedback do not resolve the problem of discrete guidance and, thus, guessing of BVI users plays an important role in navigation. Consequently, the sense of reliability and security of BVI users significantly suffers.

Raw ergonomic user experience. For action control, the acoustics are essential but difficult to follow. For better adoption of designs, the essential vibrations must be improved or replaced.

Bulky. Although the volume and complexity of sensory composition is not a scientific problem, it significantly influences the usability and the device's potential adoption. According to References [3,40], a number of recent studies compensated for capability with bulk. This also led to higher prices and lower robustness in most cases, which prevents the future commercial versions from being widely adopted by price-sensitive BVI users.

3.2. *Define Stage*

After refining the research and design challenges, it was concluded that there is a grand demand of feasible action control mechanisms and guidance devices.

3.2.1. Orientation Guidance in a BVI Human–Machine System

Following insights by Long [49,50], in this work, we define orientation as the knowledge of one's direction relative to egocentric frames and the ability to keep track of the spatial relationships in motion. Orientation guidance is provided by a certain device or service through multimodal feedback or interaction. The goal is to allow BVI users to access orientation-related information or cues to support decisions and actions in real time.

3.2.2. Synthesis Design Opportunities

Human body tactile sensitivity map

According to Zeagler [51], tactile feedback may be used to support BVI navigation. For orientation guidance at the action control level, tactile stimuli can be mapped onto an azimuth egocentric frame, which is, hence, a primary choice. As shown in Figure 3, a body tactile sensitivity map must be considered while choosing a wearable design (data were taken from Reference [51]). Specifically, the two-point discrimination sensitivity test finds the distance needed to distinguish two compass points simultaneously applied to the skin [52]. In most cases, the two-point discrimination map reflects the reaction sensitivity of the skin.

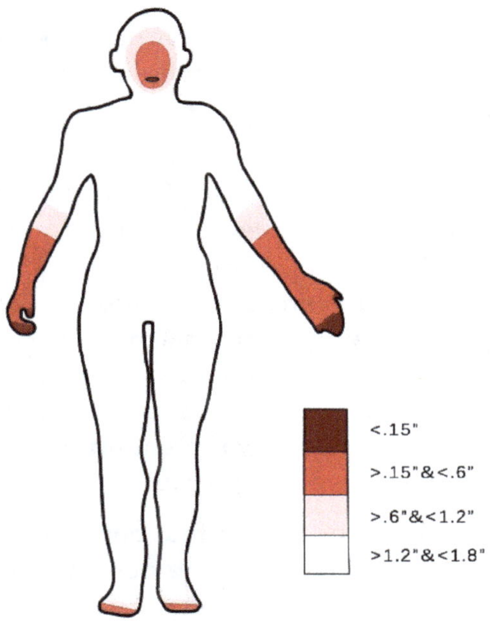

Figure 3. Average distance in two-point discrimination sensitivity test on body locations; data were taken from the associated website of Reference [51].

BVI human–machine systems

For any orientation guidance module, the human–machine navigation system must have a supporting main system. By considering applicability and functionality, we chose the ARCore-based navigation system [53] as the main system providing extra sensors, power, and multimodal interactions.

Spatial perception rehabilitation for BVI

Schinazi and Majerova's study [54,55] indicated that BVI people face difficulties in spatial perception and imagination, especially in performing dead reckoning in strange places. An advanced level of design seeks an orientation guidance that provides a convenient way to train and strengthen the spatial perception of BVI people.

3.3. Develop Stage

Usability and adoptability are the basis of product design. Usability design focuses on product functionality. Nielsen divided it into five evaluation dimensions: learnability, memorability, efficiency, fault tolerance, and user satisfaction [56]. Hartson analyzed usability from the two levels of usefulness and ease of use [57]. The international standard ISO-9241 (International Organization for Standardization-9241) defines it as "the effectiveness, efficiency, and satisfaction of a particular user in achieving a particular goal in a particular scenario" [58]. Like developments in industrial design, usability-oriented product design cannot fully fulfill demands; meanwhile, the multi-dimensional experience-oriented design is highly reputed. Experience design is especially concerned with the subjective feelings that products bring to users. Tom Wood believes that experience design is a design practice that focuses on both process and outcome, specifically the relevance of experience to user needs and context.

In navigation, orientation guidance cooperates with cognitive modules such as sensory distance directors, computer visual cognition modules, anchor-based re-localization modules, and radio frequency positioning modules to guide movements. As an essential component of the cooperative cognition in human–machine systems, orientation guidance is supposed to be concisely developed under specified conditions that fit the demands of BVI navigation.

According to the tactile sensitivity body map in Figure 3, designs are chosen to be attached to the hand or forearm [29], foot [59], or tongue [60]. Moreover, the design improves the limitations of existing studies presented above.

Tactile feedback is delivered in real time to guide the BVI user, which means that the perception of feedback should be as simple as possible to ease the burden of perceiving feedback. A polar steering style is preferred since it can be projected onto egocentric azimuth orientation maps. The sliding tactile feedback is chosen to instruct upcoming motion directions continuously. Meanwhile, one specific direction is clearly presented at any given time. This also guarantees clear and reliable orientation cues. Making the instructions simple and matching human natural instincts and habits are important to lessen the learning burden and the possibility of misunderstanding. More importantly, the straightforward steering style makes the navigation pleasant instead of annoying. Since the guidance is no longer discrete, the path planning is free from waypoint finding. This simple yet efficient feedback style also allows the design to be inexpensive and portable.

Based on the above conceptual ideation, two independent designs were derived. To avoid distraction, the non-essential steps and procedures are described only briefly. The first design is a guidance glove that works on palms and is sensitive to pressure, as shown in Figure 4. The sliding pressure contactor driven by a steering gear is applied to indicate orientation guidance. A coordination projection between the palm and egocentric frame is applied, whereby a scaled-down virtual user standing on the palm of a left hand is facing toward the middle finger of the palm. The real-time contactor's pointing direction indicates the suggested direction for forthcoming movements.

Typical application scenarios of the guidance glove are shown in Figure 5. The cognitive translation from tactile feedback to egocentric spatial perception is intuitive, which alleviates the burdens associated with learning and perception.

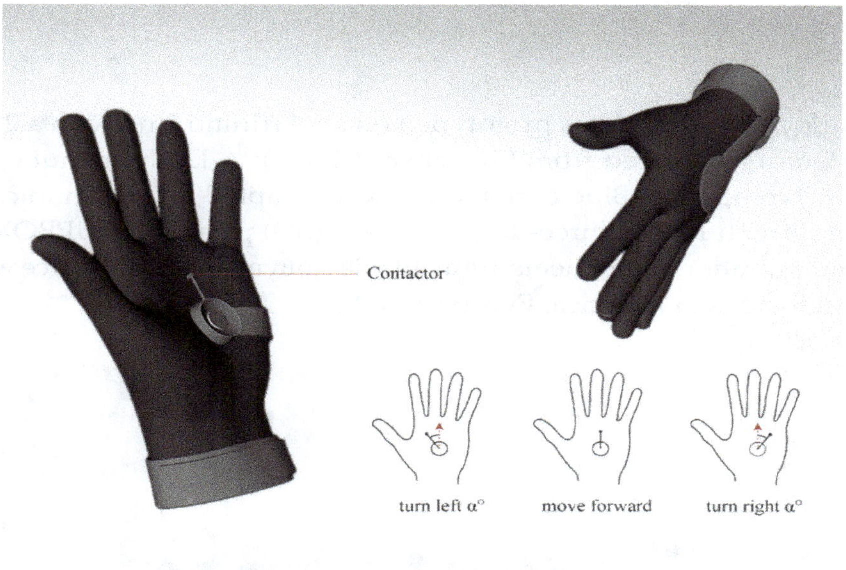

Figure 4. The design concept of the guidance glove.

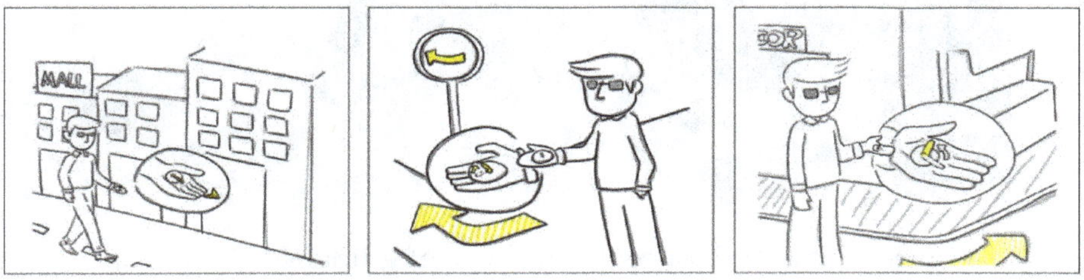

Figure 5. Typical application scenarios of guidance glove.

The second design is a guidance wristband that uses a steering-style pressure contactor on the wrists to indicate the instructed motion direction to BVI users, as shown in Figure 6. A coordination projection between the wrist frame and egocentric frame is applied, whereby a scaled-down virtual user is standing on the wrist of a left hand, and the egocentric frame and the wristband frame are coincident. The real-time contactor's pointing direction indicates the suggested direction for upcoming movements.

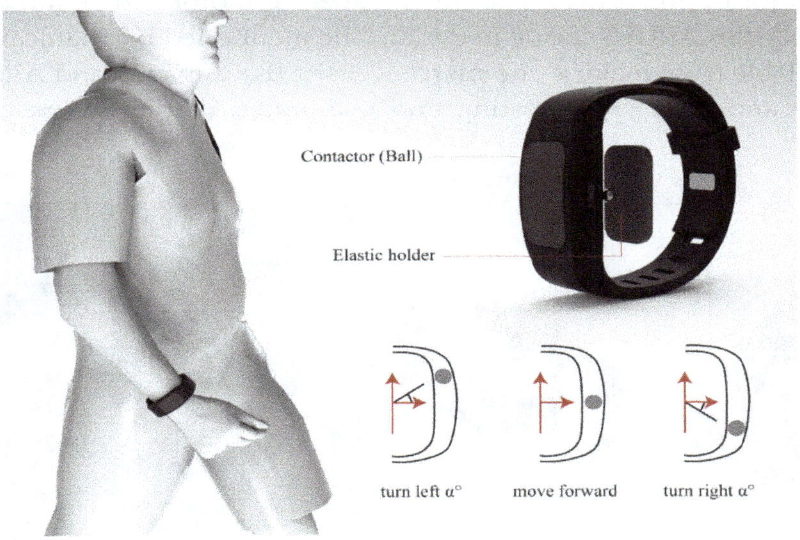

Figure 6. The design concept of the guidance wristband.

3.4. *Deliver Stage*

3.4.1. Prototyping

The guidance glove (Figure 7) was prototyped on an Arduino Uno with a 28BYJ-48 step motor manufactured by (Quason, sourced from Shenzhen, China.) A Dofly manufactured HC-05 MCU (Microcontroller Unit) compatible Bluetooth module was adapted for communication, and the main body supporting the structure was three-dimensionally (3D) printed by UPBOX+. The mentioned mechanical and communication components are available from major e-commerce website like Amazon and Alibaba, in most regions in America, Europe and Asia.

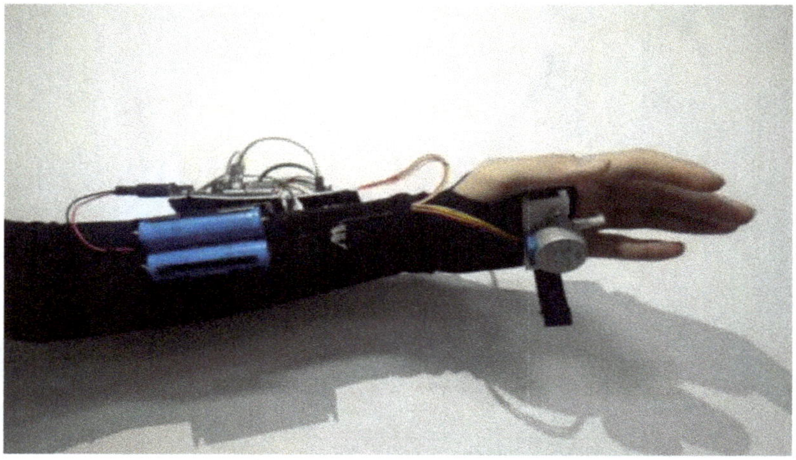

Figure 7. Proof of concept prototype of guidance glove [53].

This prototype was tested with four blindfolded and four BVI volunteers; part of the development and testing was conducted in our previous study [53]. Compared with conventional vibration feedback, the guidance glove guides the user smoothly, and the sensing experience is natural and pleasant. However, according to the subjects, some features heavily impair the experience. Firstly, the device occupies the palm, which is essential for conducting daily activities. Secondly, the palm is not always flat, which results in inadequate contact between the contactor and the palm.

The guidance wristband (Figure 8) was prototyped on an Arduino Uno with either an SG90 standard steering motor or an AFRC D1015 linear steering motor. The main body was 3D printed by UPBOX+ with Poly-flex TPU95 elastic material. The mentioned mechanical and communication components are available from major e-commerce website like Amazon and Alibaba, in most regions in America, Europe and Asia. The testing and evaluation of the design are illustrated in the experimental section.

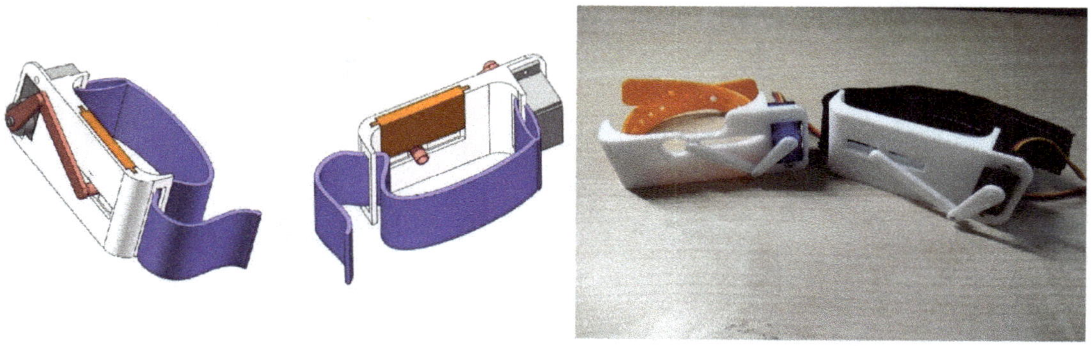

Figure 8. Proof-of-concept prototype of guidance wristband.

3.4.2. Bezier-Curve Based Planning

Continuous orientation guidance requires motion planning unlike that used in conventional waypoint finding mechanisms. Instead of seeking the shortest or most inexpensive solution, the planning pursues smooth and collision-free motions. The smoothness is generally expressed in terms of continuity [61], i.e., geometric continuity or parametric continuity. In this work, the smoothness is expressed by geometric continuity. To achieve geometric continuity of motion, we used a Bezier curve-based algorithm [62] to plan the guidance. A Bezier curve of degree n is defined as

$$P(t) = \sum_{i=0}^{n} B_i^n(t) P_i, \tag{1}$$

where P_i denotes the control points, and $B_i^n(t)$ is a Bernstein polynomial.

$$B_i^n(t) = \binom{n}{i} \left(\frac{t_1 - t}{t_1 - t_0}\right)^{n-i} \left(\frac{t - t_0}{t_1 - t_0}\right)^{i} \quad i \in \{0, 1, \ldots, n\}. \tag{2}$$

The paths generated by the Bezier curve have the following merits:

They always pass through the starting point P_0 and ending point P_k.

They are always tangent to the lines connecting consequential control point pairs.

They form curves to avoid the collision area surrounded by control points.

They form straight lines if there is no collision area.

The orientation guidance module aims to guide the BVI user according to the planned navigation path. In other words, given a predefined path, it makes efforts to generate sub-level path planning to follow the predefined path. In simpler terms, it guides the BVI user toward selected far-ahead points on the path.

Given a path H, the designed sub-level path begins from P_0 and ends at P_k, where $|P_0P_k| = \alpha{\cdot}r$, $P_k \in \mathrm{H}$, $\overrightarrow{P_0P_k}{\cdot}\overrightarrow{\mathrm{H}} > 0$. The purpose of the curve is to generate a path that avoids collision spaces C. It is easy to find an external point P_{ext} such that the hull defined by P_0P_{ext} and $P_{ext}P_k$ fully covers C. Taking Figure 9 as an example, to avoid collisions with C, a curve that connects P_0P_k is formed. As long as P_0P_{ext} and $P_{ext}P_k$ have no intersection point with C, a Bezier curve passing, P_0, P_{ext}, and P_k forms a trajectory that meets the requirements. To form the curve, the absent control point P_C can be calculated via

$$P_C = P_{ext} - \frac{1}{2}\sqrt{|P_0 - P_{ext}||P_k - P_{ext}|}\left[\frac{P_0 - P_{ext}}{|P_0 - P_{ext}|} + \frac{P_k - P_{ext}}{|P_k - P_{ext}|}\right]. \tag{3}$$

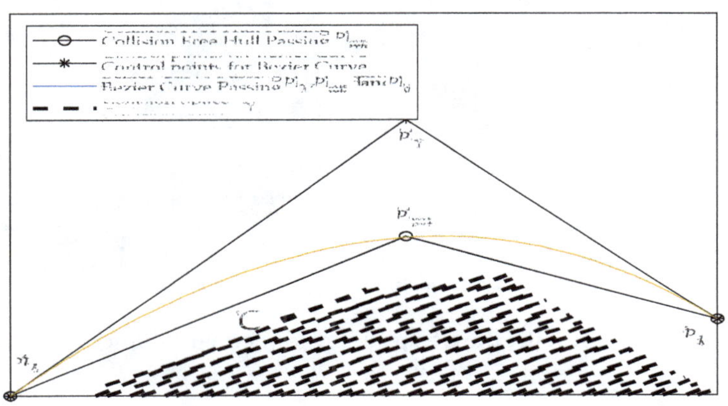

Figure 9. A Bezier curve passing P_0, P_{ext}, and P_k, defined by control points P_0, P_C, and P_k.

4. Experiment and Evaluation

4.1. Orientation Guidance Tests in Virtual Test-Fields

We designed a desktop testbed to observe participants' path-following behavior in virtual test-fields. In the test, the designed orientation guidance wristband was used to provides tactile feedback to the person under test, and a flight control game joystick (PXN-2113 Pro) was used for the participant to provide real-time feedback regarding perceived orientations. Virtual paths were generated on test-fields in Matlab, while a virtual character was placed at the given position of the test-field.

Four blindfolded volunteers (A, B, C, D) and four BVI volunteers (E, F, G, H) participated in the virtual field test. The participants all reported no irregularities with wrist and hand tactile perception. All of them were informed of the purpose of the test in advance, but none of them were aware of the details of the experiments before the tests. The research procedure and protocol obeyed the local human-related research ethics regulations.

In the test, a participant sat down in front of the testbed, wearing the proposed orientation guidance wristband on the left wrist. The joystick was held by the right hand, and the primary trigger button was under the control of the right index finger, as shown in Figure 10. The purpose of this set-up was to let the participant echo their perception regarding the orientation guidance introduced by the wristband. In the test, the real-time orientation guidance aiming to follow the pre-defined path was delivered to the participant via wristband, and the virtual character in the test field behaved as instructed by the joystick. A motion scaler that moderated the turning speed was arbitrarily set to 3%.

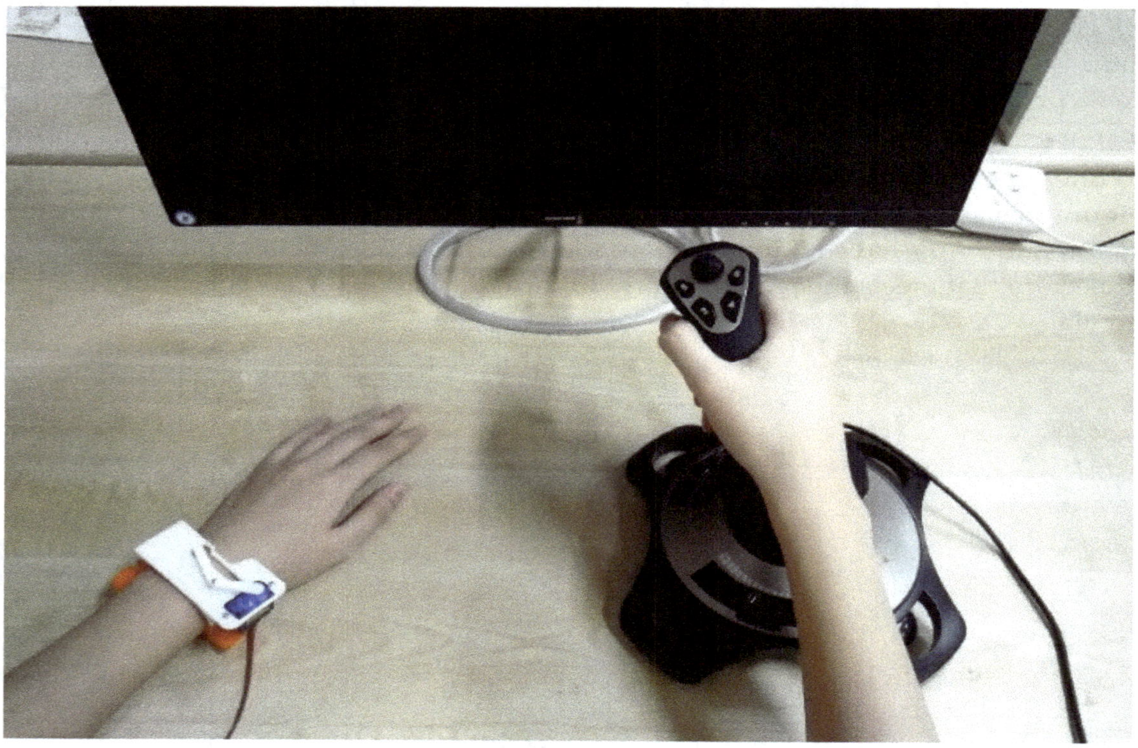

Figure 10. Virtual field test with the designed guidance wristband and feedback joystick.

A standard sinusoidal path was applied as the predefined path, as shown in Figure 11. Two sets of tests (test α and β) were launched accordingly. In test α, participants received 15 min of training in virtual fields before entering the task. In test β, participants received training and practice in virtual fields until they felt confident in guidance.

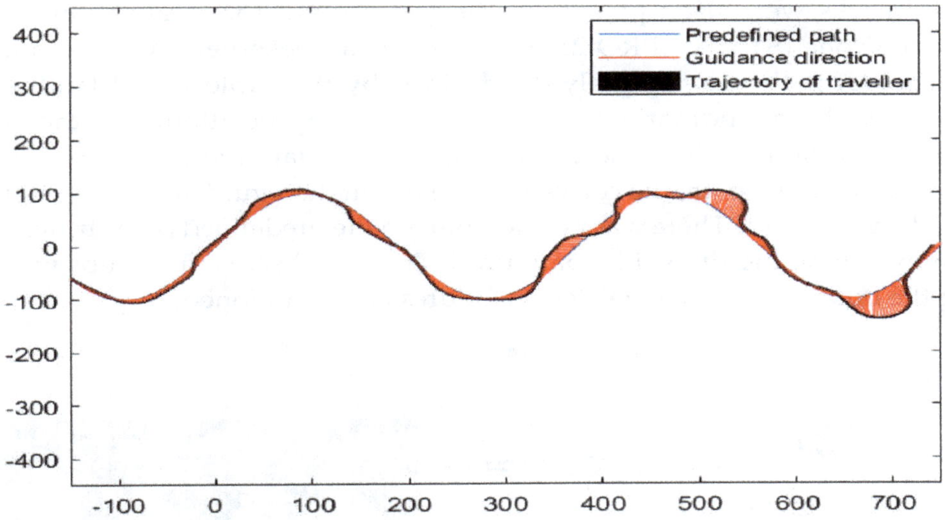

Figure 11. Predefined path, guiding force, and trajectory of traveler in virtual fields tests.

The displacements of participants to the predefined path were collected as shown in Figure 12. In test α, although the concept of following orientation guidance was simple, most participants were unable to steadily control the virtual character on the virtual test-fields by exclusively receiving orientation guidance from the designed wristband. One reason was that the controlled character always turned excessively, especially right after sharp turns. In the test, participant E reported that the sliding tactile feedback was difficult to perceive, causing a relatively larger displacement than other participants in test α. To deal with this, we adjusted the tightness of wristband. Thus, their displacement in test β was closer to the others. However, participant E reported an uncomfortable feeling after adjusting the tightness of the wristband. This phenomenon may have been caused by the diversity of each person's skin tactile sensitivities. In general, the displacements in test β were smaller than those in test α, indicating that a series of training and practice sessions allows participants to rapidly adapt to the guidance tools and rules.

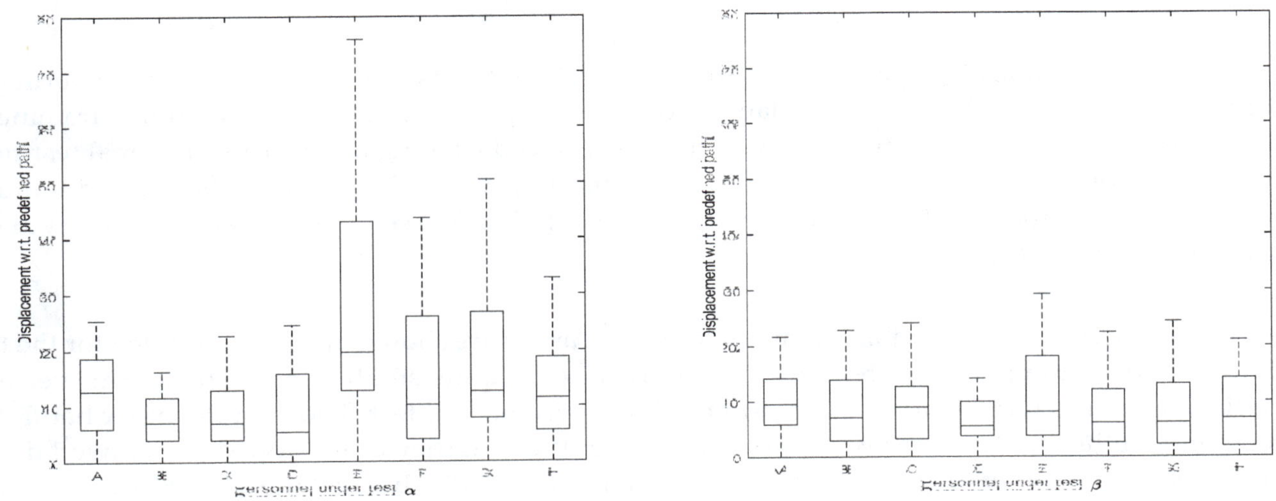

Figure 12. Displacement to predefined path in virtual field tests.

4.2. Orientation Guidance Tests in Real Test-Fields

To evaluate the design in practice, we conducted field tests in obstacle-free real test-fields In the experiment, the Arduino-driven tactile wristband was mounted on the left wrist of the participant to provide orientation guidance, a Bluetooth module was used to receive real-time guidance messages, triple visual landmarks were used placed on the test ground for localization purposes, and an overlooking mode drone (SYMA XPRO 25) was used as an observer. As shown in Figure 13, the pre-defined sinusoidal path was uniquely determined by the triple visual landmarks, where the mid-point of the dual blue landmarks was set as the starting position, and the amplitude of the sinusoidal path was equal to half of the distance between dual blue landmarks. By matching the participant's location with the path, the corresponding orientation guidance instruction was calculated and delivered to the wristband. There was no end point on the predefined path. Instead, the participant was guided to move along the sinusoidal path until 100 valid discrete data clips were collected. Test trials exceeding the boundary were regarded as failures and abandoned.

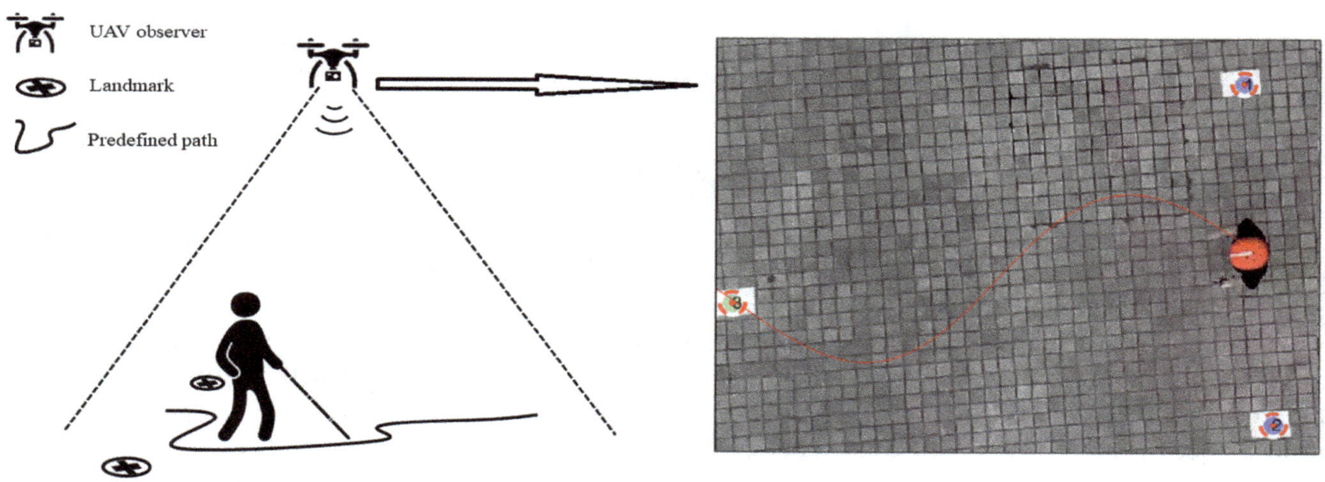

Figure 13. Field test scene. Left, an overlook mode unmanned aerial vehicle (UAV) is used to capture and transmit the positioning status of the participant and landmarks to the server to calculate the guiding direction. Right, the image from the UAV camera is shown, in addition to the auto-marked landmarks and the predefined path.

Note that the same eight participants in the virtual field tests took part in the field experiment. Three sets of tests (test γ, Δ, and θ) were launched. In test γ, participants received 15 min of training in a real test-field before the test. In test Δ, participants received training and practice in a real test-field until they felt confident. Test θ was conducted 24 h after test Δ, and the participants received training and practice in a virtual test-field until they felt confident. The five set of tests were conducted in the following sequence: α, γ, β, Δ, and θ.

The displacements of each participant in tests γ, Δ, and θ are shown in Figure 14. Even for the test without much training experience, the displacements were quite small. On one hand, this verified the efficiency of the wristband in orientation guidance in the real test-field. On the other hand, the participants in the real test-field were more careful. In the test, they often stopped or slowed down their movement for better orientation perception. Participant E still obtained the largest drift, implying that the personal skin tactile sensitivity features significantly influenced the adoption of the designed device. Apparently, after a short learning and practice period in real test-fields, the participants rapidly mastered the skill of following the guidance provided by the wristband. Test θ indicates that the training in virtual fields benefited participants using the wristband in real test-fields.

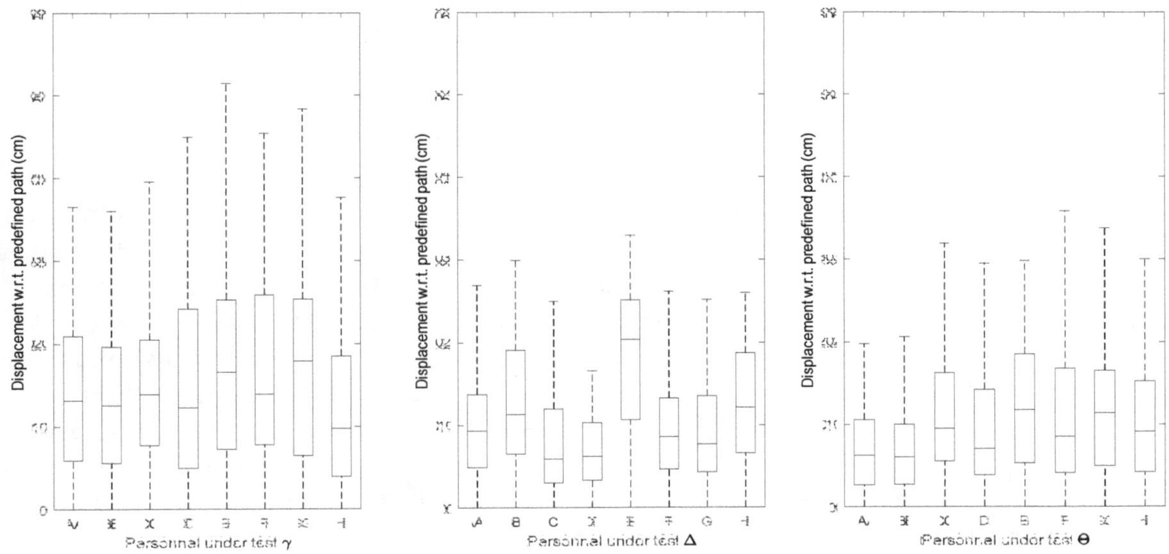

Figure 14. Displacement to predefined path in field tests.

5. Discussion

The advances of machine intelligence and sensor technology significantly expanded the imagination space of modern scientific services and rehabilitation therapy for BVI people. Currently, the multimodal representation of the external world in the absence of a primary sensory capability requires not only a theoretical contribution but also human-centric design thinking solutions.

5.1. The Design Thinking in BVI Navigation Systems

BVI human–machine systems require more than task-fulfilling execution. Some navigation tasks easy for robots may be challenging for BVI users. On one hand, the ability to maintain a stable body reference in egocentric tasks is challenging for BVI users. On the other hand, the inherent mental status, involving the feeling of safety, pride, comfort, and fear, may affect distinct human cognition and behaviors. The design thinking double-diamond model is human-centered, whereby the needs of humans and objective factors are the main determinants of its design and delivery. Simple yet efficient, the design of the wristband provides continuous and reliable instructions in navigation, while distributing the cognitive load from hearing to tactile.

5.2. Motion Behavior Style Differences between subjects in Virtual Test-Field and Real Test-Field

By observing the tests on virtual test-fields and real test-fields, we realized that the real motion behaviors of BVI pedestrians were quite different from those in virtual field tests. Firstly, the subject in virtual fields always moved forward, while the frontal orientation changed over time. In contrast, the BVI pedestrians in real test-fields moved with more freedom, whereby they did not have to turn before moving or keep moving forward. In other words, the well-adapted game motion styles may not perfectly represent pedestrian motion styles in the real world. However, this kind of motion style may suit BVI semi-automatic driving perfectly, e.g., a BVI user driving a semi-automatic electric scooter.

5.3. Adaptive Tactile Stimulation and Reactions

The skin tactile sensing capability varied, especially for the wristband sliding tactile pressure. In the test, the subjects reported losing track of touch to varying degrees with the guidance wristband contactor. Fortunately, by gently pressing down the surface of the wristband, they were capable to retrack the pressure from the wristband contactor, since the contactor was pressed toward the wrist skin. However, this is not a long-term solution. Thus, a vibration supplement might be added to enhance the contactor sensation. Moreover, by monitoring, recording, and learning from individual specifications regarding skin sensibility, a customized tactile stimulation mechanism would be helpful for assisting BVI users in travel. For example, users with more wrist fat tend to receive stronger tactile stimulation.

5.4. Orientation Finding and Spatial Perception Rehabilitation

The inner clock orientation exercise is the most popular orientation finding training method for BVI people. The proposed design of the wristband borrowed insight from spatial perception training, and it was developed to help enhance the capability of orientation finding in locomotion. In the experiments, we found that the blindfolded participants performed better than the BVI participants in virtual test-fields. One of the reasons is that the blind-folded participants had a similar experience when controlling virtual characters in video games. However, when it came to the real test-field, the performances of the blindfolded and BVI participants showed inconspicuous differences. The extensive training in virtual fields also benefited the experience in real test-fields, which implies that testing in a virtual scenario may potentially be a usefully tool in spatial perception rehabilitation.

6. Conclusions

In this work, we presented a novel orientation guidance design for a BVI navigation system. The design followed the double-diamond design model and achieved human-centric innovation while ensuring technical feasibility and economic viability. It provided continuous and smooth instructions via a sliding tactile sensor, to overcome the numerous limitations of existing acoustic and vibration orientation guidance solutions. We also presented a Bezier curve-based path-following algorithm to support the orientation guidance. To verify the efficiency, we prototyped and tested the design in both virtual test-fields and real test-fields. The results confirmed the efficiency of the design, and also implied that extensive training in a virtual test-field also benefits users in real test-fields. The testbed of the virtual field test may potentially be useful in the spatial perception rehabilitation of BVI people.

The prototyped design has an approximate weight of 50 g and a cost of about $2 United States dollars (USD) plus the wireless communication module. Such a lightweight and commercially affordable design has the potential to become a ubiquitous guiding accessory for general BVI smart navigation systems.

In future work, the restriction of the weak tactile stimulation will be resolved without negatively influencing the usability and user experience. Moreover, a comprehensive experimental user statistical study in a larger area and in a crowded urban area will be conducted to evaluate the capability of the orientation guidance tool and its impact on BVI people's daily life and behavior.

Author Contributions: Conceptualization, X.Z.; data curation, H.Z.; formal analysis, X.Z.; funding acquisition, F.H.; investigation, F.H.; methodology, Y.Z.; project administration, F.H.; software, H.Z. and L.Z.; validation, H.Z.; visualization, Y.Z.; writing—original draft, X.Z.; writing—review and editing, L.Z.

Acknowledgments: The authors would like to thank Jizhong Xiao, Yi Sun, Bing Li, and the anonymous reviewers for their insightful suggestions regarding this research. We thank LetPub for its linguistic assistance during the preparation of this manuscript.

References

1. Rra, B.; Flaxman, S.R.; Braithwaite, T.; Cicinelli, M.V.; Das, A.; Jonas, J.B.; Keeffe, J.; Kempen, J.H.; Leasher, J.; Limburg, H.J.L.G.H. Magnitude, temporal trends, and projections of the global prevalence of blindness and distance and near vision impairment: A systematic review and meta-analysis. *Lancet Glob. Health* **2017**, *5*, e888–e897.
2. World Health Organization. *Blindness and Vision Impairment*; WHO: Geneva, Switzerland, 2018.

3. Islam, M.M.; Sadi, M.S.; Zamli, K.Z.; Ahmed, M.M. Developing walking assistants for visually impaired people: A review. *IEEE Sens. J.* **2019**, *19*, 2814–2828. [CrossRef]
4. Bhowmick, A.; Hazarika, S.M. An insight into assistive technology for the visually impaired and blind people: State-of-the-art and future trends. *J. Multimodal User Interfaces* **2017**, *11*, 149–172. [CrossRef]
5. Kulkarni, A.; Wang, A.; Urbina, L.; Steinfeld, A.; Dias, B. Robotic assistance in indoor navigation for people who are blind. In Proceedings of the 11th ACM/IEEE International Conference on Human-Robot Interaction (HRI), Christchurch, New Zealand, 7–10 March 2016; pp. 461–462.
6. Pacaux-Lemoine, M.-P.; Trentesaux, D.; Rey, G.Z.; Millot, P. Designing intelligent manufacturing systems through Human-Machine Cooperation principles: A human-centered approach. *Comput. Ind. Eng.* **2017**, *111*, 581–595. [CrossRef]
7. Li, B.; Munoz, J.P.; Rong, X.; Xiao, J.; Tian, Y.; Arditi, A. ISANA: Wearable context-aware indoor assistive navigation with obstacle avoidance for the blind. In Proceedings of the European Conference on Computer Vision 2016, Amsterdam, The Netherlands, 8–10 and 15–16 October 2016; pp. 448–462.
8. Henry, P.; Krainin, M.; Herbst, E.; Ren, X.; Fox, D. RGB-D mapping: Using depth cameras for dense 3D modeling of indoor environments. In *Experimental Robotics*; Springer: Berlin/Heidelberg, Germany, 2014; pp. 477–491.
9. Guerreiro, J.; Ohn-Bar, E.; Ahmetovic, D.; Kitani, K.; Asakawa, C. How context and user behavior affect indoor navigation assistance for blind people. In Proceedings of the Internet of Accessible Things, Lion, France, 23–25 April 2018; p. 2.
10. Hafting, T.; Fyhn, M.; Molden, S.; Moser, M.-B.; Moser, E.I. Microstructure of a spatial map in the entorhinal cortex. *Nature* **2005**, *436*, 801. [CrossRef]
11. Pissaloux, E.; Velázquez, R. On Spatial Cognition and Mobility Strategies. In *Mobility of Visually Impaired People: Fundamentals and ICT Assistive Technologies*; Pissaloux, E., Velazquez, R., Eds.; Springer: Cham, Switzerland, 2018; pp. 137–166.
12. Katz, B.F.; Kammoun, S.; Parseihian, G.; Gutierrez, O.; Brilhault, A.; Auvray, M.; Truillet, P.; Denis, M.; Thorpe, S.; Jouffrais, C. NAVIG: Augmented reality guidance system for the visually impaired. *Virtual Real.* **2012**, *16*, 253–269. [CrossRef]
13. Zhang, X. A Wearable Indoor Navigation System with Context Based Decision Making for Visually Impaired. *Int. J. Adv. Robot. Autom.* **2016**, *1*, 1–11. [CrossRef]
14. Ahmetovic, D.; Gleason, C.; Kitani, K.M.; Takagi, H.; Asakawa, C. NavCog: Turn-by-turn smartphone navigation assistant for people with visual impairments or blindness. In Proceedings of the 13th Web for All Conference, Montreal, Canada, 11–13 April 2016; pp. 90–99.
15. Li, B.; Munoz, J.P.; Rong, X.; Chen, Q.; Xiao, J.; Tian, Y.; Yousuf, M. Vision-based Mobile Indoor Assistive Navigation Aid for Blind People. *IEEE Trans. Mob. Comput.* **2019**, *18*, 702–714. [CrossRef]
16. Nair, V.; Budhai, M.; Olmschenk, G.; Seiple, W.H.; Zhu, Z. ASSIST: Personalized Indoor Navigation via Multimodal Sensors and High-Level Semantic Information. In Proceedings of the Computer Vision—ECCV 2018 Workshops, Munich, Germany, 8–14 September 2019; pp. 128–143.
17. Apostolopoulos, I.; Fallah, N.; Folmer, E.; Bekris, K.E. Integrated online localization and navigation for people with visual impairments using smart phones. *ACM Trans. Interact. Intell. Syst.* **2014**, *3*, 21. [CrossRef]
18. Maurer, M.; Gerdes, J.C.; Lenz, B.; Winner, H. *Autonomous Driving*; Springer: Berlin/Heidelberg, Germany, 2016; pp. 973–978.
19. Jiao, J.; Yuan, L.; Deng, Z.; Zhang, C.; Tang, W.; Wu, Q.; Jiao, J. A Smart Post-Rectification Algorithm Based on an ANN Considering Reflectivity and Distance for Indoor Scenario Reconstruction. *IEEE Access* **2018**, *6*, 58574–58586. [CrossRef]
20. Joseph, S.L.; Xiao, J.; Zhang, X.; Chawda, B.; Narang, K.; Rajput, N.; Mehta, S.; Subramaniam, L.V. Being aware of the world: Toward using social media to support the blind with navigation. *IEEE Trans. Hum. Mach. Syst.* **2015**, *45*, 399–405. [CrossRef]
21. Ganz, A.; Schafer, J.M.; Tao, Y.; Wilson, C.; Robertson, M. PERCEPT-II: Smartphone based indoor navigation system for the blind. In Proceedings of the 36th Annual International Conference of the IEEE Engineering in Medicine and Biology Society, Chicago, IL, USA, 26–30 August 2014; pp. 3662–3665.
22. Fernandes, H.; Costa, P.; Filipe, V.; Paredes, H.; Barroso, J. A review of assistive spatial orientation and navigation technologies for the visually impaired. *Univers. Access Inf. Soc.* **2019**, *18*, 155–168. [CrossRef]

23. Paden, B.; Cap, M.; Yong, S.Z.; Yershov, D.; Frazzoli, E. A Survey of Motion Planning and Control Techniques for Self-driving Urban Vehicles. *IEEE Trans. Intell. Veh.* **2016**, *1*, 33–55. [CrossRef]
24. O'Brien, E.E.; Mohtar, A.A.; Diment, L.E.; Reynolds, K.J. A detachable electronic device for use with a long white cane to assist with mobility. *Assist. Technol.* **2014**, *26*, 219–226. [CrossRef] [PubMed]
25. Rizvi, S.T.H.; Asif, M.J.; Ashfaq, H. Visual impairment aid using haptic and sound feedback. In Proceedings of the International Conference on Communication, Computing and Digital Systems (C-CODE), Islamabad, Pakistan, 8–9 March 2017; pp. 175–178.
26. Sohl-Dickstein, J.; Teng, S.; Gaub, B.M.; Rodgers, C.C.; Li, C.; DeWeese, M.R.; Harper, N.S. A device for human ultrasonic echolocation. *IEEE Trans. Biomed. Eng.* **2015**, *62*, 1526–1534. [CrossRef] [PubMed]
27. Bai, J.; Lian, S.; Liu, Z.; Wang, K.; Liu, D. Virtual-blind-road following-based wearable navigation device for blind people. *IEEE Trans. Consum. Electron.* **2018**, *64*, 136–143. [CrossRef]
28. Patil, K.; Jawadwala, Q.; Shu, F.C. Design and construction of electronic aid for visually impaired people. *IEEE Trans. Hum. -Mach. Syst.* **2018**, *48*, 172–182. [CrossRef]
29. Amemiya, T.; Sugiyama, H. Design of a Haptic Direction Indicator for Visually Impaired People in Emergency Situations. In Proceedings of the International Conference on Computers Helping People with Special Needs. Berlin, 9–11 July 2008; pp. 1141–1144.
30. Kaushalya, V.; Premarathne, K.; Shadir, H.; Krithika, P.; Fernando, S. 'AKSHI': Automated help aid for visually impaired people using obstacle detection and GPS technology. *Int. J. Sci. Res. Publ.* **2016**, *6*, 579–583.
31. Cardillo, E.; Di Mattia, V.; Manfredi, G.; Russo, P.; De Leo, A.; Caddemi, A.; Cerri, G. An electromagnetic sensor prototype to assist visually impaired and blind people in autonomous walking. *IEEE Sens. J.* **2018**, *18*, 2568–2576. [CrossRef]
32. Brown, T. Design thinking. *Harv. Bus. Rev.* **2008**, *86*, 84.
33. Przybilla, L.; Klinker, K.; Wiesche, M.; Krcmar, H. A Human-Centric Approach to Digital Innovation Projects in Health Care: Learnings from Applying Design Thinking. In Proceedings of the PACIS, Yokohama, Japan, 26–30 June 2018; p. 226.
34. Kaler, J. Morality and strategy in stakeholder identification. *J. Bus. Ethics* **2002**, *39*, 91–100. [CrossRef]
35. Porter, M.E. Industry structure and competitive strategy: Keys to profitability. *Financ. Anal. J.* **1980**, *36*, 30–41. [CrossRef]
36. Kotler, P. *Marketing Management*; Prentice Hall: Englewood Cliffs, NJ, USA, 2000.
37. The Design Process: What Is the Double Diamond. Available online: http://www.designcouncil.org.uk/news-opinion/design-process-what-double-diamond (accessed on 26 October 2019).
38. Nielsen, J. Enhancing the Explanatory Power of Usability Heuristics. In Proceedings of the SIGCHI Conference on Human Factors in Computing Systems, Boston, MA, USA, 24–28 April 1994; pp. 152–158.
39. Nassar, V.J.W. Common criteria for usability review. *Work* **2012**, *41* (Suppl. 1), 1053–1057. [PubMed]
40. Ilas, C. Electronic sensing technologies for autonomous ground vehicles: A review. In Proceedings of the 8th International Symposium on Advanced Topics in Electrical Engineering (ATEE), Bucharest, Romania, 23–25 May 2013; pp. 1–6.
41. Miao, M.; Spindler, M.; Weber, G. Requirements of indoor navigation system from blind users. In Proceedings of the Symposium of the Austrian HCI and Usability Engineering Group, Graz, Austria, 25–26 November 2011; pp. 673–679.
42. Lock, J.C.; Cielniak, G.; Bellotto, N. A Portable Navigation System with an Adaptive Multimodal Interface for the Blind. In Proceedings of the AAAI Spring Symposium Series, Stanford, CA, USA, 27–29 March 2017.
43. Joseph, S.L.; Zhang, X.; Dryanovski, I.; Xiao, J.; Yi, C.; Tian, Y. Semantic indoor navigation with a blind-user oriented augmented reality. In Proceedings of the IEEE International Conference on Systems, Man, and Cybernetics, Manchester, UK, 13–16 October 2013; pp. 3585–3591.
44. Bujacz, M.; Strumiłło, P. Sonification: Review of auditory display solutions in electronic travel aids for the blind. *Arch. Acoust.* **2016**, *41*, 401–414. [CrossRef]
45. Balan, O.; Moldoveanu, A.; Moldoveanu, F. Navigational audio games: An effective approach toward improving spatial contextual learning for blind people. *Int. J. Disabil. Hum. Dev.* **2015**, *14*, 109–118. [CrossRef]
46. Yang, K.; Wang, K.; Bergasa, L.; Romera, E.; Hu, W.; Sun, D.; Sun, J.; Cheng, R.; Chen, T.; López, E. Unifying terrain awareness for the visually impaired through real-time semantic segmentation. *Sensors* **2018**, *18*, 1506. [CrossRef]

47. Cheraghi, S.A.; Namboodiri, V.; Walker, L. GuideBeacon: Beacon-based indoor wayfinding for the blind, visually impaired, and disoriented. In Proceedings of the IEEE International Conference on Pervasive Computing and Communications (PerCom), Kona, HI, USA, 13–17 March 2017; pp. 121–130.
48. Mekhalfi, M.L.; Melgani, F.; Zeggada, A.; De Natale, F.G.; Salem, M.A.-M.; Khamis, A. Recovering the sight to blind people in indoor environments with smart technologies. *Expert Syst. Appl.* **2016**, *46*, 129–138. [CrossRef]
49. Long, R.G.; Hill, E. Establishing and maintaining orientation for mobility. *Found. Orientat. Mobil.* **1997**, *1*, 49–62.
50. Pawluk, D.T.; Adams, R.J.; Kitada, R. Designing haptic assistive technology for individuals who are blind or visually impaired. *IEEE Trans. Haptics* **2015**, *8*, 258–278. [CrossRef]
51. Zeagler, C. Where to wear it: Functional, technical, and social considerations in on-body location for wearable technology 20 years of designing for wearability. In Proceedings of the ACM International Symposium on Wearable Computers, Maui, Hawaii, USA, 11–15 September 2017; pp. 150–157.
52. Mendoza, J.E. Two-Point Discrimination. In *Encyclopedia of Clinical Neuropsychology*; Kreutzer, J.S., DeLuca, J., Kreutzer, B., Eds.; Springer: New York, NY, USA, 2011.
53. Zhang, X.; Yao, X.; Zhu, Y.; Hu, F. An ARCore Based User Centric Assistive Navigation System for Visually Impaired People. *Appl. Sci.* **2019**, *9*, 989. [CrossRef]
54. Schinazi, V.R.; Thrash, T.; Chebat, D.R. Spatial navigation by congenitally blind individuals. *WIREs Cogn. Sci.* **2016**, *7*, 37–58. [CrossRef] [PubMed]
55. Majerova, H. The aspects of spatial cognitive mapping in persons with visual impairment. *Procedia Soc. Behav. Sci.* **2015**, *174*, 3278–3284. [CrossRef]
56. Nielsen, J. *Usability Engineering*; Academic Press: Boston, MA, USA, 1993.
57. Hartson, H.R. Human–computer interaction: Interdisciplinary roots and trends. *J. Syst. Softw.* **1998**, *43*, 103–118. [CrossRef]
58. International Organization for Standardization. *Ergonomics of Human-System Interaction: Part. 210: Human-Centred Design for Interactive Systems*; ISO: Geneva, Switzerland, 2010.
59. Velázquez, R.; Pissaloux, E.; Rodrigo, P.; Carrasco, M.; Lay-Ekuakille, A.J.A.S. An Outdoor Navigation System for Blind Pedestrians Using GPS and Tactile-Foot Feedback. *Appl. Sci.* **2018**, *8*, 578. [CrossRef]
60. Danilov, Y.; Tyler, M. Brainport: An alternative input to the brain. *J. Integr. Neurosci.* **2005**, *4*, 537–550. [CrossRef]
61. Continuity Issues. Available online: http://pages.mtu.edu/~{}shene/COURSES/cs3621/NOTES/curves/continuity.html (accessed on 26 October 2019).
62. Bartels, R.H.; Beatty, J.C.; Barsky, B.A. *An Introduction to Splines for Use in Computer Graphics and Geometric Modeling*; Morgan Kaufmann: Berlington, MA, USA, 1995.

2

Fusion of Heart Rate, Respiration and Motion Measurements from a Wearable Sensor System to Enhance Energy Expenditure Estimation

Ke Lu [1,*], Liyun Yang [1,2], Fernando Seoane [3,4,5], Farhad Abtahi [1,2], Mikael Forsman [1,2] and Kaj Lindecrantz [2,4]

1. School of Engineering Sciences in Chemistry, Biotechnology and Health, KTH Royal Institute of Technology, Hälsovägen 11C, 141 57 Huddinge, Sweden; liyuny@kth.se (L.Y.); farhad.abtahi@ki.se (F.A.); mikael.forsman@ki.se (M.F.)
2. Institute of Environmental Medicine, Karolinska Institutet, Solnavägen 1, 171 77 Solna, Sweden; kaj.lindecrantz@ki.se
3. Department of Clinical Science, Intervention and Technology, Karolinska Institutet, Hälsovägen 7, 141 57 Huddinge, Sweden; fernando.seoane@ki.se
4. Swedish School of Textiles, University of Borås, Allégatan 1, 501 90 Borås, Sweden
5. Department of Biomedical Engineering, Karolinska University Hospital, 1, 171 76 Solna, Sweden

* Correspondence: kelu@kth.se

Abstract: This paper presents a new method that integrates heart rate, respiration, and motion information obtained from a wearable sensor system to estimate energy expenditure. The system measures electrocardiography, impedance pneumography, and acceleration from upper and lower limbs. A multilayer perceptron neural network model was developed, evaluated, and compared to two existing methods, with data from 11 subjects (mean age, 27 years, range, 21–65 years) who performed a 3-h protocol including submaximal tests, simulated work tasks, and periods of rest. Oxygen uptake was measured with an indirect calorimeter as a reference, with a time resolution of 15 s. When compared to the reference, the new model showed a lower mean absolute error (MAE = 1.65 mL/kg/min, R^2 = 0.92) than the two existing methods, i.e., the flex-HR method (MAE = 2.83 mL/kg/min, R^2 = 0.75), which uses only heart rate, and arm-leg HR+M method (MAE = 2.12 mL/kg/min, R^2 = 0.86), which uses heart rate and motion information. As indicated, this new model may, in combination with a wearable system, be useful in occupational and general health applications.

Keywords: energy expenditure; wearable device; accelerometer; impedance pneumography; neural network

---

1. Introduction

The energy expenditure (EE), as an indicator of metabolic state and physical activity level, provides valuable information that can be used for occupational health and safety design [1], exercise, and daily life management, and prevention and treatment of health problems such as obesity and diabetes [2]. Direct measurement methods of EE or oxygen consumption (VO_2), a commonly-used indicator of EE, requires expensive and sophisticated equipment, such as the direct calorimetry using metabolic chamber, the double labeled water method, and indirect calorimetry with a face mask, which are not suitable for daily free-living use [3]. Therefore, indirect measurement techniques using wearable sensors are desired, and have attracted significant attention in the last two decades; consequently, considerable effort has been allocated to the issue [4–32].

Heart rate (HR) monitoring is often used to estimate EE, as it has a good linearity with oxygen consumption in a large range of aerobic work [13,21]. The relationship between HR and EE at an individual level can be established through a calibration procedure, i.e., maximal or submaximal tests performed with a treadmill or cycle ergometer, which requires time and resources [33]. However, the poor relationship between HR and EE in resting and low intensity activities is an important limiting factor [24]. The HR-VO_2 relation can vary in different activities [19], e.g., difference has been reported between upper body and lower body activities [34]. In addition, HR is affected by several factors that are not directly related to metabolism e.g., mental stress, emotions, and medication [16].

Accelerometry is also a popular tool to estimate physical activity related EE in free-living conditions. With count-based methods [11,35], the activity count is calculated using acceleration, and then directly linked to EE, while the type of activity being performed is not considered [6]. In activity related methods [4,7,12], firstly, the activity recognition is preformed, then the EE is estimated through a look-up table or by using the activity specified EE model [6]. The acceleration (ACC) measurement directly reflects the movement information. However, it lacks the information about the effort of the movements, which limits its effectiveness for assessing complex activities involving interaction with other objects, such as manual handling. Several methods that utilize HR and ACC have been proposed, which improves the estimation of EE by the sole use of HR or ACC [9,36].

Respiration is another factor that is related to EE [14]. Several studies have demonstrated that pulmonary ventilation (V_E) has better linearity with EE compared to the HR [37,38]. As an accurate V_E measurement requires devices with facemasks or mouthpieces, the real application is very limited in free-living conditions. Recent developments in wearable technologies, such as impedance pneumography (IP), inductive plethysmography, and piezoresistive pneumography integrated in smart clothing [39–43], give new opportunities to use portable respiration measurement devices for EE estimation in a free-living setting, and preliminary studies have been carried out [15,18].

The purpose of this study was to develop and test a method that uses a combination of information from measurements of heart rate, respiration, and accelerations to estimate energy expenditure. The measurements were acquired through a wearable sensor system, and integrated by a model based on neural network. The wearable sensor system was developed under our research projects towards automatic risk assessment at work [44,45]. A lab experiment was implemented to support the development of the model and evaluate the developed system and estimation model. The proposed method was compared with two existing methods: HR-flex [28], a HR based method that uses a bi-linear model to improve the estimation in low intensity, and Arm-Leg HR+M [29,36], a method which uses combined HR and ACC measurements, with independent arm and leg calibration. The results showed improved accuracy over the two existing methods. In addition, the proposed method does not require complex lab calibration, which can dramatically improve the usability of such a system in field settings.

2. Materials and Methods

2.1. The Wearable Sensor System

The wearable sensor system and the sensor placement are shown in Figure 1. The vest, reported in [40,46], includes four textile electrodes made by conductive fabric. One pair of electrodes was used for IP current injection, and the other was used for electric potential sensing for IP and ECG. A compact recorder, ECGZ2 (Z-Health Technologies AB, Borås, Sweden), for ECG and electrical bioimpedance was connected to the vest and placed in a pocket on the shoulder strap of the vest. The frequency of the injection current for impedance measurement was 50 kHz. ECG and IP signals were recorded with sampling rates of 250 Hz and 100 Hz, respectively. Four 3-axis accelerometers (AX3, Axivity Ltd., Newcastle, UK) were placed on both wrists, using rubber wristbands, and on the thighs, using trousers with specially designed pockets to hold the accelerometer units. The acceleration was recorded at 100 Hz.

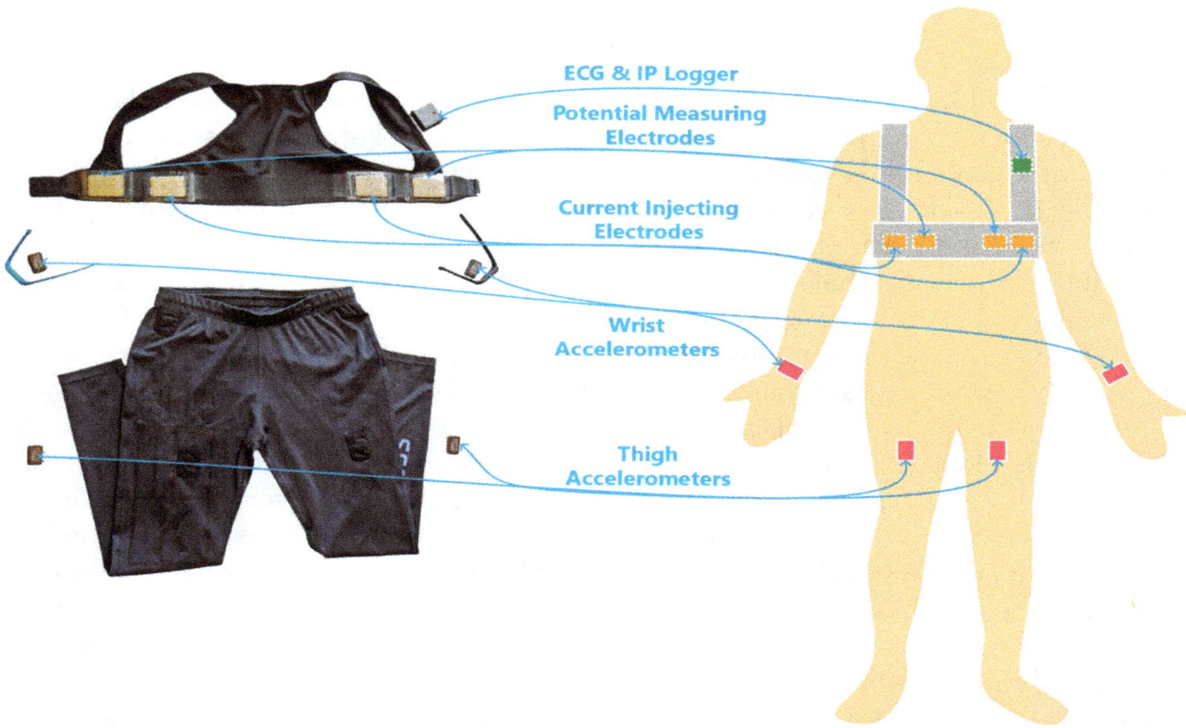

Figure 1. The wearable sensor system and its placement. The system includes a vest with textile electrodes, a wireless ECG and IP recording unit, 4 accelerometers, rubber wristbands, and trousers with specially designed pockets.

2.2. Data Collection

2.2.1. Participants

Nine men and three women participated in the laboratory experiment implemented in GIH, the Swedish School of Sport and Health Sciences, Stockholm, Sweden. The subjects consisted of a homogeneous group with young male subjects, and a heterogeneous group with both male and female participants in different age groups. Data from one subject was removed from the analysis because of the lack of a vest with a suitable size for the participant, which resulted in poor ECG and IP signal quality. The detailed characteristics of the included participants are shown in Table 1. All participants provided written informed consent. Ethical approval for the study was obtained from the Regional Ethical Review Board in Stockholm (Dnr 2016/724-31/5).

Table 1. Characteristics of included participants (median [range]).

	Men (N = 9)	**Women (N = 2)**	**All (N = 11)**
Age (year)	27 [21–65]	43 [25–61]	27 [21–65]
Height (cm)	181 [171–199]	169 [165–173]	177 [165–199]
Weight (kg)	77 [51–89]	60 [58–62]	75 [51–89]
BMI (kg/m^2)	22.8 [17.4–25.6]	20.9 [20.7–21.2]	22.6 [17.4–25.6]
$VO_{2\,max}$ (mL/min/kg)	42.9 [32.1–54.6]	35.6 [30.9–40.3]	40.3 [30.9–54.6]

2.2.2. Experiment Protocol

The participants were asked to avoid intense physical activity for 1 day before the experiment, and to refrain from eating, smoking, drinking tea, coffee, or alcohol for at least 2 h beforehand. The experiment process took about 3 h. During the experiment, VO_2 was measured by a computerized metabolic system (Jaeger Oxycon Pro, VIASYS Healthcare GmbH, Würzburg, Germany), where a facemask was worn by the participants. The experiment protocol consisted of three categories of activities: resting, simulated working tasks, and submaximal tests. The list of performed tasks and corresponding VO_2 levels measured in the experiment is presented in Table 4 under the result section. After each task, the subject had a break for 5 to 25 min, until the HR returned to within 10 percent of the resting HR.

The resting test included resting in three postures: 20 min in lying, 5 min in sitting and 5 min in standing. During the resting test, the resting energy expenditure (REE) was measured. Five different working tasks, with different intensity levels and active muscle groups, were performed afterwards. Each of the tasks lasted 8–10 min. The office work required the participant to type on a computer while sitting beside a table. The painting work required the participant to simulate painting a wall at their own pace using a painting pole. The postal delivery work was performed by cycling at a cycle ergometer with 0.75 kg resistance. The meat cutting work was simulated by pulling a resistance band repetitively. The construction work included arm and whole body lifting tasks. The submaximal tests session consisted of 3 tests. The first was the Chester step test [47], with maximal 5 levels of incremental stepping pace. The second was a walking pace treadmill test as described in [36]. Each level of the treadmill test lasted three minutes. The speed was increased after the first level. From the second level, the inclination was raised by 2% between each stage. The third test was an arm ergometer test with a constant cadence while the resistance increased between each level [36]. All the submaximal tests were terminated when the HR of the subject reached the 80% of the age-predicted maximal HR (220 − age).

2.3. *The Model for VO_2 Estimation*

The process of the estimation is shown in Figure 2. A multilayer perceptron neural network (MLPNN) with four input units, five hidden units, and one output unit was used to construct the model. The activation function of the hidden layer was hyperbolic tangent sigmoid function, and linear function for the output layer. All features and the output are listed in Table 2. All data were analyzed with 15-s non-overlapping windows. Four features were used that represent HR, V_E, arm motion and leg motion, respectively. HR, V_E, and VO_2 were normalized by corresponding individual characteristics before being used as the inputs and output of the MLPNN to train a network with good genericization that learns characteristics at the group level.

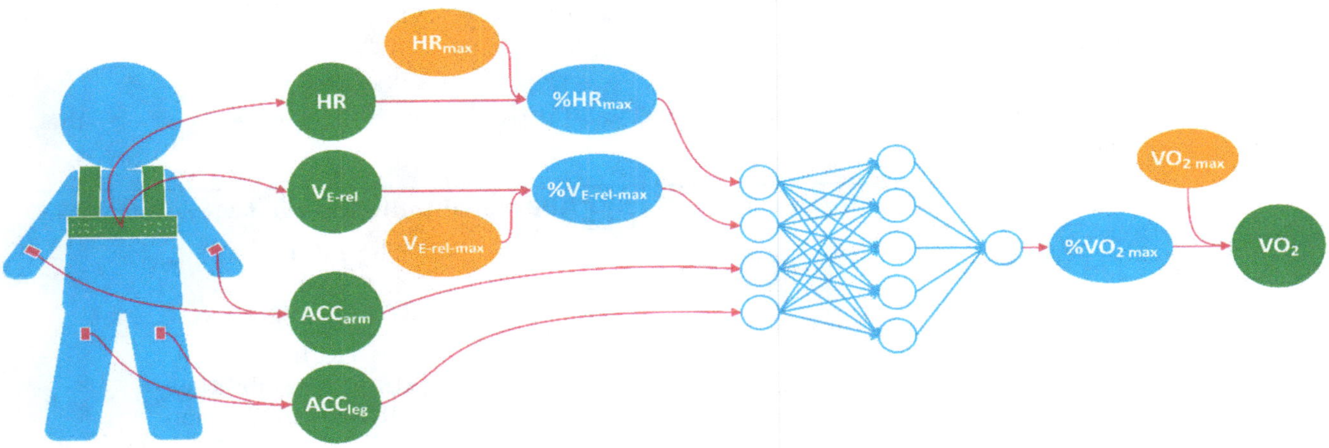

Figure 2. A demonstration of the flow of the oxygen consumption (VO_2) process. The input and output are explained in Table 2.

Table 2. Summary of the input features and the output of the neural network.

Input Features	% HR_{max}	HR normalized by age predicted HR_{max}
	% $V_{E\text{-rel max}}$	$V_{E\text{-rel}}$ normalized by estimated $V_{E\text{-rel max}}$
	ACC_{arm}	Mean absolute value of wrist acceleration
	ACC_{leg}	Mean absolute value of thigh acceleration
Output	% $VO_{2\ max}$	VO_2 normalized by estimated $VO_{2\ max}$

The VO_2 measurements were normalized by the individual maximal oxygen uptake ($VO_{2\ max}$), which was estimated through the Chester step test with pre-estimated VO_2 level on each stage [47]. The HR was normalized by individual maximal HR (HR_{max}), calculated by $HR_{max} = 220 - \text{age}$. The relative tidal volume ($V_{T\text{-rel}}$) of each breath was represented by the impedance difference in peak and valley pairs of the filtered IP signal. The relative ventilation ($V_{E\text{-rel}}$) during each 15-s epoch was acquired by the sum of the $V_{T\text{-rel}}$ values in the window. A quadratic relationship between HR and $V_{E\text{-rel}}$ was established for each subject by the least square method using measured HR and $V_{E\text{-rel}}$ during the experiment. The maximal relative ventilation ($V_{E\text{-rel max}}$) was then estimated by applying the HR_{max} to the HR-$V_{E\text{-rel}}$ relationship. $V_{E\text{-rel}}$ was then normalized by the $V_{E\text{-rel max}}$ and fed to the network. The acceleration data was first band pass filtered with a 0.25−6 Hz passband; then, the mean absolute acceleration was computed for each 15-s epoch. For the arm and leg acceleration, the higher value from the right and the left sides of each epoch was picked.

2.4. Model Training and Cross Validation

The so-called Leave one subject out (LOSO) validation method was used. In repeated trials, all data except one subject was used for training the model; the data of that subject was used for testing the model. The LOSO method avoids test results that are overfitted to individual characteristics. The overall performance of the network was evaluated by combining test results from all LOSO cross validation. The training data was split for training and validation set with a ratio of 6:4, and the Levenberg-Marquardt backpropagation was used for the training process.

2.5. Comparision to Published Methods

Results from our method were compared with two published methods, i.e., HR-flex [28], one of the mostly used HR based method in the field, and Arm-Leg HR+M method [29,36], a method showed improved accuracy during occupational tasks in our previous evaluation [48]. The inputs and calibration requirements of all methods are listed in Table 3.

Table 3. A comparison of requirements of input data and personalized measurement among the three methods.

Methods	Input Data	Additional Individualized Measurements
Flex-HR	HR	Flex HR Point REE HR-VO_2 Calibration
Arm-Leg HR+M	HR, ACC_{leg}, ACC_{arm}	REE Leg HR-VO_2 Calibration Arm HR-VO_2 Calibration
Proposed	HR, ACC_{leg}, ACC_{arm}, $V_{E\text{-rel}}$	$VO_{2\ max}$

The flex-HR method [28] considers the nonlinearity in HR-EE relation in low intensity. It uses REE when the HR is below the flex point, and a linear HR-EE relationship when the HR is above the flex point. For the comparison, we chose to use step test data with pre-estimated VO_2 levels on each stage for calibration, as it required the same level of test equipment as the new method. The REE was measured during the resting test. The flex-point was chosen as the average of the highest HR during rest and the lowest HR during walking on treadmill test.

The Arm-Leg HR+M method [29,36] accounts for the difference in HR-EE response between the upper and the lower body. It uses the level of arm and leg ACC and their ratio to determine the arm specified HR-EE equation, the leg specified HR-EE equation, or the REE for EE estimation. We used a treadmill test and arm ergometer test data to establish the arm and leg calibration respectively, together with a simultaneously measured VO_2 level. The calibration requires a treadmill, an arm ergometer, and indirect calorimetry. Thresholds for the ACC level and ratio were re-adapted to our measurement data, as a different accelerometer and acceleration signal processing procedure were used in comparison to the original study.

2.6. Statistics

Estimated VO_2 in 15-s epochs were compared to the criterion measurements. Bias, the mean absolute error (MAE), the root-mean-square-error (RMSE) and the coefficient of determination (R^2) were calculated to evaluate the performance. Paired *t*-tests were performed to compare the absolute errors between the new method and each of the two published methods. Bland-Altman plots with error histograms were plotted to assess the agreement and the error distribution.

3. Results

The mean levels of measured VO_2 for performing each task during the experiment are listed in Table 4.

Table 4. A summary of tasks performed during the experiments and corresponding mean VO_2 level (mL/min/kg) of the 11 subjects.

Group	Task	VO_2 Level (Mean ± SD)
Resting	Lying	3.78 ± 0.96
	Sitting	3.82 ± 1.16
	Standing	4.01 ± 0.41
Work Tasks	Office Work	4.01 ± 1.42
	Painting Work	8.51 ± 1.68
	Postal Delivery Work	14.04 ± 2.37
	Meat Cutting Work	7.62 ± 1.89
	Construction Work	12.24 ± 4.56
Submaximal Tests	Step Test	22.23 ± 7.71
	Treadmill Test	22.88 ± 8.05
	Arm Ergometer Test	11.06 ± 4.98

The training and testing results (%$VO_{2\,max}$) on each subject, as well as the averaged results from the LOSO validation, are shown in Table 5. The RMSE and R^2 level from training and testing results were very close, which indicates the method has a good generalization among the participants. The averaged group bias was very low (−0.16%). However, a relatively lager bias (maximal 2.71%) can be found on individual level in few occasions. No strong relationship was found between the estimation errors and the personal characteristics, such as gender, age, and aerobic capacity.

The results of overall performance in VO_2 estimation, measured by individual bias (IB), group bias (GB), MAE, RMSE, and R^2 of three methods, are shown in Table 6. The proposed method showed a more accurate estimation (IB = 0.42 mL/kg/min, GB = −0.01 mL/kg/min, MAE = 1.65 mL/kg/min) compared to the flex-HR method (IB = 1.11 mL/kg/min, GB = 0.69 mL/kg/min, MAE = 2.83 mL/kg/min), where estimation error, individual bias, and group bias were significantly reduced ($p < 0.001$). The proposed method also showed a significant improvement ($p < 0.001$) in estimation error over the arm-leg HR+M method (MAE = 2.12 mL/kg/min).

Table 5. Results of the cross validation of the relative VO_2 (%$VO_{2\,max}$) from the neural network.

Gender	Age (Year)	Weight (kg)	Height (cm)	BMI (kg/m^2)	$VO_{2\,max}$ (mL/kg/min)	%$VO_{2\,max}$					
						Train			Test [1]		
						Bias	RMSE	R^2	Bias	RMSE	R^2
M	65	80	188	22.6	32.7	−0.03	5.26	0.92	−2.03	5.74	0.88
M	21	77	176.5	24.7	54.6	0.07	5.54	0.90	−0.35	5.40	0.92
F	61	62	173	20.7	30.9	0.10	5.06	0.92	−1.19	8.03	0.84
F	25	58	165.5	21.2	40.3	−0.01	5.39	0.91	0.11	4.55	0.93
M	27	88.5	199	22.3	47.8	0.04	5.33	0.91	0.18	4.69	0.94
M	27	51	171	17.4	39.6	0.14	5.21	0.92	−0.36	6.61	0.87
M	25	79.8	176.5	25.6	43.6	0.05	5.35	0.91	1.84	4.60	0.93
M	29	88.9	190	24.6	42.9	−0.03	5.54	0.91	−0.51	4.07	0.95
M	42	75	177	23.9	32.1	0.03	5.26	0.92	2.71	5.93	0.88
M	26	75	181.5	22.8	37.2	0.06	5.28	0.91	−0.68	4.86	0.92
M	26	68.5	184	20.2	44.8	0.08	5.30	0.91	−1.47	5.76	0.90
Average Mean (SD)									−0.16 (1.38)	5.47 (1.13)	0.91 (0.03)

[1] In each row, the data for the specific subject was excluded in the training and used for the testing.

Table 6. Comparison of VO_2 estimation results among flex-HR, arm-leg HR+M, and proposed method (mL/kg/min).

Methods	Individual Bias [1]	Group Bias	MAE	RMSE	R^2
Flex-HR	1.11	0.69	2.83	4.00	0.75
Arm-Leg HR+M	0.60	−0.09	2.12	2.95	0.86
Proposed	0.42	−0.07	1.65	2.28	0.92

[1] Mean absolute value of individual biases.

The Bland-Altman plots and the error rate histograms of three methods are shown in Figure 3. The proposed method shows a large improvement in the low intensity region. The mean estimation error rate was also reduced (28.1%) compared to the other methods (44.1% and 38.4% respectively).

The errors with each specific activity are shown in Table 7, where for each activity, the worst performance among the three methods is shown in bold and italic. The proposed method has a good overall generalization over different kinds of activities, except that a large bias on the simulated construction work can be found. Comparing to the flex-HR method, the error caused by different HR response to arm and leg activity was reduced in the proposed method by learning from group characteristics without arm calibration, which can be seen from the arm ergometer results, as well as from the top right corner of the Bland-Altman plot in Figure 3.

Table 7. Comparison of task specific errors among three methods (mL/kg/min).

	Resting	Office Work	Painting	Postal Delivery	Meat Cutting	Construction Work	Step	Treadmill	Arm Ergometer
Flex-HR									
Bias	−0.05	−0.29	−0.47	***−2.42***	***1.84***	1.05	−1.05 [1]	***−0.81***	***4.18***
RMSE	0.90	0.84	***3.89***	***4.15***	***4.33***	3.90	***2.85*** [1]	***2.92***	***5.91***
Arm-Leg HR+M									
Bias	***−1.42***	***−0.93***	***−1.90***	−1.59	−0.16	−1.09	***−0.38***	−0.01 [2]	0.00 [2]
RMSE	***2.50***	***2.09***	2.55	2.57	1.56	***4.44***	2.53	1.82 [2]	1.14 [2]
Proposed									
Bias	0.02	0.17	−0.47	−0.46	0.55	***−2.01***	−1.08 [3]	0.44	0.06
RMSE	0.93	0.86	1.69	2.36	1.62	3.88	2.83 [3]	2.71	1.69

The bold and italic numbers indicate the largest error in each activity. [1] Data used for individual calibration, with pre-estimated VO_2 level. [2] Data used for individual calibration, with measured VO_2 level. [3] Data used for VO_{2max} estimation, with pre-estimated VO_2 level.

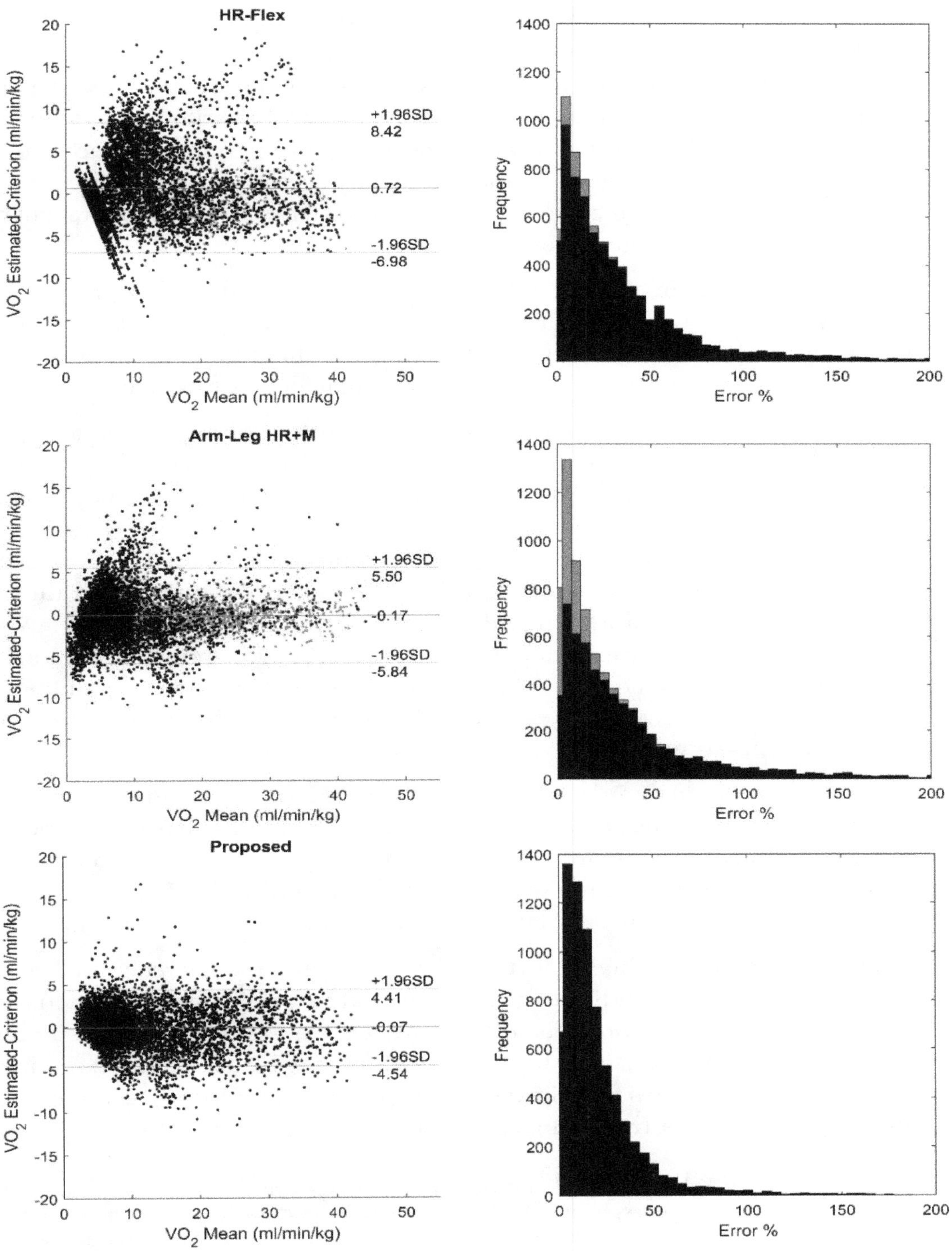

Figure 3. Bland-Altman plots and error rate histograms of flex-HR, arm-leg HR+M, and proposed methods against the criterion measurement. Data used in individual calibration are plotted in grey.

4. Discussion and Conclusions

In this study, we have demonstrated a method for free-living energy expenditure estimation that combines the HR, respiration, and motion information using nonlinear data driven modeling. In the experiment, the method showed improved accuracy over two established methods, based on HR and HR combined with ACC.

The method has also improved the usability by avoiding a complex laboratory calibration. The Chester step test used for $VO_{2\,max}$ estimation only requires a step with designed height, and takes only 6 to 10 min, which can be easily applied in the field. For certain ergonomic applications that use per cent maximum aerobic capacity (%$VO_{2\ max}$) as a measure of physical workload, the output of the network can be used directly without the need of multiplying individual $VO_{2\ max}$ value; hence, no calibration procedure is required. The wearable system used in the study is light-weight and easy to wear, which opens up the possibility for long-term, unobtrusive monitoring in different contexts. However, different contexts will come with different needs regarding number of accelerometers and their placement. The most versatile system would have many accelerometers at different sites on the body, but many sensors will increase the overall price of the system. Obviously, there will be trade-off between versatility, complexity, and cost.

A method using neural network based model to estimate EE from HR has been reported previously in [31,32]. This method uses not only the HR, but also heart rate variability derived respiration rate, and HR 'on and off dynamics' as input features. However, very limited information has been shown about the implementation. Hence, we were not able to compare our method with it.

In previous studies [15,18], which used portable indirect respiration monitoring devices to estimate EE, the measured physical quantities such as transthoracic impedance and thoracic circumference distance were converted into flow or volume through a personal calibration process using a spirometer. In this study, a rough calibration of the personalized impedance level was acquired by using simultaneously-measured HR values. How much data is needed to establish a reliable relationship and the durability of the relationship should be further studied. In the experiment, we found our $V_{E\text{-}rel}$ measurement through IP did not have very high linearity with the V_E measured by the indirect calorimetry. Possible causes for this discrepancy include the configuration of electrode position, posture change that alters the shape of ribcage [49], and motion artifacts. Applying optimized IP electrodes position [50] and advanced processing methods will have the potential to improve the IP measurement hence the EE estimation.

Limitations of this study include a small sample size (11 subjects), and the fact that limited activity types were performed under laboratory condition. The method has not yet been validated for complex real free-living scenarios, and the trained network could be overfitted to the activities that were performed in the experiment. The experiment has not taken into consideration many nonmetabolic-related factors that may alter HR or V_E, such as mental stress and temperature.

Since the new model showed a higher level of agreement with the reference methods compared to two existing methods, this study indicates a high potential for applying information fusion of HR, respiration, and motion data in combination with a nonlinear statistical learning method in the field of unobtrusive energy expenditure estimation. The solution may be used both in occupational and general health applications. Studies with improved respiration monitoring techniques and varied populations with larger size under free-living conditions are suggested in future development.

Author Contributions: L.Y. and K.L. conceived and designed the experiments in collaboration with the other authors; L.Y. and K.L. performed the experiments; K.L. analyzed the data; F.S. contributed with wearables; all authors participated in the discussion of results; K.L. drafted the paper; all authors revised the paper.

References

1. Wu, H.C.; Wang, M.J. Relationship between Maximum Acceptable Work Time and Physical Workload. *Ergonomics* **2002**, *45*, 280–289. [CrossRef] [PubMed]

2. Colberg, S.R.; Sigal, R.J.; Yardley, J.E.; Riddell, M.C.; Dunstan, D.W.; Dempsey, P.C.; Horton, E.S.; Castorino, K.; Tate, D.F. Physical Activity/Exercise and Diabetes: A Position Statement of the American Diabetes Association. *Diabetes Care* **2016** *39*, 2065–2079. [CrossRef] [PubMed]

3. Shephard, R.J.; Aoyagi, Y. Measurement of Human Energy Expenditure, with Particular Reference to Field Studies: An Historical Perspective. *Eur. J. Appl. Physiol.* **2012**, *112*, 2785–2815. [CrossRef] [PubMed]

4. Albinali, F.; Intille, S.; Haskell, W.; Rosenberger, M. Using Wearable Activity Type Detection to Improve Physical Activity Energy Expenditure Estimation. In Proceedings of the 12th ACM International Conference on Ubiquitous Computing, Copenhagen, Denmark, 26–29 September 2010.
5. Altini, M.; Penders, J.; Amft, O. Energy Expenditure Estimation Using Wearable Sensors: A New Methodology for Activity-Specific Models. In Proceedings of the Conference on Wireless Health, San Diego, CA, USA, 23–25 October 2012.
6. Altini, M.; Penders, J.; Vullers, R.; Amft, O. Estimating Energy Expenditure Using Body-Worn Accelerometers: A Comparison of Methods, Sensors Number and Positioning. *IEEE J. Biomed. Health Inform.* **2015**, *19*, 219–226. [CrossRef] [PubMed]
7. Bonomi, A.G.; Plasqui, G.; Goris, A.H.; Westerterp, K.R. Improving Assessment of Daily Energy Expenditure by Identifying Types of Physical Activity with a Single Accelerometer. *J. Appl. Physiol.* **2009**, *107*, 655–661. [CrossRef] [PubMed]
8. Bouten, C.V.; Westerterp, K.R.; Verduin, M.; Janssen, J.D. Assessment of Energy Expenditure for Physical Activity Using a Triaxial Accelerometer. *Med. Sci. Sports Exerc.* **1994**, *23*, 21–27. [CrossRef]
9. Brage, S.; Brage, N.; Franks, P.W.; Ekelund, U.; Wong, M.Y.; Andersen, L.B.; Froberg, K.; Wareham, N.J. Branched Equation Modeling of Simultaneous Accelerometry and Heart Rate Monitoring Improves Estimate of Directly Measured Physical Activity Energy Expenditure. *J. Appl. Physiol.* **2004**, *96*, 343–351. [CrossRef] [PubMed]
10. Brage, S.; Westgate, K.; Franks, P.W.; Stegle, O.; Wright, A.; Ekelund, U.; Wareham, N.J. Estimation of Free-Living Energy Expenditure by Heart Rate and Movement Sensing: A Doubly-Labelled Water Study. *PLoS ONE* **2015**, *10*, e0137206. [CrossRef] [PubMed]
11. Crouter, S.E.; Churilla, J.R.; Bassett, D.R. Estimating Energy Expenditure Using Accelerometers. *Eur. J. Appl. Physiol.* **2006**, *98*, 601–612. [CrossRef] [PubMed]
12. Ellis, K.; Kerr, J.; Godbole, S.; Lanckriet, G.; Wing, D.; Marshall, S. A Random Forest Classifier for the Prediction of Energy Expenditure and Type of Physical Activity from Wrist and Hip Accelerometers. *Physiol. Meas.* **2014**, *35*, 2191. [CrossRef] [PubMed]
13. Eston, R.G.; Rowlands, A.V.; Ingledew, D.K. Validity of Heart Rate, Pedometry, and Accelerometry for Predicting the Energy Cost of Children's Activities. *J. Appl. Physiol.* **1998**, *84*, 362–371. [CrossRef] [PubMed]
14. Gastinger, S.; Donnelly, A.; Dumond, R.; Prioux, J. A Review of the Evidence for the Use of Ventilation as a Surrogate Measure of Energy Expenditure. *J. Parenteral Enteral Nutr.* **2014**, *38*, 926–938. [CrossRef] [PubMed]
15. Gastinger, S.; Nicolas, G.; Sorel, A.; Sefati, H.; Prioux, J. Energy Expenditure Estimate by Heart-Rate Monitor and a Portable Electromagnetic-Coil System. *Int. J. Sport Nutr. Exerc. Metab.* **2012**, *22*, 117–130. [CrossRef] [PubMed]
16. Hiilloskorpi, H.; Fogelholm, M.; Laukkanen, R.; Pasanen, M.; Oja, P.; Mänttäri, A.; Natri, A. Factors Affecting the Relation between Heart Rate and Energy Expenditure During Exercise. *Int. J. Sports Med.* **1999**, *20*, 438–443. [CrossRef]
17. Jang, Y.; Jung, M.W.; Kang, J.; Kim, H.C. An Wearable Energy Expenditure Analysis System Based on the 15-Channel Whole-Body Segment Acceleration Measurement. In Proceedings of the 2005 27th Annual International Conference of the Engineering in Medicine and Biology Society, Shanghai, China, 1–4 September 2005.
18. Lu, K.; Yang, L.; Abtahi, F.; Lindecrantz, K.; Rödby, K.; Seoane, F. Wearable Cardiorespiratory Monitoring System for Unobtrusive Free-Living Energy Expenditure Tracking. In Proceedings of the World Congress on Medical Physics and Biomedical Engineering 2018, Prague, Czech Republic, 3–8 June 2018.
19. Li, R.; Deurenberg, P.; Hautvast, J.G. A Critical Evaluation of Heart Rate Monitoring to Assess Energy Expenditure in Individuals. *Am. J. Clin. Nutr.* **1993**, *58*, 602–607. [CrossRef] [PubMed]
20. Lin, C.W.; Yang, Y.T.; Wang, J.S.; Yang, Y.C. A Wearable Sensor Module with a Neural-Network-Based Activity Classification Algorithm for Daily Energy Expenditure Estimation. *IEEE Trans. Inform. Technol. Biomed.* **2012**, *16*, 991–998.
21. Livingstone, M.B. Heart-Rate Monitoring: The Answer for Assessing Energy Expenditure and Physical Activity in Population Studies? *Br. J. Nutr.* **1997**, *78*, 869–871. [CrossRef] [PubMed]

22. Livingstone, M.B.; Prentice, A.M.; Coward, W.A.; Ceesay, S.M.; Strain, J.J.; McKenna, P.G.; Nevin, G.B.; Barker, M.E.; Hickey, R. Simultaneous Measurement of Free-Living Energy Expenditure by the Doubly Labeled Water Method and Heart-Rate Monitoring. *Am. J. Clin. Nutr.* **1990**, *52*, 59–65. [CrossRef] [PubMed]
23. Lu, K.; Yang, L.; Abtahi, F.; Lindecrantz, K.; Rödby, K.; Seoane, F. *Wearable Cardiorespiratory Monitoring System for Unobtrusive Free-Living Energy Expenditure Tracking*; Springer: Singapore, 2019.
24. Luke, A.; Maki, K.C.; Barkey, N.; Cooper, R.; McGEE, D.A. Simultaneous Monitoring of Heart Rate and Motion to Assess Energy Expenditure. *Med. Sci. Sports Exerc.* **1997**, *29*, 144–148. [CrossRef] [PubMed]
25. Meijer, G.A.; Westerterp, K.R.; Koper, H.A. Assessment of Energy Expenditure by Recording Heart Rate and Body Acceleration. *Med. Sci. Sports Exerc.* **1989**, *21*, 343–347. [CrossRef] [PubMed]
26. Montoye, H.J.; Washburn, R.I.; Servais, S.T.; Ertl, A.N.; Webster, J.G.; Nagle, F.J. Estimation of Energy Expenditure by a Portable Accelerometer. *Med. Sci. Sports Exerc.* **1983**, *15*, 403–407. [CrossRef] [PubMed]
27. Murakami, H.; Kawakami, R.; Nakae, S.; Nakata, Y.; Ishikawa-Takata, K.; Tanaka, S.; Miyachi, M. Accuracy of Wearable Devices for Estimating Total Energy Expenditure: Comparison with Metabolic Chamber and Doubly Labeled Water Method. *JAMA Internal Med.* **2016**, *176*, 702–703. [CrossRef] [PubMed]
28. Spurr, G.B.; Prentice, A.M.; Murgatroyd, P.R.; Goldberg, G.R.; Reina, J.C.; Christman, N.T. Energy Expenditure from Minute-by-Minute Heart-Rate Recording: Comparison with Indirect Calorimetry. *Am. J. Clin. Nutr.* **1988**, *48*, 552–559. [CrossRef] [PubMed]
29. Strath, S.J.; Bassett, J.D.; Thompson, D.L.; Swartz, A.M. Validity of the Simultaneous Heart Rate-Motion Sensor Technique for Measuring Energy Expenditure. *Med. Sci. Sports Exerc.* **2002**, *34*, 888–894. [CrossRef] [PubMed]
30. Swartz, A.M.; Strath, S.J.; Bassett, D.R.; O'brien, W.L.; King, G.A.; Ainsworth, B.E. Estimation of Energy Expenditure Using Csa Accelerometers at Hip and Wrist Sites. *Med. Sci. Sports Exerc.* **2000**, *32*, S450–S456. [CrossRef] [PubMed]
31. Pulkkinen, A.; Kettunen, J.; Martinmäki, K.; Saalasti, S.; Rusko, H.K. On-and Off Dynamics and Respiration Rate Enhance the Accuracy of Heart Rate Based Vo2 Estimation. In Proceedings of the 51st Annual Meeting of the American College of Sports Medicine, Indianapolis, IN, USA, 2–5 June 2004.
32. Pulkkinen, A.; Saalasti, S.; Rusko, H.K. Energy Expenditure Can Be Accurately Estimated from Hr without Individual Laboratory Calibration. In Proceedings of the 52nd Annual Meeting of the American College of Sports Medicine, Nashville, TN, USA, 1–4 June 2005.
33. Brage, S.; Ekelund, U.; Brage, N.; Hennings, M.A.; Froberg, K.; Franks, P.W.; Wareham, N.J. Hierarchy of Individual Calibration Levels for Heart Rate and Accelerometry to Measure Physical Activity. *J. Appl. Physiol.* **2007**, *103*, 682–692. [CrossRef] [PubMed]
34. Vokac, Z.H.; Bell, H.; Bautz-Holter, E.; Rodahl, K. Oxygen Uptake/Heart Rate Relationship in Leg and Arm Exercise, Sitting and Standing. *J. Appl. Physiol.* **1975**, *39*, 54–59. [CrossRef] [PubMed]
35. Crouter, S.E.; Kuffel, E.; Haas, J.D.; Frongillo, E.A.; Bassett, D.R., Jr. A Refined 2-Regression Model for the Actigraph Accelerometer. *Med. Sci. Sports Exerc.* **2010**, *42*, 1029. [CrossRef] [PubMed]
36. Strath, S.J.; Brage, S.Ø.; Ekelund, U. Integration of Physiological and Accelerometer Data to Improve Physical Activity Assessment. *Med. Sci. Sports Exerc.* **2005**, *37*, S563–S571. [CrossRef] [PubMed]
37. Gilgen-Ammann, R.; Koller, M.; Huber, C.; Ahola, R.; Korhonen, T.; Wyss, T. Energy Expenditure Estimation from Respiration Variables. *Sci. Rep.* **2017**, *7*, 15995. [CrossRef] [PubMed]
38. Gastinger, S.; Sorel, A.; Nicolas, G.; Gratas-Delamarche, A.; Prioux, J. A Comparison between Ventilation and Heart Rate as Indicator of Oxygen Uptake During Different Intensities of Exercise. *J. Sports Sci. Med.* **2010**, *9*, 110–118. [PubMed]
39. Loriga, G.; Taccini, N.; de Rossi, D.; Paradiso, R. Textile Sensing Interfaces for Cardiopulmonary Signs Monitoring. In Proceedings of the 27th Annual International Conference of the Engineering in Medicine and Biology Society, New York, NY, USA, 31 August–3 September 2006.
40. Seoane, F.; Ferreira, J.; Alvarez, L.; Buendia, R.; Ayllón, D.; Llerena, C.; Gil-Pita, R. Sensorized Garments and Textrode-Enabled Measurement Instrumentation for Ambulatory Assessment of the Autonomic Nervous System Response in the Atrec Project. *Sensors* **2013**, *13*, 8997–9015. [CrossRef] [PubMed]
41. De Rossi, D.; Carpi, F.; Lorussi, F.; Mazzoldi, A.; Paradiso, R.; Scilingo, E.P.; Tognetti, A. Electroactive Fabrics and Wearable Biomonitoring Devices. *AUTEX Res. J.* **2003**, *3*, 180–185.

42. Lanatà, A.; Scilingo, E.P.; Nardini, E.; Loriga, G.; Paradiso, R.; De-Rossi, D. Comparative Evaluation of Susceptibility to Motion Artifact in Different Wearable Systems for Monitoring Respiratory Rate. *IEEE Trans. Inform. Technol. Biomed.* **2010**, *14*, 378–386. [CrossRef] [PubMed]
43. Młyńczak, M.C.; Niewiadomski, W.; Żyliński, M.; Cybulski, G.P. Ambulatory Impedance Pneumography Device for Quantitative Monitoring of Volumetric Parameters in Respiratory and Cardiac Applications. In Proceedings of the Computing in Cardiology Conference (CinC), Cambridge, MA, USA, 7–10 September 2014.
44. Abtahi, F.; Yang, L.; Lindecrantz, K.; Seoane, F.; Diaz-Olivazrez, J.A.; Ke, L.; Eklund, J.; Teriö, H.; Mediavilla Martinez, C.; Tiemann, C. Big Data & Wearable Sensors Ensuring Safety and Health@ Work. In Proceedings of the GLOBAL HEALTH 2017, The Sixth International Conference on Global Health Challenges, Barcelona, Spain, 12–16 November 2017.
45. Yang, L.; Lu, K.; Diaz-Olivares, J.A.; Seoane, F.; Lindecrantz, K.; Forsman, M.; Abtahi, F.; Eklund, J.A. Towards Smart Work Clothing for Automatic Risk Assessment of Physical Workload. *IEEE Access* **2018**, *6*, 40059–40072. [CrossRef]
46. Mohino-Herranz, I.; Gil-Pita, R.; Ferreira, J.; Rosa-Zurera, M.; Seoane, F. Assessment of Mental, Emotional and Physical Stress through Analysis of Physiological Signals Using Smartphones. *Sensors* **2015**, *15*, 25607–25627. [CrossRef] [PubMed]
47. Sykes, K.; Roberts, A. The Chester Step Test—A Simple yet Effective Tool for the Prediction of Aerobic Capacity. *Physiotherapy* **2004**, *90*, 183–188. [CrossRef]
48. Yang, L.; Lu, K.; Forsman, M.; Lindecrantz, K.; Seoane, F.; Ekblom, Ö.; Eklund, J. Development of Smart Wearable Systems for Physiological Workload Assessment Using Heart Rate and Accelerometry. Unpublished work. 2018.
49. Seppa, V.P.; Viik, J.; Hyttinen, J. Assessment of Pulmonary Flow Using Impedance Pneumography. *IEEE Trans. Biomed. Eng.* **2010**, *57*, 2277–2285. [CrossRef] [PubMed]
50. Seppä, V.P.; Hyttinen, J.; Uitto, M.; Chrapek, W.; Viik, J. Novel Electrode Configuration for Highly Linear Impedance Pneumography. *Biomed. Eng.* **2013**, *58*, 35–38. [CrossRef] [PubMed]

3

A Novel Adaptive Recursive Least Squares Filter to Remove the Motion Artifact in Seismocardiography

Shuai Yu [1] **and Sheng Liu** [1,2,3,*]

1 School of Mechanical Science and Engineering, Huazhong University of Science and Technology, 1037 Luoyu Road, Wuhan 430074, China; yushuai91@hust.edu.cn
2 Key Lab for Hydropower Transients of Ministry of Education, School of Power and Mechanical Engineering, Wuhan University, 8 East Lake South Road, Wuhan 430072, China
3 Institute of Technological Sciences, Wuhan University, 8 East Lake South Road, Wuhan 430072, China
* Correspondence: shengliu@whu.edu.cn

Abstract: This paper presents a novel adaptive recursive least squares filter (ARLSF) for motion artifact removal in the field of seismocardiography (SCG). This algorithm was tested with a consumer-grade accelerometer. This accelerometer was placed on the chest wall of 16 subjects whose ages ranged from 24 to 35 years. We recorded the SCG signal and the standard electrocardiogram (ECG) lead I signal by placing one electrode on the right arm (RA) and another on the left arm (LA) of the subjects. These subjects were asked to perform standing and walking movements on a treadmill. ARLSF was developed in MATLAB to process the collected SCG and ECG signals simultaneously. The SCG peaks and heart rate signals were extracted from the output of ARLSF. The results indicate a heartbeat detection accuracy of up to 98%. The heart rates estimated from SCG and ECG are similar under both standing and walking conditions. This observation shows that the proposed ARLSF could be an effective method to remove motion artifact from recorded SCG signals.

Keywords: adaptive recursive least squares filter (ARLSF); Seismocardiography (SCG); motion artifact; Electrocardiogram (ECG); heart rate

---

1. Introduction

Seismocardiography (SCG) is a non-invasive measurement that records the local vibrations of the chest wall in response to the heartbeat [1]. SCG was first discovered in 1961 [1], and its first clinical application was used 30 years later in 1991 [2]. With the development of an accelerometer with high-sensitivity, low-noise, small-size, high-efficiency, and high-robustness signal-processing technology, SCG has shown its great potential to be used by wearables. Consequently, it is now feasible to use the information in clinical applications [3,4].

However, there are still some limitations in SCG measurements and assessments. Motion artifact is one of the major limitations. As a result, SCG research on motion artifact has been very active in recent years. Motion artifact is usually irregular and it is mixed with the heartbeat signals in the time and frequency domains. The mixture makes it difficult to separate the heartbeat signal from the mixed signal [3–5]. Some researchers tried to use multiple sensors to remove the motion artifact from the recorded signals [6–9]. The tri-axis acceleration data collected from a chest-worn accelerometer were utilized to remove motion artifact in an electrocardiogram (ECG) signal in 2003 [6], 2008 [7] and 2010 [8]. An independent component analysis approach and a normalized least means square (NLMS) adaptive filter to motion artifact cancellation of the SCG signal using two accelerometers were developed in [9] and [10], respectively. In these studies, one accelerometer was placed at the center of the sternum and the other was attached to the right side of the back of the subjects. The results were promising, but multiple sensors used in the experiments increased the complexity of the SCG measurement and assessment.

Meanwhile, other researchers developed several algorithms to remove motion artifact from the SCG signal by using only one accelerometer [11–17]. An ensemble empirical mode decomposition method was developed to remove white noise from a synthetic vibrocardiographic signal in [11] and the same method was successfully utilized to reduce the motion artifacts generated due to walking at normal and moderately fast speeds at a treadmill [12]. However, SCG signal could not be well recovered from corrupted signal. Rienzo et al. utilized an accelerometer to record a 24-hour SCG signal from freely moving subjects [13]. A movement-free SCG was extracted from the recorded accelerometer data using a continuous 5-second segment-based method. The results were promising, but the physiological parameters were not extracted from the signal. Pandia et al. designed a Savitzky Golay-based polynomial smoothing algorithm to extract the primary heart sound from the accelerometer data during walking [14]. The primary heart sound detection rate was up to 99.36%, but the graph of the extracted SCG signal could not be recovered. In another approach, the motion-free SCG signal was successfully extracted using a time delay-based normalized least mean square (NLMS) adaptive filter [17]. However, an extra moving average method was utilized to obtain the heart rate as the primary heart sound graph was not clear in the extracted motion-free SCG signal.

To solve this problem, we present a novel adaptive recursive least squares filter (ARLSF) for motion artifact removal in the SCG signal that was obtained by one accelerometer. The primary heartbeat signal graph is very clear in the motion artifact removed SCG signal without any other signal-processing procedures.

In Section 2 of this paper, the main idea of ARLSF is introduced and two major parameters of ARLSF are discussed. The measurement system including the hardware system, experimental setup and software system are discussed in Section 3. Section 4 shows the results and Section 5 concludes this paper.

2. Theory of Adaptive Recursive Least Squares Filter (ARLSF)

2.1. The Principle of Adaptive Recursive Least Squares Filter

Figure 1 illustrates the block diagram of ARLSF. An RLS filter is a finite impulse response (FIR) filter of length M with coefficients $\mathbf{w}(n)$ [18,19]. The input vector $\mathbf{u}(n)$ is passed through the FIR filter to produce the output vector $y(n)$. At each time-step, the coefficients are updated through the adaptive control unit using the input vector $\mathbf{u}(n)$. The prior estimation error $\xi(n)$ is described in Figure 2. All the parameters are defined in Equations (1)–(4) where $d(n)$ is the desired signal.

$$\mathbf{w}(n) = [w_0(n), w_1(n), \cdots, w_{M-1}(n)]^T \tag{1}$$

$$\mathbf{u}(n) = [u(n), u(n-1), \cdots, u(n-M+1)]^T \tag{2}$$

$$y(n) = \mathbf{w}^H(n-1)\mathbf{u}(n) \tag{3}$$

$$\xi(n) = d(n) - y(n) \tag{4}$$

The adaptive control unit updates the coefficients using the input vector and the prior estimation error. The detailed information can be described in Equation (5):

$$\hat{\mathbf{w}}(n) = \hat{\mathbf{w}}(n-1) + \mathbf{k}(n)\xi(n) \tag{5}$$

where $\mathbf{k}(n)$ is the gain vector that is described in Equation (6):

$$\mathbf{k}(n) = \frac{\lambda^{-1}\mathbf{P}(n-1)\mathbf{u}(n)}{1 + \lambda^{-1}\mathbf{u}^H\mathbf{P}(n-1)\mathbf{u}(n)} \tag{6}$$

where λ is the forgetting factor and $\mathbf{P}(n)$ is a covariance matrix of the noise which can be updated by Equation (7):

$$\mathbf{P}(n) = \lambda^{-1}\mathbf{P}(n-1) - \lambda^{-1}\mathbf{k}(n)\mathbf{u}(n)\mathbf{P}(n-1) \tag{7}$$

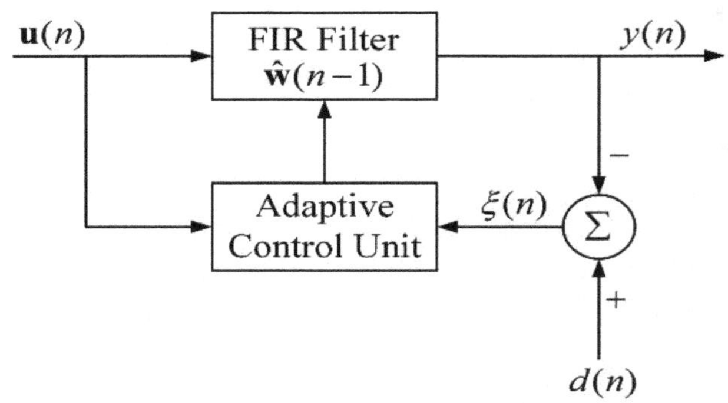

Figure 1. Block diagram of adaptive recursive least squares filter (ARLSF).

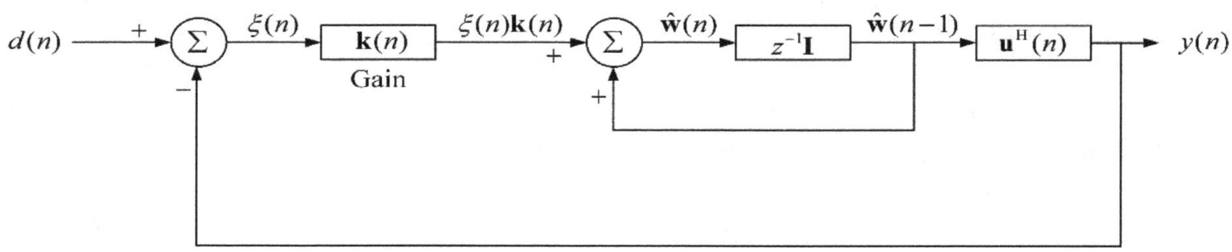

Figure 2. Signal-flow graph of ARLSF.

2.2. Discussion of the Desired Signal

The design of the desired signal is very important in the RLS filter when the desired signal cannot be directly obtained from an aiding sensor. The RLS filter works under the premise that the desired signal is linearly correlated to the input signal and orthogonal to the estimation error. The RLS filter will perform better with the higher linear correlation and the stronger orthogonality mentioned above [18,19].

The desired signal and the estimation error are the motion artifact and the SCG signal, respectively. They are collected from a single accelerometer simultaneously and they are aliased in the frequency domain with different frequency characteristics. The collected acceleration data contains the heartbeat signal, the motion artifact, the respiratory component, the noise of the hardware system and sounds from the other organs. The frequency of the respiratory component is less than 1 Hz [20,21], and the frequency of the heartbeat signal can be up to 25 Hz [22,23]. As a result, the collected acceleration data is band-pass filtered from 1 to 25 Hz with a 32th order FIR filter to remove the gravity component, the respiratory component and the high frequency noise, and the filtered data composed of the expected SCG signal and motion artifact within a frequency range from 1 to 25 Hz can be set as the input of ARLSF.

In addition, the maximum heart rate of a healthy adult is less than 210 beats per minute (bpm) [24–26] which illustrate the maximum frequency of an adult's heart rate is 3.5 Hz. In order to further analyze the frequency of the motion signal and the heartbeat signal, a similar experiment has been conducted to record the motion signal and the heartbeat signal [9]. Firstly, the SCG recorder system is attached to the chest wall of the subject to record the heartbeat signal under the condition of stand-up without moving as shown in Figure 3a; z-axis acceleration data is collected at a sampling rate of 800 Hz for about 120 s. Afterward, the same SCG recorder system is placed at the right side of the back of the same subject to record the motion artifact at a sampling rate of 800 Hz as shown in Figure 3b. The subject is asked to walk on a treadmill that works at a low speed (3–5 km/h) and the tri-axis acceleration data are collected for about 120 s. Four continuous 60-second signals are selected from the middle of each recorded acceleration data respectively and they are analyzed in time and frequency domain. Figure 4a illustrates that the heart rate frequency (1.2 Hz) lies in the low-frequency range(<3.5 Hz) while high frequency heart sound signal lies in the range from 4 Hz to 25 Hz. An obvious low-frequency point (1.82 Hz) representing the footsteps frequency is marked in Figure 5b, and the high-frequency component of the motion concentrates on the range from 4 Hz to 10 Hz [15,27]. It can be observed that the heartbeat signal and the motion signal are overlapped in the frequency domain and cannot be separated by bandpass filters.

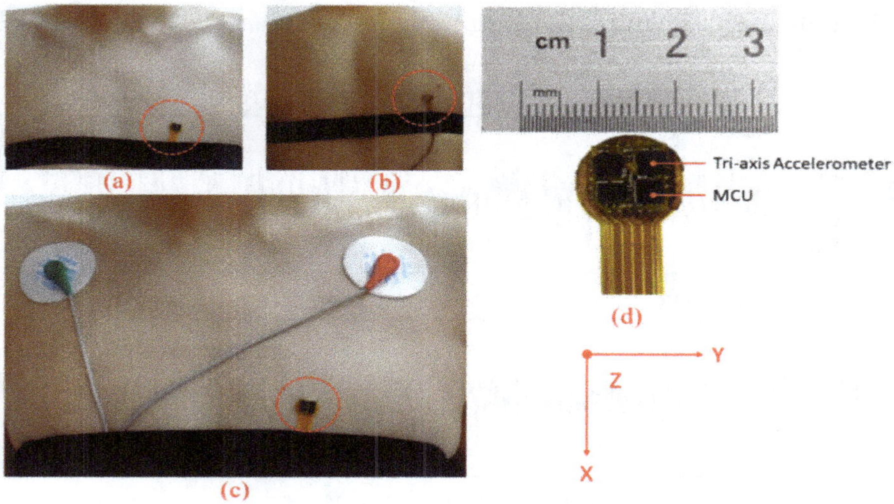

Figure 3. (**a**,**b**) Seismocardiography (SCG) recorder system placement for measuring heartbeat signal and motion signals, respectively. (**c**) A pair of electrocardiogram (ECG) lead I electrodes placement and SCG recorder system placement. (**d**) An image of the SCG recorder system which shows the dimensions. *X*-axis, *y*-axis and *z*-axis describe the head to foot, shoulder to shoulder and dorsoventral direction, respectively.

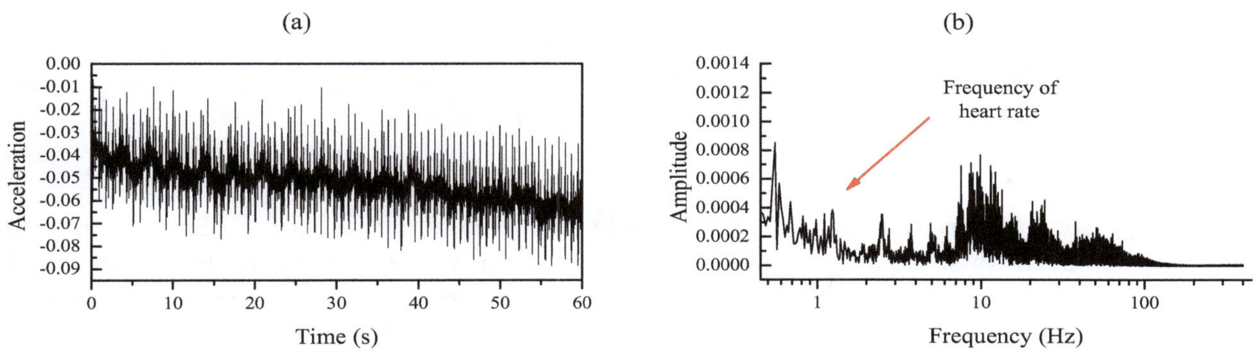

Figure 4. (**a**,**b**) Time plot and frequency plot of heartbeat signal respectively.

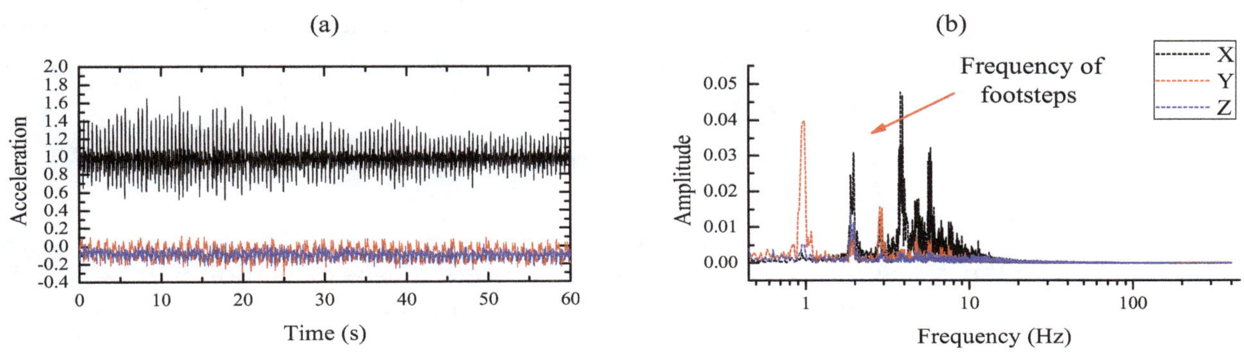

Figure 5. (**a**,**b**) Time plot and frequency plot of the tri-axis motion signal respectively.

Further process procedures including bandpass filtering and correlation analyzation are performed on the z-axis of the motion signal and the heartbeat data. The z-axis of the motion signal and heartbeat signal are bandpass filtered from 1 Hz to 25 Hz, and the filtered signals are plotted in Figure 6a,c respectively. Figure 6b represents the filtered signal of the z-axis of the motion signal through the FIR bandpass filter of the same type as Figure 6a,c, but at different cutoff frequencies from 3.5 Hz to 25 Hz. Meanwhile, the correlation coefficient between signals in Figure 6a,b is calculated to be 0.99978 and the counterpart between signals in Figure 6a,c is 0.15374, which proved well the high linear correlation of the signals in Figure 6a,b, and the strong orthogonality of the signals in Figure 6a,c [28]. Therefore, the desired signal can be obtained by bandpass filtering the recorded acceleration signal from 3.5 to 25 Hz.

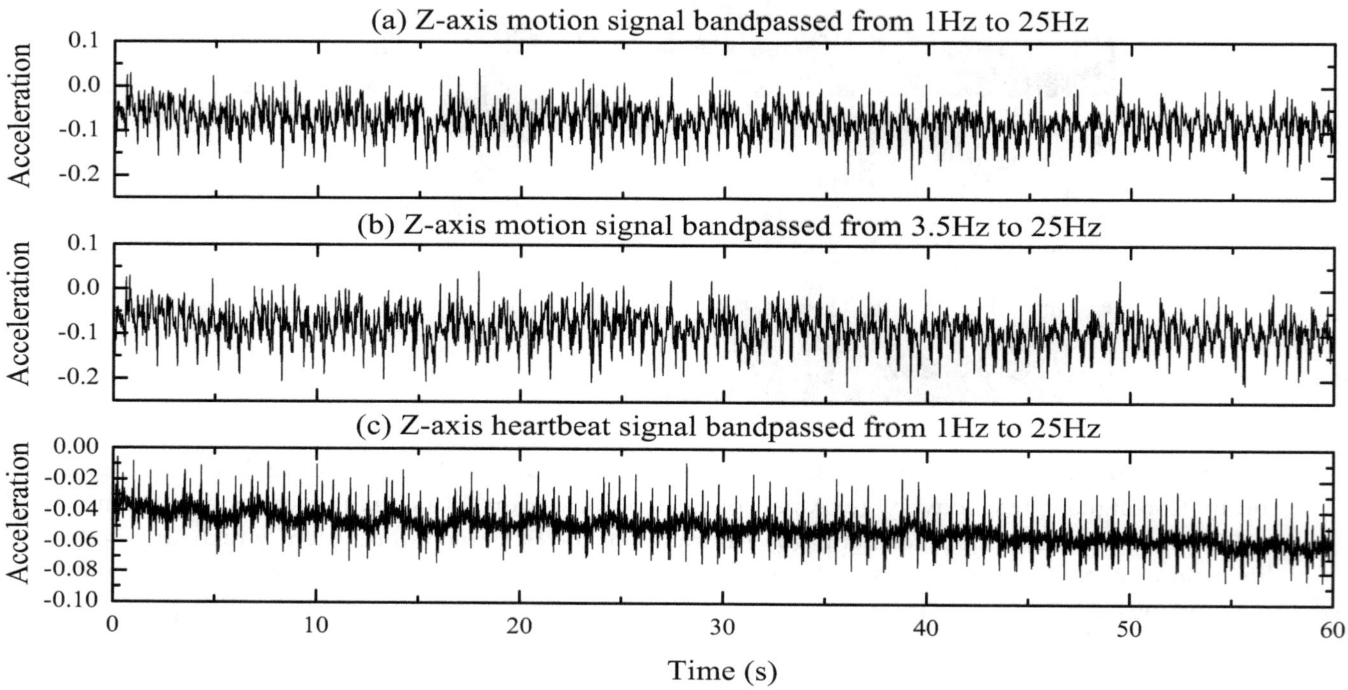

Figure 6. (**a**) Z-axis motion signal band passed from 1 to 25 Hz. (**b**) The Z-axis motion signal band passed from 3.5 to 25 Hz. (**c**) The Z-axis heartbeat signal band passed from 1 to 25 Hz.

2.3. Discussion of the Forgetting Factor

The forgetting factor plays an important role in the behavior of the RLS algorithm under non-stationary conditions. In a classical RLS algorithm, the value of the forgetting factor is fixed between 0 and 1. For the value of the forgetting factor closer to 0, the RLS algorithm has not only a smaller memory length and fast-tracking ability but also a reduced convergence speed and stability. On the other hand, when the forgetting factor is closer to 1, the RLS algorithm has fast convergence and good stability, but the tracking ability suffers and the memory length becomes longer [18,19]. In order to meet the conflicting requirements in non-stationary conditions, the forgetting factor is set between 0.98 and 1.0 [29,30]. In theory, the optimal value of the forgetting factor in non-stationary conditions can be defined by Equation (8) [19]:

$$\lambda \approx 1 - \frac{1}{\sigma_v}\left(\frac{tr[R_\omega]}{tr[R_u^{-1}]}\right)^{1/2} \tag{8}$$

where σ_v^2, R_ω, R_u are the measurement noise variance, process noise correlation matrix, and input vector correlation matrix respectively, $tr[\cdot]$ denotes the trace of the matrix.

3. Measurement Technique

3.1. Hardware System

Figure 3d shows the prototype of the SCG Recorder System (SRS), which integrates a commercial tri-axis accelerometer (ICM-20602 manufactured by InvenSense) and a microprocessor (STM32F411CEY6 manufactured by STMicroelectronics). The size of the device is less than 1 cm^2. The tri-axis accelerometer is used to capture acceleration data including SCG signal and motion information within a range of ±2g. The micro controller unit (MCU) collects the acceleration data from the accelerometer via a serial peripheral interface (SPI) at a rate of 800 Hz. The SRS is attached to the chest wall and placed at the left of the sternum as shown in Figure 3c. The z-axis of SRS describes the dorsoventral direction of the subject, and the x-axis and y-axis describe the head to foot direction and the shoulder to shoulder direction respectively.

In addition to the acceleration data captured by the tri-axis accelerometer, a standard ECG system simultaneously collects a standard ECG lead I signal at a rate of 512 Hz. The two electrodes are placed at the right arm and the left arm, respectively, as shown in Figure 3c. Both the SCG Recorder System and ECG system are connected to a host PC via serial cables for data transmission and synchronization.

3.2. Experiment Setup

The hardware system described above was used on sixteen subjects whose ages ranged from 24 to 35. The experiment was conducted on a treadmill and the subjects were asked to keep standing for at least 120 s before walking at least 180 s. After walking, the subjects stood for at least 60 s. The subjects could breathe freely during the whole experiment. The walking speed of the subjects was limited to less than 1.5 m/s by setting the treadmill at a low speed (3–5 km/h). The SCG and ECG signals including sampling time and sensor data were collected and transmitted to the PC for further analyzation in MATLAB (R2016a).

3.3. Software System

MATLAB (R2016a) was used to analyze all the data. The processing procedure consists of three parts: signal preprocessing to obtain the primary and reference channel of the ARLSF, the ARLSF and feature extraction.

3.3.1. Signal Preprocessing

The collected acceleration data is a mixed collection of signals in both the time and frequency domains, which contain the heartbeat signal, the motion artifact, the respiratory component, the noise of the hardware system and sounds from the other organs.

Firstly, the collected acceleration data is bandpass filtered from 1 to 25 Hz with a 32th order FIR filter to remove the gravity component, the respiratory component and the high-frequency noise. This procedure leaves the expected SCG signal and motion artifact within a frequency range from 1 to 25 Hz in the filtered signal, which is fed to the primary channel of the ARLSF.

The second filtered signal is obtained by bandpass filtering the acceleration data from 3.5 to 25 Hz with the same order and type of FIR filter. The correlation coefficient between the filtered signal of the primary channel and the second filter signal is calculated to be 0.987 which proved well the high linear correlation of these two filtered signals as discussed in Section 2.2. Therefore, the second filtered signal can be fed into the reference channel of the ARLSF. The raw data of the collected acceleration data, the primary channel obtained, and the reference channel are plotted in Figure 7a–c, respectively.

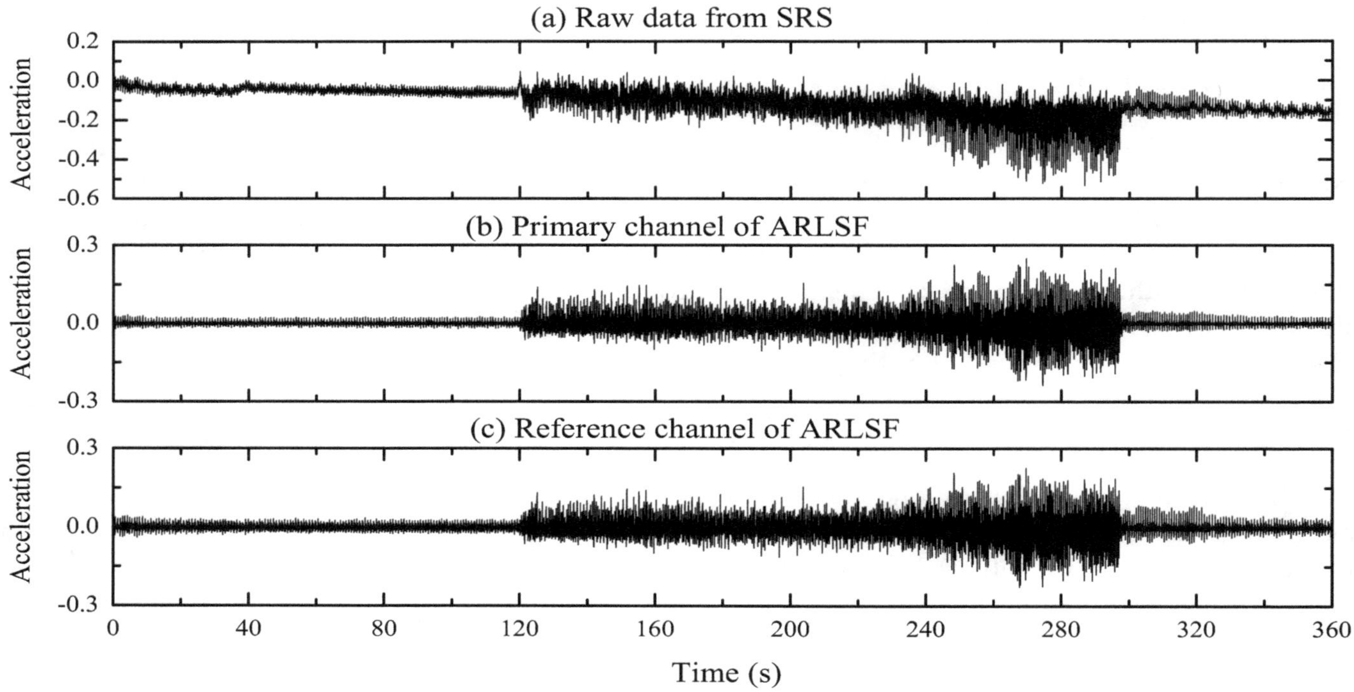

Figure 7. (**a**) Raw data from SCG Recorder System (SRS). (**b**,**c**) The primary and reference channel of ARLSF respectively.

3.3.2. ARLSF

The same order and same type of FIR filter used in signal preprocessing section creates the same delay to both the primary channel and the reference channel. As a result, the primary channel and the reference channel are synchronized in the time domain. In addition, the forgetting factor is calculated to be 0.9908 based on Equation (8). The variable $\xi(n)$ described in Equation (4) is the estimated heartbeat signal.

3.3.3. Feature Extraction

Features extracted from the ECG signal and filtered SCG signal are R peaks and aortic valve opening (AO) peaks, respectively. R peaks can be extracted from the ECG signal using the classical Pan Tompkin algorithm [31], while the extraction algorithm for AO peaks is different. The formula is described in Equations (9) and (10):

$$[loc\_min, val\_min] = \min(\xi(t-0.3:t)) \tag{9}$$

$$[loc\_max, val\_max] = \max(\xi(t-0.3:t)) \tag{10}$$

The estimated heartbeat signal $\xi(n)$ is divided into several segments with a length of 0.3s [32]. $\xi(t-0.3:t)$ is the segment at time t and *loc_min*, *val_min*, *loc_max* and *val_max* are the timestamp of the minimum value, the minimum value, the timestamp of maximum value and the maximum value of the segment at time t respectively. In addition, some constraints are used to avoid incorrect extracted AO peaks:

$$\begin{cases} val\_min < -0.007 \\ val\_max > 0.01 \\ |loc\_max - loc\_min| < 0.02 \end{cases} \tag{11}$$

A continuous 0.3 s segment including a correct AO peak is picked from the estimated heartbeat signal and plotted in Figure 8. *val_max* represents the magnitude of the AO peak and *val_min* represents the magnitude of the successive isovolumic moment (IM) peak or maximum acceleration (MA) peak.

Constant values -0.007 and 0.01 in Equation (11) are the maximum amplitude of the IM envelope peaks and minimum amplitude of the AO envelope peaks respectively [32]. In addition, the time interval between *val_max* and *val_min* should be restricted shorter than 0.02s [33]. When *loc_min*, *val_min*, *loc_max* and *val_max* meet the restrictions in Equation (11), *loc_max* and *val_max* are the timestamp and the value of the extracted AO peak respectively. For further analysis, the heart rate can be calculated from the R–R and AO–AO interval.

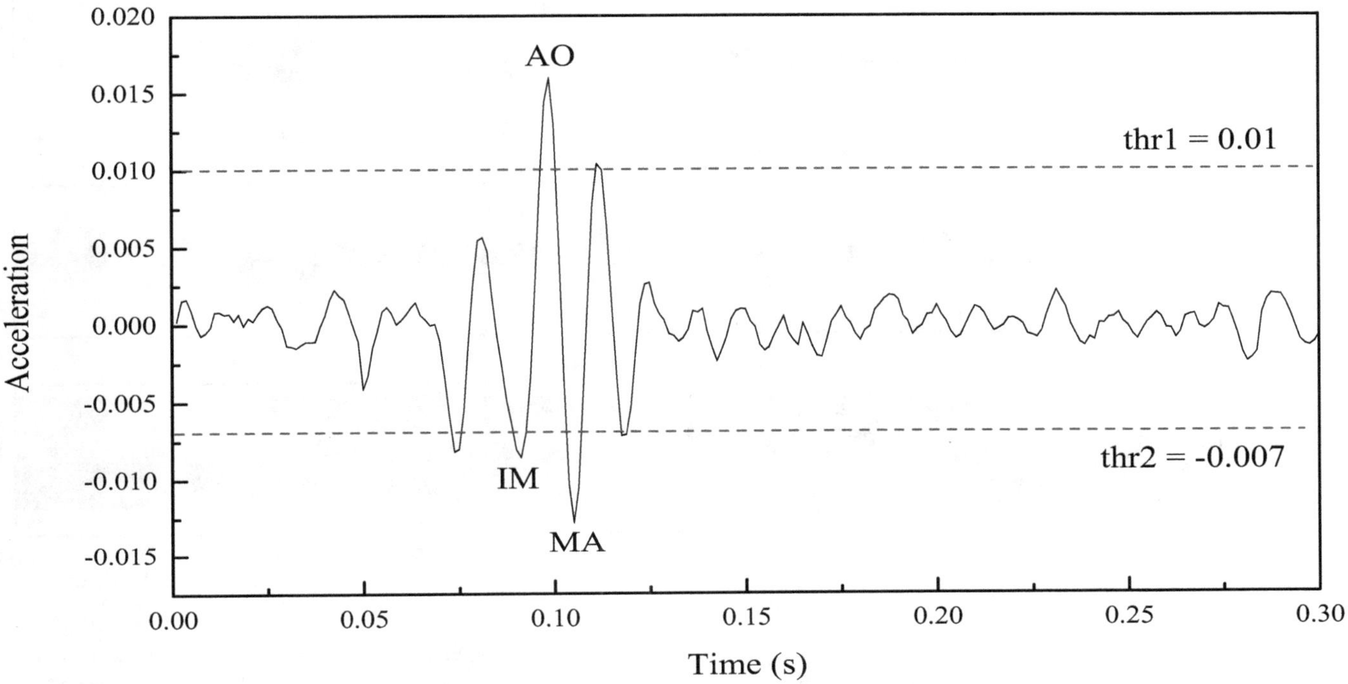

Figure 8. A correct aortic valve opening (AO) peak from a continuous 0.3s segment.

4. Results

Figure 9 displays the raw data and processing results. Figure 9a shows the raw acceleration data collected from the SRS. The data show that the heartbeat signals are contaminated by the motion artifact, and the features and graphs of the heartbeat signals cannot be identified during the walking period. Figure 9b,c show the extracted heartbeat signals using Savitzky Golay-based polynomial smoothing [14] and ARLSF. Features and graphs of heartbeat signals are not clear from 120 s to 300 s in Figure 9b. It can be observed that the proposed ARLSF outperforms the Savitzky Golay-based polynomial smoothing. For better visualization, six segmented signals selected from the standing period before walking, transitions from standing to walking, the first half of walking, the second half of walking, transitions from walking to standing, and standing after walking are plotted in Figure 10a–f respectively. It is obvious that the features and graphs of the heartbeat signals are visually noticeable after ARLSF. Thus, any other signal-processing procedures are unnecessary on the heartbeat signals.

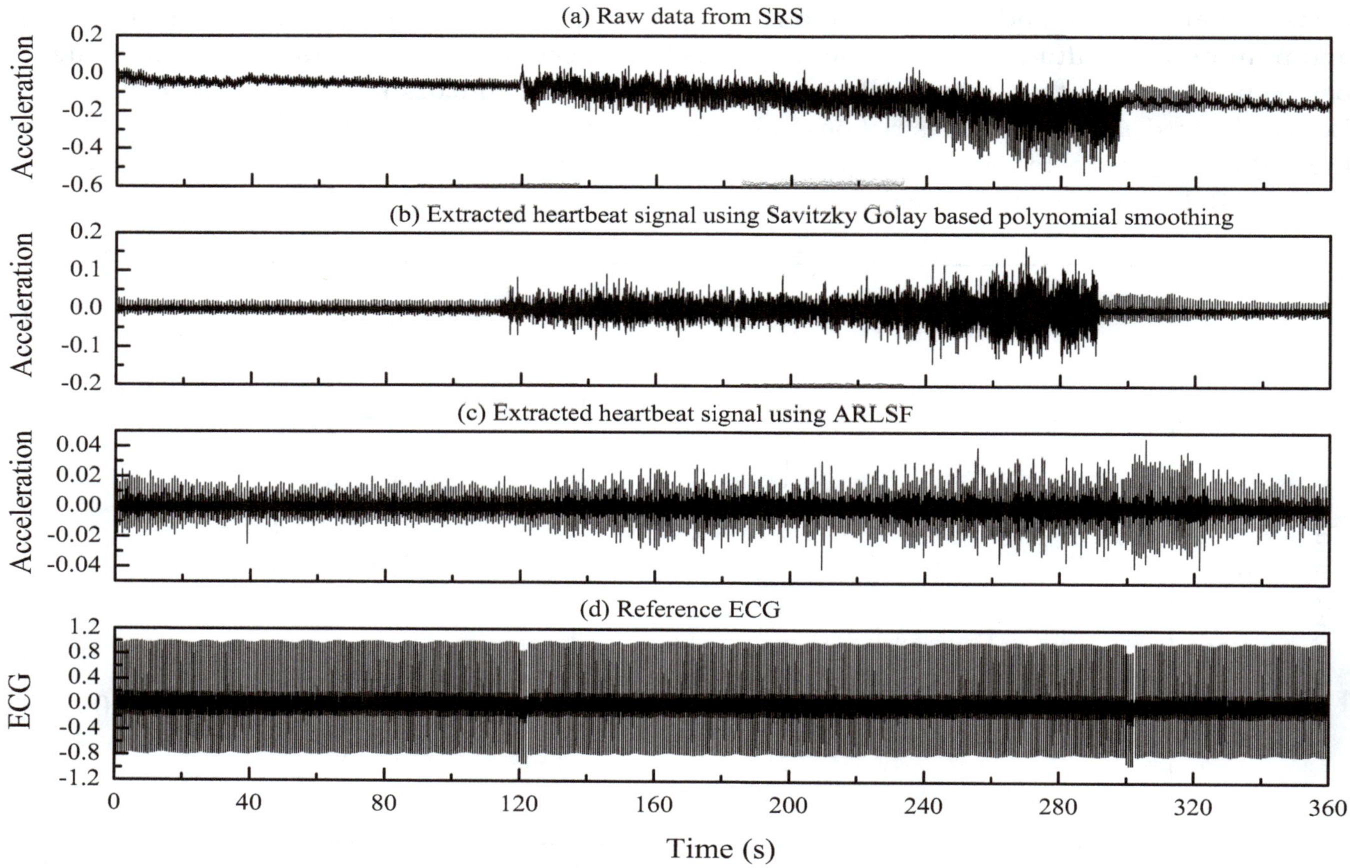

Figure 9. (**a**) Raw data from SRS. (**b**) Extracted heartbeat signal using Savitzky Golay filter. (**c**) Extracted heartbeat signal using ARLSF. (**d**) The reference ECG lead I signal. (The units of acceleration and ECG are g and mV, respectively.)

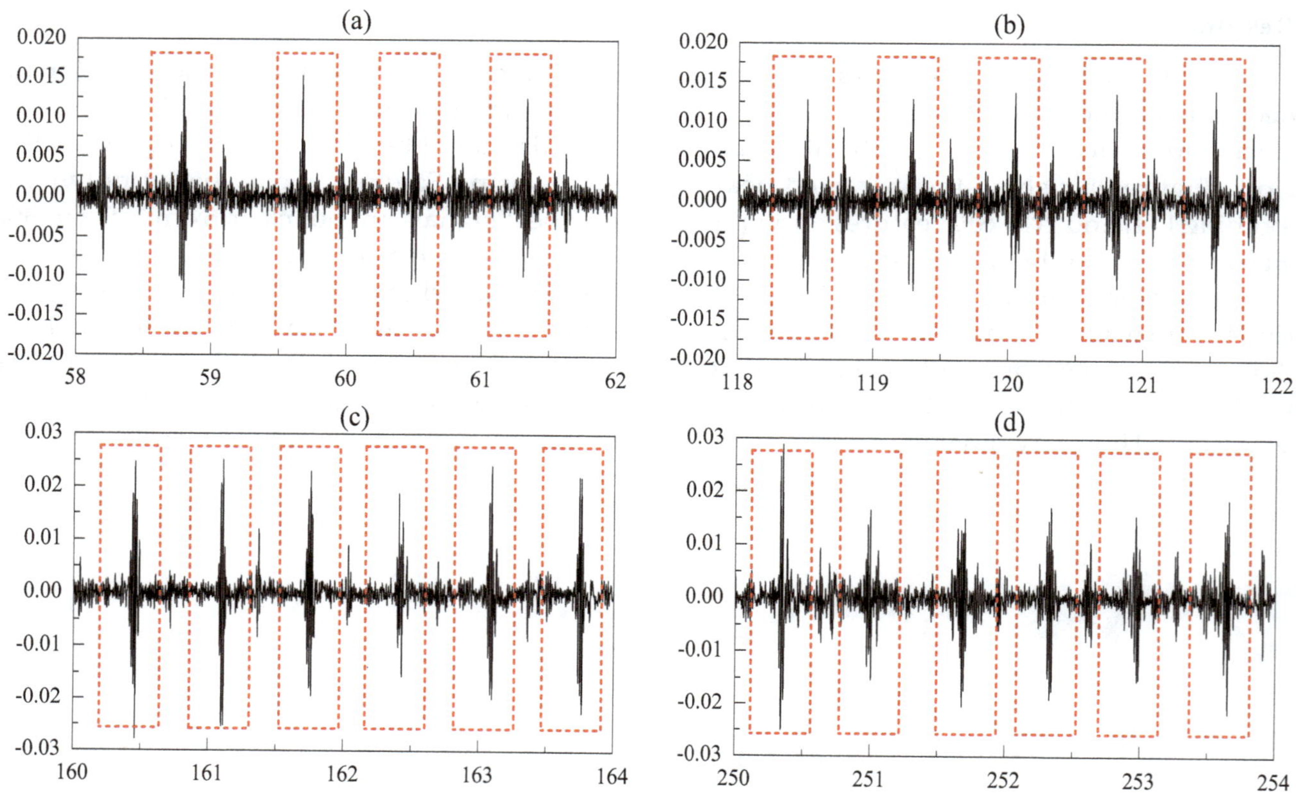

Figure 10. *Cont.*

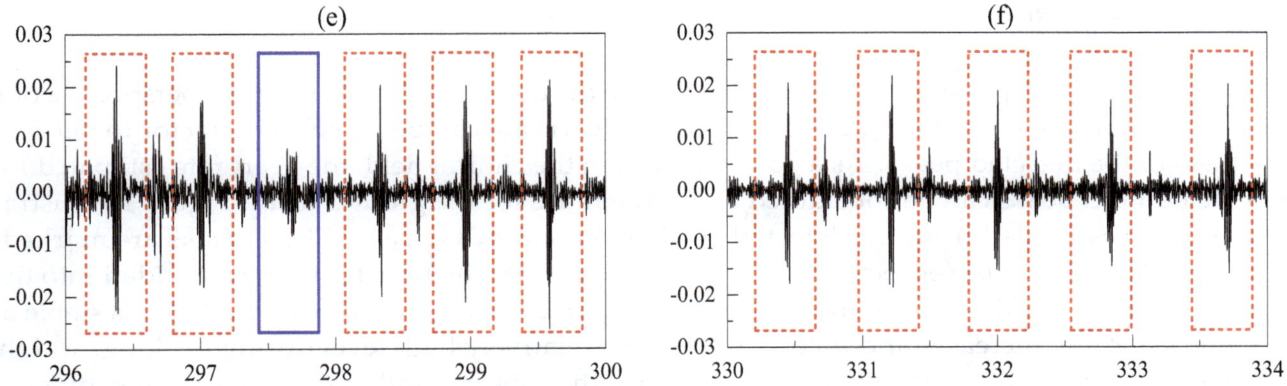

Figure 10. (**a–f**) Segmented signal during standing before walking, transitions from standing to walking, the first half of walking, the second half of walking, transitions from walking to standing, standing after walking. (The x-axis and y-axis are time in seconds and acceleration in gravity respectively.)

4.1. Heartbeat Detection Accuracy

The standard ECG lead I recordings are the baseline references for heartbeat signals. Heartbeat detection accuracy is defined as the ratio of the detected SCG peaks divided by the detected ECG peaks. The detected SCG peaks are visually noticeable and marked with the red dotted line in Figure 11. In addition, the missing SCG peaks are also considered to give a more precise estimate of detection accuracy. These peaks represent the undetected and false-positive detected SCG peaks. The blue rectangular, which is marked in Figure 10, can be considered as an undetected SCG peak using the rule of feature extraction described previously. This method is used even though the features and graphs of the signal are visually noticeable. Numbers in the brackets represent the missing peaks that occur at the beginning and end of walking in Table 1. It can be observed that above 60% of the missing SCG peaks occur at the beginning and end of walking when MA changes rapidly. The detection rates, which are shown in Table 1, are higher than 98%.

Table 1. Heartbeat detection accuracy.

Subject No.	ECG Peaks Detected	SCG Peaks Detected	SCG Peaks Missing	Accuracy
1	483	478	5(2)	98.9%
2	475	468	7(4)	98.5%
3	472	468	4(3)	99.1%
4	480	475	5(3)	98.9%
5	488	483	5(3)	98.9%
6	478	473	5(2)	98.9%
7	492	483	9(6)	98.1%
8	501	496	5(2)	99.0%
9	495	490	5(2)	98.9%
10	490	486	4(1)	99.1%
11	477	471	6(5)	98.7%
12	486	483	3(2)	99.3%
13	496	491	5(3)	98.9%
14	491	489	2(2)	99.5%
15	485	477	8(4)	98.3%
16	482	474	8(6)	98.3%

4.2. Heart Rate Estimations

The detected SCG peaks and ECG peaks evaluate the heartbeat signals from the perspective of the signal graph without considering the correctness. Heart rate can be an effective factor to verify the correctness of the detected peaks. As a gold standard in the clinical field, the heart rate estimated from the detected ECG peaks can be considered as the reference for the ground truth. Figure 11 illustrates the heart rates estimated from the detected SCG peaks and ECG peaks. These peaks are marked as black stars and red points, respectively. The x-axis represents the time that can be divided into three regions: standing, walking and return to standing. It can be observed that the heart rate is stable and low while standing, increases and then stabilizes at a relatively high level during walking, and then decreases to a stable and similar low magnitude when the subject stands again. The detailed difference between the heart rates from ECG and SCG with a mean value of 0.08 bpm and a standard deviation value of 2.08 bpm is plotted in Figure 12. It can be observed that the heart rates estimated from the detected SCG peaks and ECG peaks match very well.

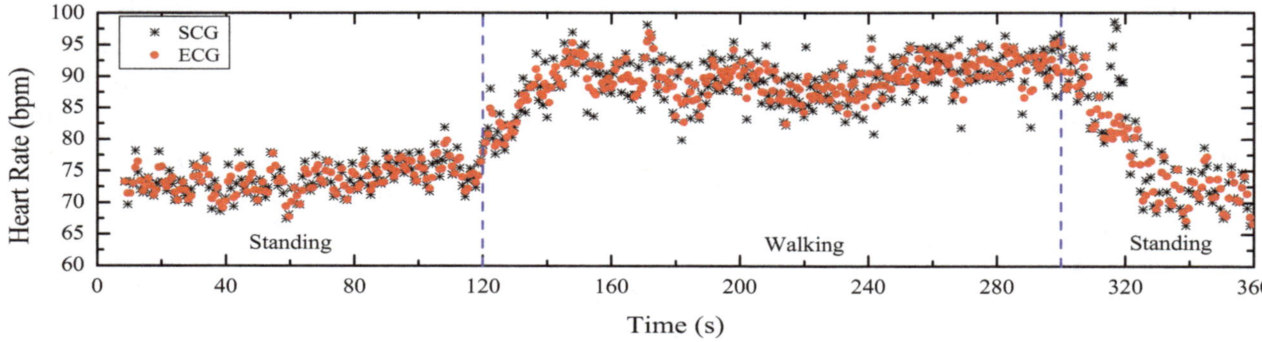

Figure 11. Heart rates estimated from ECG and SCG.

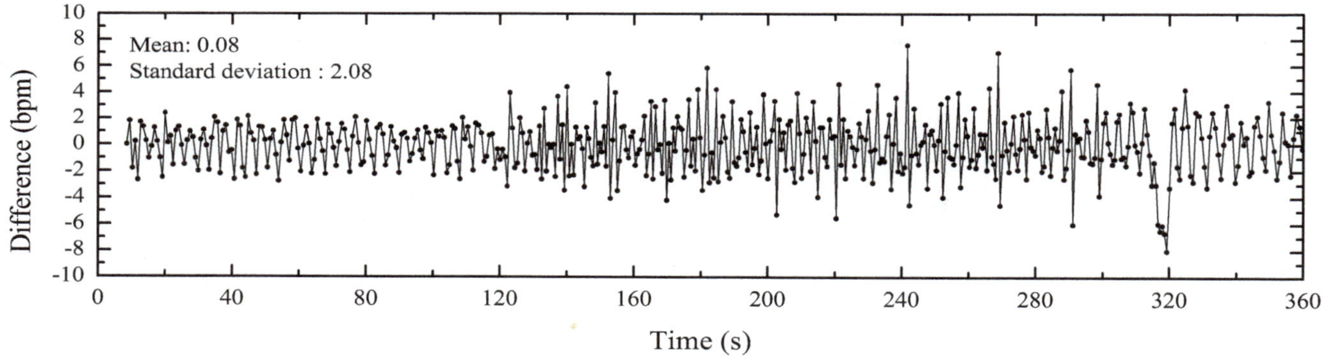

Figure 12. Heart rate difference between ECG and SCG.

4.3. Bland–Altman Analyzation

To further analyze the agreement between the heart rates estimated from the detected SCG peaks and ECG peaks, a Bland–Altman plot [34] is used and shown in Figure 13. Based on the definition of a Bland–Altman plot, the x-axis represents the average heart rates from SCG and ECG, and the y-axis represents their differences. A 95% confidence region is marked with blue dashed lines that have an upper threshold of 4.9 and a lower threshold of –4.6. It is observed that there are a few outliers, but overall most measurements lie in the 95% confidence region.

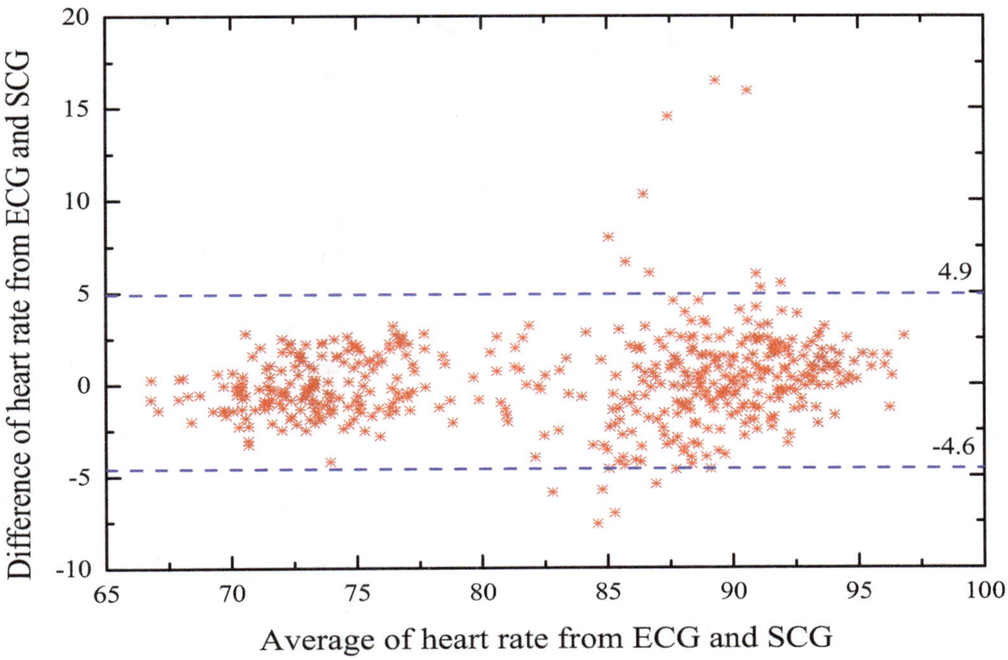

Figure 13. Bland–Altman plot of the heart rate measurements from ECG and SCG.

5. Discussion and Conclusions

In this paper, we proposed a novel method based on an adaptive recursive least squares filter to remove the motion artifact of the acceleration data recorded by only one accelerometer. The primary channel of ARLSF containing the heartbeat signal and motion artifact signal within a frequency range of 1 to 25 Hz was obtained by bandpass filtering the recorded acceleration data from 1Hz to 25Hz. Then the same acceleration data was bandpass filtered from 3.5 to 25 Hz to remove the heart rate frequency and footsteps frequency component from the heartbeat and motion artifact signals, respectively. The filtered signal and the signal of the primary channel were proved to have high correlation, and the heartbeat and motion artifact signal were proved to have strong orthogonality, which proved well that the filtered data could be fed into the reference channel of the ARLSF. The heartbeat signal graph of the extracted SCG signal was very clear without the need for any other signal recovery procedures. The heartbeat detection accuracy was up to 98% and heart rates estimated from the SCG and ECG matched well under both the standing and walking conditions.

At present these results are limited by a particularly rapidly changing motion artifact which will lead to missing SCG peaks' detection. The forgetting factor is set at a fixed value at a balance of the convergency, stability and tracking ability which leads to good convergency and stability but poor tracking ability of the proposed ARLSF. Moreover, the forgetting factor calculated by Equation (8) was a globally optimal solution but not a locally optimal solution especially when motion artifact changes rapidly. To obtain better performance, future work on the ARLSF proposed in this paper will focus on the optimization of the forgetting factor by using an adaptive method. That method will change the forgetting factor in real time according to the changes of the motion and promote the performance of ARLSF.

In addition, the experimental setup will be improved in future work. More subjects with a wider range of age and different health conditions, and more dynamic conditions including jumping and running, will be considered to evaluate the filter performance. In order to simplify the sensor placement before experiment and sensor data collection during the experiment, a miniature system-integrated SCG sensor, ECG sensor, MCU-embedded real-time filter algorithm and Bluetooth module will be developed in the future.

Author Contributions: S.Y. proposed the signal processing algorithm, developed the homemade prototype of SCG recorder system, designed the experiments and wrote this paper; S.L. gave some valuable suggestions and revised the paper. All authors have read and agreed to the published version of the manuscript.

References

1. Bozhenko, B.S. Seismocardiography—a new method in the study of functional conditions of the heart. *Ter Arkh* **1961**, *33*, 55–64.
2. Salerno, D.M.; Zanetti, J. Seismocardiography for monitoring changes in left ventricular function during ischemia. *Chest J.* **1991**, *100*, 991–993. [CrossRef]
3. Inan, O.T.; Migeotte, P.F.; Park, K.S.; Etemadi, M.; Tavakolian, K.; Casanella, R.; Zanetti, J.; Tank, J.; Funtova, I.; Prisk, G.K.; et al. Ballistocardiography and seismocardiography: A review of recent advances. *IEEE J. Biomed. Health Inform.* **2014**, *19*, 1414–1427. [CrossRef]
4. Taebi, A.; Solar, B.E.; Bomar, A.J.; Sandler, R.H.; Mansy, H.A. Recent Advances in Seismocardiography. *Vibration* **2019**, *2*, 5. [CrossRef]
5. Lee, H.; Lee, H.; Whang, M. An enhanced method to estimate heart rate from seismocardiography via ensemble averaging of body movements at six degrees of freedom. *Sensors* **2018**, *18*, 238. [CrossRef]
6. Ng, J.; Sahakian, A.V.; Swiryn, S. Accelerometer-based body- position sensing for ambulatory electrocardiographic monitoring. *Biomed Instrum. Technol.* **2003**, *37*, 338–346.
7. Yoon, S.; Min, S.; Yun, Y.; Lee, S.; Lee, M. Adaptive motion artifacts reduction using 3-axis accelerometer in e-textile ecg measurement system. *J. Med. Syst.* **2008**, *2*, 101–106. [CrossRef]
8. Liu, S.H. Motion artifact reduction in electrocardiogram using adaptive filter. *J. Med. Bio Log. Eng.* **2011**, *31*, 67–72. [CrossRef]
9. Yang, C.; Tavassolian, N. An Independent Component Analysis Approach to Motion Noise Cancelation of Cardio-Mechanical Signals. *IEEE Trans. Biomed. Eng.* **2019**, *3*, 66. [CrossRef]
10. Yang, C.; Tavassolian, N. Motion noise cancellation in seismocardiogram of ambulant subjects with dual sensors. In Proceedings of the International Conference of the IEEE Engineering in Medicine and Biology Society, Orlando, FL, USA, 16–20 August 2016; pp. 5881–5884.
11. Taebi, A.; Mansy, H.A. Noise cancellation from vibrocardiographic signals based on the ensemble empirical mode decomposition. *J. Appl. Biotechnol. Bioeng.* **2017**, *2*, 49–54. [CrossRef]
12. Javaid, A.Q.; Ashouri, H.; Dorier, A.; Etemadi, M.; Heller, J.A.; Roy, S.; Inan, O.T. Quantifying and Reducing Motion Artifacts in Wearable Seismocardiogram Measurements During Walking to Assess Left Ventricular Health. *IEEE Trans. Biomed. Eng.* **2017**, *64*, 1277–1286. [CrossRef]
13. Di Rienzo, M.; Meriggi, P.; Vaini, E.; Castiglioni, P.; Rizzo, F. 24h seismocardiogram monitoring in ambulant subjects. In Proceedings of the International Conference of the IEEE Engineering in Medicine and Biology Society, San Diego, CA, USA, 28 August–1 September 2012; pp. 5050–5053.
14. Pandia, K.; Ravindran, S.; Cole, R.; Kovacs, G.; Giovangrandi, L. Motion artifact cancellation to obtain heart sounds from a single chest-worn accelerometer. In Proceedings of the IEEE International Conference on Acoustics, Speech and Signal Processing, Dallas, TX, USA, 14–19 March 2010; pp. 590–593.
15. Kumar Jain, P.; Kumar Tiwari, A. A novel method for suppression of motion artifacts from the seismocardiogram signal. In Proceedings of the IEEE International Conference on Digital Signal Processing, Beijing, China, 16–18 October 2016; pp. 6–10.
16. Choudhary, T.; Sharma, L.N.; Bhuyan, M.K. Heart Sound Extraction from Sternal Seismocardiographic Signal. *IEEE Signal Process. Lett.* **2018**, *25*, 482–486. [CrossRef]
17. Yang, C.; Tavassolian, N. Motion artifact cancellation of seismocardiographic recording from moving subjects. *IEEE Sens. J.* **2016**, *16*, 5702–5708. [CrossRef]
18. Diniz, P.S.R. *Adaptive Filtering: Algorithms and Practical Implementation*, 4th ed.; Springer: New York, NY, USA, 2013; pp. 209–248.
19. Haykin, S.O. *Adaptive Filter Theory*, 5th ed.; Pearson: Upper Saddle River, TX, USA, 2013; pp. 449–472.
20. Reinvuo, T.; Hannula, M.; Sorvoja, H.; Alasaarela, E.; Myllyla, R. Measurement of respiratory rate with high-resolution accelerometer and emfit pressure sensor. In Proceedings of the IEEE Sensors Applications Symposium, Houston, TX, USA, 22–25 October 2006; pp. 192–195.

21. Morillo, D.S.; Ojeda, J.L.R.; Foix, L.F.P.; Jimenez, A.L. An accelerometer-based device for sleep apnea screening. *IEEE Trans. Inf. Technol. Biomed.* **2010**, *14*, 491–499. [CrossRef]
22. Marcus, F.; Sorrell, V.; Zanetti, J.; Bosnos, M.; Baweja, G.; Perlick, D.; Ott, P.; Indik, J.; He, D.S.; Gear, K. Accelerometer-derived time intervals during various pacing modes in patients with biventricular pacemakers: Comparison with normals. *PACE* **2007**, *30*, 1476–1481. [CrossRef]
23. Zanetti, J.M.; Tavakolian, K. Seismocardiography: Past, present and future. In Proceedings of the International Conference of the IEEE Engineering in Medicine and Biology Society, Osaka, Japan, 3–7 July 2013; pp. 7004–7007.
24. Roskamm, H. Optimum patterns of exercise for healthy adults. *Can. Med. Assoc. J.* **1967**, *96*, 895–900.
25. Robergs, R.A.; Landwehr, R. The surprising history of the "HRmax=220-age" equation. *J. Exerc. Physiol. Online* **2002**, *5*, 1–10.
26. Tanaka, H.; Monahan, K.D.; Seals, D.R. Age-predicted maximal heart rate revisited. *J. Am. Coll. Cardiol.* **2001**, *37*, 153–156.
27. Pachi, A.; Ji, T. Frequency and velocity of people walking. *Struct. Eng.* **2005**, *83*, 36–40.
28. Ratner, B. The correlation coefficients: Its values range between or do they? *J. Target. Meas. Anal. Mark.* **2009**, *17*, 139–142. [CrossRef]
29. Suresh, H.N. New Technique for Recursive Least Square Adaptive Algorithm for Acoustic Echo Cancellation of Speech signal in an auditorium. *Int. Research J. Eng. Technol.* **2015**, *36*, 110–117.
30. LabVIEW 2013 System Identification Toolkit Help. Available online: http://zone.ni.com/reference/en-XX/help/372458D-01/lvsysidconcepts/recursive_ls/ (accessed on 28 February 2020).
31. Pan, J.; Tompkins, W.J. A Real-Time QRS Detection Algorithm. *IEEE Trans. Biomed. Eng.* **1985**, *32*, 230–236. [CrossRef] [PubMed]
32. Khosrow, K.F.; Tavakolian, K.; Menon, C. Moving toward automatic and standalone delineation of seismocardiogram signal. In Proceedings of the International Conference of the IEEE Engineering in Medicine and Biology Society (EMBC), Milan, Italy, 25–29 August 2015; pp. 7163–7166.
33. Sørensen, K.; Schmidt, S.E.; Jensen, A.S. Definition of Fiducial Points in the Normal Seismocardiogram. *Sci. Rep.* **2018**, *8*, 15455. [CrossRef] [PubMed]
34. Bland, J.M.; Altman, D.G. Measuring agreement in method comparison studies. *Stat. Methods Med. Res.* **1999**, *8*, 135–160. [CrossRef] [PubMed]

4

Detection of Talking in Respiratory Signals: A Feasibility Study Using Machine Learning and Wearable Textile-Based Sensors

Andreas Ejupi and Carlo Menon *

Menrva Research Group, Schools of Mechatronic Systems & Engineering Science at Simon Fraser University (SFU), Burnaby, BC V5A 1S6, Canada; andreas@ejupi.at

* Correspondence: cmenon@sfu.ca

Abstract: Social isolation and loneliness are major health concerns in young and older people. Traditional approaches to monitor the level of social interaction rely on self-reports. The goal of this study was to investigate if wearable textile-based sensors can be used to accurately detect if the user is talking as a future indicator of social interaction. In a laboratory study, fifteen healthy young participants were asked to talk while performing daily activities such as sitting, standing and walking. It is known that the breathing pattern differs significantly between normal and speech breathing (i.e., talking). We integrated resistive stretch sensors into wearable elastic bands, with a future integration into clothing in mind, to record the expansion and contraction of the chest and abdomen while breathing. We developed an algorithm incorporating machine learning and evaluated its performance in distinguishing between periods of talking and non-talking. In an intra-subject analysis, our algorithm detected talking with an average accuracy of 85%. The highest accuracy of 88% was achieved during sitting and the lowest accuracy of 80.6% during walking. Complete segments of talking were correctly identified with 96% accuracy. From the evaluated machine learning algorithms, the random forest classifier performed best on our dataset. We demonstrate that wearable textile-based sensors in combination with machine learning can be used to detect when the user is talking. In the future, this approach may be used as an indicator of social interaction to prevent social isolation and loneliness.

Keywords: wearable sensors; machine learning; smart textiles; healthcare; talking detection

---

1. Introduction

Social isolation and loneliness are important health risk factors and known to negatively influence wellbeing. It has been reported that up to 50% of older people suffer from a low level of social interaction [1]. The causes can be diverse including general health issues, disabilities and certain life events such as the loss of a spouse or a change in residence [2,3]. On a positive note, research has shown that social isolation and loneliness can be prevented. Intervention programs such as in-person support activities or phone-mediated groups have shown promising results [3]. However, due to the limited health care resources, it would be warranted to accurately identify people who are in need of targeted interventions. Traditional approaches rely on the self-reports using questionnaires to assess the daily level of social interaction. Self-reports are often described as subjective and influenced by a recall bias [4].

One alternative approach could be to automatically identify people with a low level of social interaction by using technology. Previous work in this area has mainly focused on audio-based systems using a microphone to capture talking throughout the day [5,6]. Previous work has also investigated the use of video-based systems to monitor mouth movements as an indicator of social interaction [7,8].

Both methods look promising in terms of accuracy. However, user acceptance and portability might be a challenge [9].

There is a need for more unobtrusive and portable solutions. We propose to detect if someone is talking by using wearable textile-based sensors, which can be directly integrated into everyday clothing. Our approach does not rely on audio or video recordings; instead, it aims to detect talking by monitoring changes in the respiratory (i.e., breathing) patterns.

1.1. Detection of Talking (Speech Breathing)

Generally, breathing results in an expansion and a contraction of the chest and abdominal region. It has been found that the breathing pattern differs significantly between normal and speech breathing (i.e., talking), with the respiration more rhythmic during normal breathing [10,11]. It has been also reported that the inhalation duration and the ratio between the inhalation and exhalation time are good discriminatory indicators [12,13].

To date, only a few studies have investigated the use of wearable sensors to detect if someone is talking based on respiratory markers [10,12,14]. These studies used inductive plethysmography sensors, which consist of electrical wires embedded in elastic bands usually attached to the chest and abdominal region. By generating a magnetic field and passing it through a sinusoidal arrangement of electrical wires, the self-conductance of the coils, which is proportional to the cross-sectional area surrounded by the band, can be measured [12]. However, these sensors are primarily designed for clinical settings and mainly used for short duration recordings.

1.2. Textile-Based Sensors

In this paper, we investigate the feasibility of wearable textile-based sensors. In particular, we focus on resistive stretch sensors, which are made by a mixture of polymer (e.g., silicone, rubber) and a conductive material (e.g., carbon black). These resistive sensors act like a resistor, which means that any elongation results in a measurable change in electrical resistance. Related work in this field has investigated the use of textile-based stretch sensors in several human applications. For example, Tognetti et al. [15] investigated a textile-based sensor for posture monitoring. Similarly, Mattman et al. [16] integrated sensors into tight-fitting clothing to classify between various body postures. Papi et al. [17] explored the feasibility to discriminate between daily activities (i.e., walking, running, stair climbing) by using a stretch sensor attached to the knee. These studies suggest the preliminary feasibility of textile-based stretch sensors to monitor human motions. To the best of our knowledge, our study is the first to use this type of sensor to detect talking in respiratory signals.

The main aims of this study were to (1) investigate the feasibility of textile-based stretch sensors to monitor breathing patterns, (2) develop an algorithm using machine learning to accurately detect talking and (3) evaluate its performance in a study with 15 participants.

2. Materials and Methods

2.1. Stretch Sensor

In this paper, we investigated the feasibility of a wearable textile-based stretch sensor to detect if someone is talking. The stretch sensor has been fabricated in our research lab (Menrva) at Simon Fraser University, Canada [18], using a mixture of polymer and conductive carbon black. The sensor shows similar properties as the commercially available sensors from Adafruit (New York, NY, USA) [19] and Image SI (Staten Island, NY, USA) [20], but only has a diameter of 0.4 mm, which makes it suitable to integrate into garments (Figure 1). Previous work has shown good results in using machine learning to obtain accurate measurements from these textile-based stretch sensors [21,22] and using them for the monitoring of human movements [15,16,23].

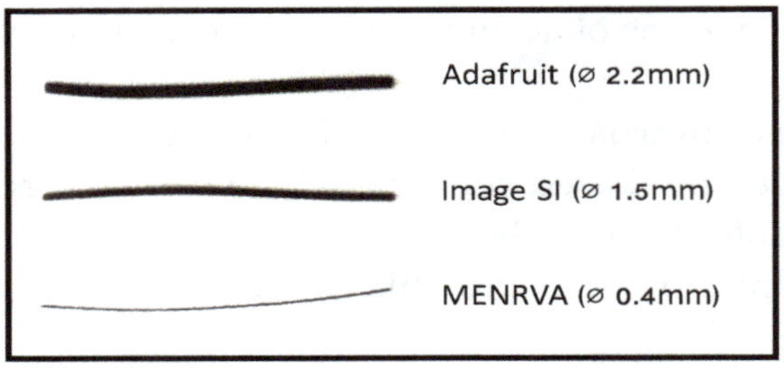

Figure 1. Comparison between the Adafruit, Image SI and Menrva sensors.

2.2. *Chest and Abdominal Bands*

The approach was to detect talking based on changes in the breathing pattern. As is known from the literature, we can differentiate between chest and abdominal breathing [24,25]. Chest breathing can be described as the drawing of air into the chest area by using the intercostal muscles. This type of breathing is more common during states of exertion. In contrast, abdominal breathing is the expansion of the belly by contracting the diaphragm. This type of breathing is common during phases of relaxation [26].

However, breathing can be quite diverse between people. Some people are more heavily chest breathers, whereas others are more so abdominal breathers [25]. To capture the expansion and contraction of the full torso, we designed three elastic bands with the stretch sensor integrated and positioned them at the abdominal, lower and upper chest region for our study (Figure 2). In the future, the sensor might be directly integrated into the clothing.

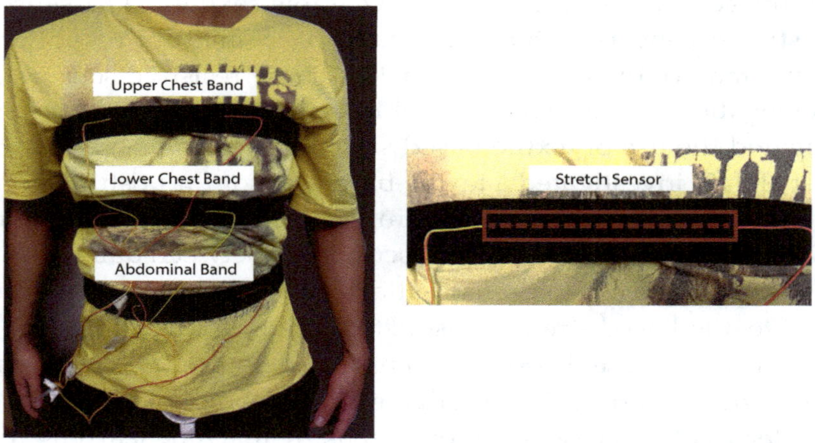

Figure 2. Three custom-made sensor bands to monitor the expansion and contraction of the torso while breathing (and talking). The red dashed line shows the positioning of the sensor.

The bands were made out of two materials. The back and side part were made out of a synthetic knit with medium elasticity. The front piece and attachment of the sensor were made of a fleece material with high elasticity. The intention was to concentrate the stretch during breathing (and talking) primarily on the sensor. Three pieces of the Menrva stretch sensor with a length of 10 cm each were integrated into the front piece of the bands (Figure 2). Sensors were laid out straight and secured with an elastic stitch on top. The wires were connected on both sides with a mixture of rubber glue and conductive ink.

2.3. *Data Acquisition Hardware*

The three bands were connected to a data acquisition system (Model NI-USB-6009, National Instruments, Austin, TX, USA) using a voltage divider circuit to measure their electrical response by connecting a 5 V DC voltage source and a resistor in series to the sensors. The resistor value was selected to match the base resistance of the stretch sensor (20 kΩ). All data were captured with a sampling rate of 100 Hz.

2.4. Study Protocol

The study protocol included three main parts with a total duration of 1.5 h per participant including the setup time. Participants were asked to wear the three custom-made sensors to monitor the expansion and contraction of the torso while talking. Sensor bands were tightly fitted, but still comfortable, for each participant. The tightness was adjusted based on the user's feedback by explaining that the bands should be similarly tight and comfortable as, for example, a tight-fitting t-shirt, usually used for exercising. Participants were asked to talk while sitting, standing and walking. We selected these activities because they are the most common activities in which people talk in daily life. Each activity lasted for 20 min and included 5 trials with 2 min of non-talking and 2 min of talking. The order of the activities was randomized. To capture sufficient data of talking during each period and activity, we asked the participants to read out the text of a news article. The article included general information about the city of Vancouver, Canada. For the walking part, participants were asked to walk on a treadmill. We used a treadmill for convenience due to the limited length of the wires, which connected the bands with the data acquisition hardware. Talking while walking usually occurs at slower speed, and therefore, we selected 2 mph for this test.

2.5. Participants

Fifteen young adults were asked to participate in this study. Participants were between 19 and 30 years old and were students at Simon Fraser University (SFU), Canada. Table 1 shows the participant characteristics. Written informed consent was obtained from all participants prior to data collection. The study was approved by the Research Ethics Board of SFU.

Table 1. Participant characteristics.

	Study Participants (n = 15)
Age (years)	23 (3.8)
Gender (F/M)	6/9
Height (cm)	169.8 (8.9)
Weight (kg)	68.5 (12.1)
BMI (kg/m^2)	23.6 (3.1)

2.6. Talking Detection Algorithm

Our main aim was to detect talking based on changes in the respiratory signals. Before talking, air usually gets inhaled fast and then exhaled slowly while talking. This results in a specific breathing pattern when compared to normal breathing (Figure 3). Our algorithm utilizes this information to detect talking.

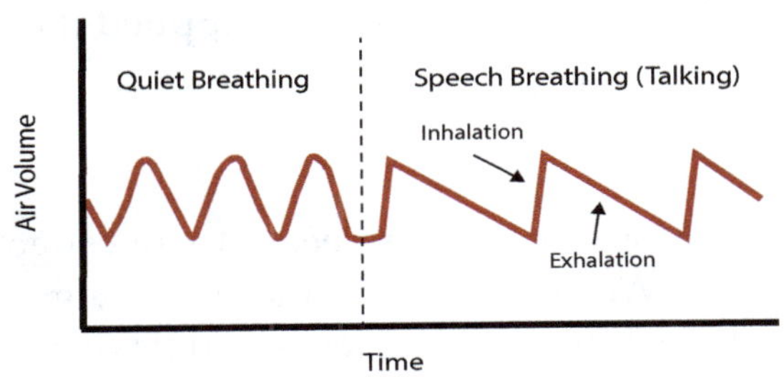

Figure 3. Changes in the air volume while talking.

Our algorithm is based on the following steps of data processing and analysis (Figure 4):

- Data input: The input data to our algorithm were the raw sensor signals (sampled with 100 Hz) of the three bands, which we converted from voltage to resistance values.
- Signal filtering: A healthy adult usually breathes between 12 and 18 times per minute at rest. For older adults, the breathing can vary between 12 and 30 times per minute [27]. We filtered the sensor signals accordingly with a bandpass filter (4th order Butterworth, lower cut-off frequency of 0.1 Hz and higher cut-off of 1.5 Hz) to account for possible drift and reduce the overall level of noise in the sensor signals.
- Breathing detection: Any inhalation of air and consequent expansion of the torso results in a peak of the stretch sensor signal. Our algorithm detects these peaks using MATLAB's peak detection algorithm with an empirically-defined parameter of 5 for the minimum peak prominence setting. The prominence of a peak measures how much the peak stands out due to its intrinsic height and its location relative to other peaks.
- Feature extraction: The detection of a peak triggers the feature extraction process. The algorithm centres a window with an empirically-found length of 3 s on each detected peak. From this time window, a set of predefined features get extracted and used as the input to a machine learning classifier.
- Classification of talking: A machine learning classifier has been trained to detect speech breathing (i.e., talking) based on the extracted features.

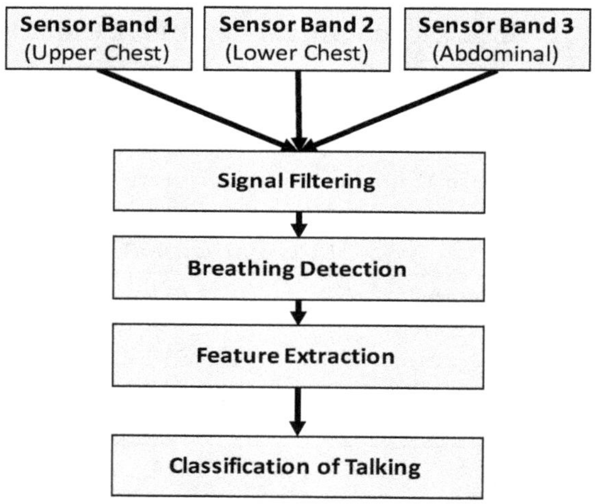

Figure 4. Design of the talking detection algorithm incorporating machine learning.

2.7. Machine Learning Approach

In the first part of the analysis, we were focused on identifying which machine learning algorithm, hyper parameters and features would generally perform best in the task of detecting talking using this kind of technology. In the second part of the analysis, we applied the selected model and calculated the accuracy for each participant.

2.7.1. Model Selection

Four machine learning algorithms have been selected to investigate their feasibility in detecting talking based on our collected data. We have selected these four algorithms because they have been commonly used in health-related machine learning tasks and have achieved promising results in the past. First, random forest is an ensemble method that operates by constructing multiple decision trees at training time and then uses the mean prediction of individual trees to estimate the target values [28]. Second, neural network is a method inspired by the biological neural network system using layers and a number of interconnected nodes to make a prediction [29]. Third, support vector machine operates by constructing a set of hyperplanes in a high- or infinite-dimensional space to estimate the target value [30]. Fourth, linear discriminant analysis uses a linear decision boundary and has been proven to work well in practice due to its low computational costs [31].

The hyper parameters for the machine learning classifiers were empirically identified. To calculate the performance of each model and select the best performing hyper parameters, we used 15-fold cross-validation. This was done on a training dataset that consisted of the first 70% of data of each participant. The model performance was evaluated using the receiver operating characteristics curve (ROC) and the associated area under the curve (AUC) metric.

For the random forest classifier, the best performance was achieved using 200 as the parameter for the number of trees (values tested between 10 and 200). For the support vector machine, the best performance was achieved with gamma set to 0.01 (tested between 0.001 and 1) and C set to 10 (tested between 1 and 100). For the neural network classifier, the best performance was achieved with a network structure of 2 hidden layers (tested from 1 to 2) and 30 neurons in the hidden layers.

2.7.2. Feature Extraction and Selection

Features were extracted with an automated feature extraction approach. Therefore, we used the Python library tsfresh [32], which calculates and tests more than 100 predefined time and frequency-domain features with various parameters. Using this approach, we extracted features from the raw and first derivate of the sensor signals of all three bands. Features were extracted using a sliding window (size of 3 s) approach. For the feature selection, we also applied 15-fold cross-validation and used the same training dataset as for the hyper parameter tuning. A tree-based approach was used to rank the best performing features based on their relevance (i.e., Gini importance [33]) for each run. Only the top 10% features among all runs were selected for the final algorithm to reduce complexity and computation time. For a detailed description of the calculation of these features, see [32]. The majority of significant features were based on the sensor signals of the upper chest and lower chest band. The features included in our final model were:

- Ratio beyond sigma: the ratio of values that are more than $r \times std(x)$ away from the mean of x (with $r = \{1,2\}$).
- Symmetry looking: the Boolean variable denoting if the distribution of x looks symmetric.
- Continues Wavelet Transform peaks: the number of peaks of the continuous wavelet transform using a Mexican hat wavelet [34].
- Skewness: the sample skewness of x (calculated with the adjusted Fisher–Pearson standardized moment coefficient G1).
- Energy ratio by chunks: the sum of squares of chunk i out of N chunks expressed as a ratio with the sum of squares over the whole (with $N = 10$).
- Augmented Dickey–Fuller: the hypothesis test that checks whether a unit root is present in x [35].
- Count above mean: the number of values in x that are higher than the mean of x.
- Count below mean: the number of values in x that are lower than the mean of x.
- Number of crossings: the number of crossings of x on m (with $m = 0$).
- Fourier coefficients: the coefficients of the one-dimensional discrete Fourier transform [36].
- Welch's spectral density: the cross power spectral density of x [37].
- Sample entropy: the sample entropy of x.
- Autoregressive coefficients: the fit of the unconditional maximum likelihood of an autoregressive $AR(k)$ process.

2.7.3. Performance Evaluation

We integrated the best performing machine learning model, features and parameters into our algorithm and evaluated its performance in detecting talking in an intra-subject analysis. The data of each participant were split into the activities of sitting, standing and walking. For each activity, we trained a model separately and evaluated it using cross-validation.

As sample-based performance metrics, accuracy (ACC), true positive rate (TPR) and false positive rate (FPR) were selected. TPR has been defined as the percentage of correctly identified speech breathing patterns. FPR has been defined as the percentage of incorrectly identified speech breathing patterns among all other breathing patterns.

$$ACC = \frac{TP + TN}{TP + TN + FP + FN} \quad (1)$$

$$TPR = \frac{TP}{TP + FN} \quad (2)$$

$$FPR = \frac{FP}{FP + TN} \quad (3)$$

Furthermore, the number of correctly identified talking segments was calculated. A talking segment was classified correctly if the majority of prediction labels in this segment predicted talking.

$$ACC_{seg} = \frac{correctly\_classified\_talking\_segments}{total\_number\_of\_talking\_segments} \quad (4)$$

2.8. Software

MATLAB (R2016b) was used for data acquisition, processing of the sensor data and algorithm development. The Python package scikit-learn [38] was used to train and evaluate the machine learning models. The Python package tsfresh [32] was used for automated feature extraction.

3. Results

One hour of sensor data was recorded from each participant with a recording time of 30 min of talking. The entire dataset included 11,924 detected breathings, which were used for further classification. We observed significant differences between normal and speech breathing in the activities of sitting, standing and walking (Figure 5). During the phases of talking, the breathing is less rhythmic with faster inhalations and slower exhalations.

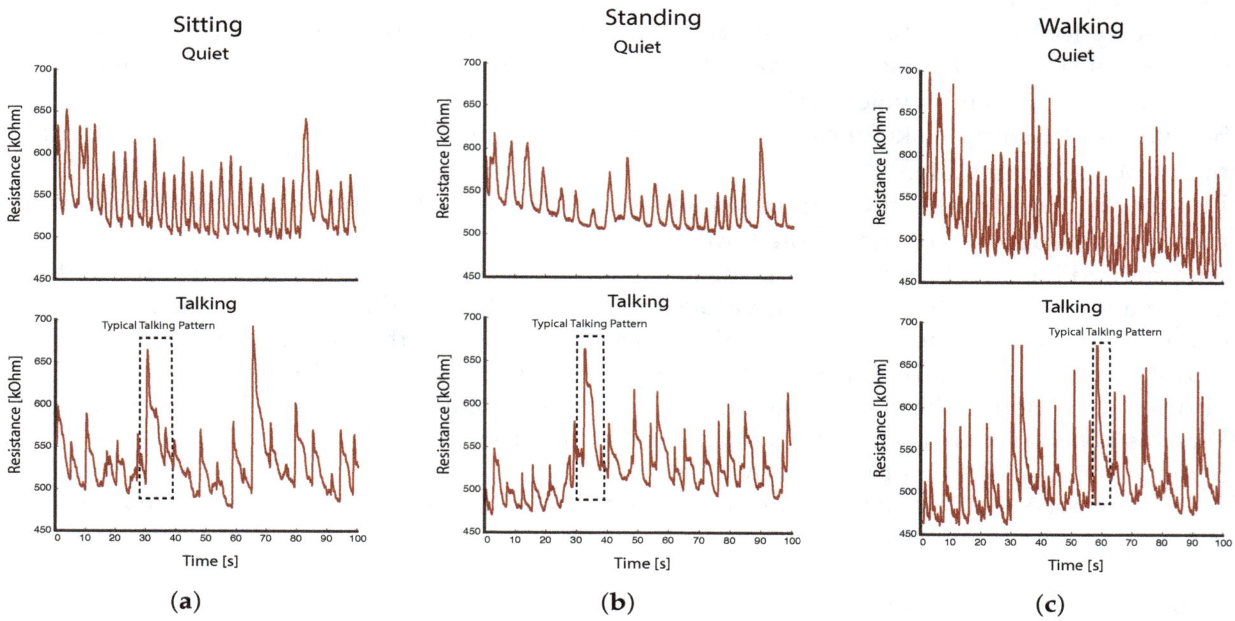

Figure 5. Comparison of the raw sensor signals (upper chest band) between quiet and speech breathing (i.e., talking) for: (**a**) sitting; (**b**) standing; and (**c**) walking.

3.1. Model Selection

Among all tested machine learning algorithms, the random forest (and support vector machine) classifier performed best on our dataset with an AUC value of 0.90, which was slightly higher compared to the performance of the neural network classifier (AUC = 0.89) and linear discriminant analysis (AUC = 0.87) (Figure 6).

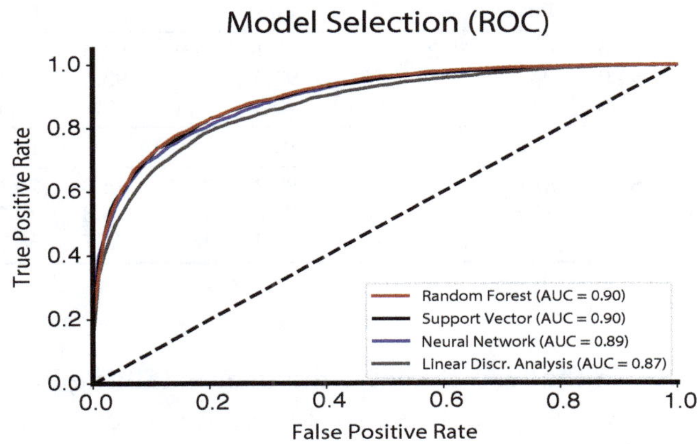

Figure 6. Comparison of the ROC curves (and the associated AUC metric) among the tested machine learning algorithms.

3.2. Accuracy of Talking Detection Algorithm

Among all participants, our algorithm utilizing the random forest classifier detected talking with an average *ACC* of 85% (*TPR*: 81.3%, *FPR*: 12.8%) (Table 2). The highest *ACC* of 88% was achieved in the sitting task and the lowest *ACC* of 80.6% in walking. Table 3 shows the results for each participant in detail with the accuracy ranging from 68.8% to 97.5%. Furthermore, segments of talking have been correctly classified with an ACC_{seg} of 96.3%. Figure 7 illustrates the exemplary prediction accuracy of our algorithm on the data of participant P10. The number of misclassifications increased from sitting, standing to walking.

Table 2. Average performance of our algorithm in detecting talking among all participants.

	Average *ACC*	Average *TPR*	Average *FPR*
Sitting	88.0 (5.4)	88.0 (6.1)	12.6 (6.9)
Standing	86.3 (7.3)	84.2 (8.6)	12.5 (7.6)
Walking	80.6 (7.7)	71.8 (12.1)	13.3 (6.5)
Average	85.0 (6.8)	81.3 (8.9)	12.8 (7.0)

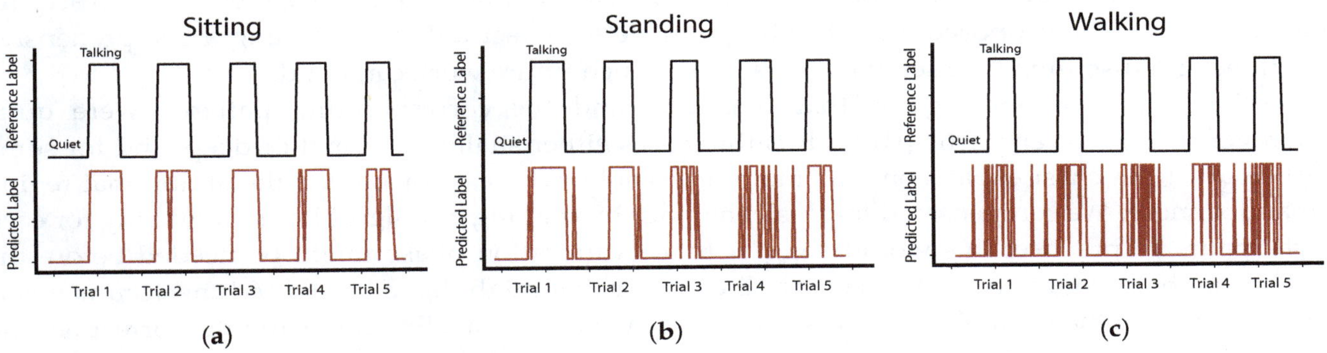

Figure 7. Exemplary detection of talking for participant P10 in activities: (**a**) sitting; (**b**) standing; and (**c**) walking.

Table 3. Performance results of our algorithm in detecting talking for each participant (P).

	P01			**P02**			**P03**			**P04**			**P05**		
	ACC	*TPR*	*FPR*	*ACC*	*TPR*	*FPR*	*ACC*	*TPR*	*FPR*	*ACC*	*TPR*	*FPR*	*ACC*	*TPR*	*FPR*
Sitting	94.3	92.3	3.9	94.8	93.5	4.2	97.5	94.9	0.9	84.9	84.9	15.0	82.9	81.2	15.6
Standing	93.9	92.2	4.4	90.5	90.0	9.1	94.2	91.5	3.7	76.1	73.1	21.3	86.0	79.1	9.9
Walking	79.6	76.4	17.6	85.2	81.0	11.6	90.2	82.4	4.4	68.8	55.3	20.7	87.2	83.6	9.8
	P06			**P07**			**P08**			**P09**			**P10**		
Sitting	81.6	87.7	24.2	88.6	95.1	20.2	93.7	93.1	5.9	89.3	93.3	14.6	92.0	90.9	7.3
Standing	82.5	79.2	14.7	94.0	94.9	7.1	95.1	92.5	2.9	93.6	96.1	8.9	87.0	81.4	9.1
Walking	71.1	70.5	28.5	87.8	84.7	9.3	95.6	90.8	1.4	79.7	75.4	17.0	81.1	68.2	11.9
	P11			**P12**			**P13**			**P14**			**P15**		
Sitting	82.7	82.0	16.7	89.8	87.0	7.9	83.5	89.3	22.7	84.3	79.1	12.6	79.3	75.0	16.7
Standing	73.9	73.8	26.1	83.3	70.8	9.0	78.7	76.2	18.8	75.8	79.5	28.2	89.8	93.2	13.9
Walking	68.3	42.5	14.8	79.4	69.4	13.5	73.0	61.3	18.6	81.7	68.2	9.9	80.0	66.9	9.9

4. Discussion

We developed an algorithm that can detect if the user is talking based on respiratory markers. In contrast to previous work, we used textile-based stretch sensors to monitor the expansion and contraction of the torso and achieved a reasonable accuracy by incorporating machine learning into our algorithm.

Previous studies have relied on either audio or video recordings to detect talking. Besides the technical challenges of these approaches, there might be also privacy concerns [9]. The aim of this study was to develop a system that is unobtrusive and portable. We selected a wearable approach, as it would allow quantifying talking throughout the day independent of the user's location. This is in alignment with a recent trend in the development of the wearable technologies for various health applications [39,40].

Our approach uses wearable textile-based sensors to monitor breathing and as a consequence detect if someone is talking. Although there were some studies that have investigated the feasibility of detecting respiratory events in the past, only a few studies have focused on the detection of talking in respiratory signals [10,12,14]. These studies have used inductive plethysmograph sensors. Conventional inductive plethysmograph sensors are primarily designed for the clinical setting and short-term recordings with possible limitations in the size of the electronics and number of sensors that can be used at the same time [41].

In terms of accuracy, Rahman et al. [10] (and Bari et al. [42]) reported 82 to 87% in speech/non-speech classification using inductive plethysmograph sensors. The reported accuracy is in alignment with what we have achieved in this study.

What differentiates this work is the use of textile-based stretch sensors in combination with the developed machine learning-based algorithm. The sensor we used is flexible with a diameter of only 0.4 mm and acts like a resistor, which makes it easy to integrate into garments and to acquire measurements. We proposed an algorithm suitable to detect talking including a comprehensive identified and discriminative set of features upon which future work can build.

What we have observed is that breathing and the corresponding patterns were quite heterogeneous between participants. Breathing was either shallow, normal or deep, and for some participants, the chest expansion was more noticeable, whereas for others, the abdominal region expanded more. We compensated for this behaviour by training our algorithm individually for each participant. In practice, this would suggest that a calibration phase might be needed before the system can be used by an individual. Another factor that might have influenced the accuracy was the sensitivity of the technology to noise due to body movements. Breathing and the corresponding expansion of the torso result in a relatively small elongation of the stretch sensor. What we have observed is that rotational and bending movements of the upper body influenced the measurements. This was especially noticeable in the task of walking, which might explain the lower accuracy in this task. Future work might combine our approach with an accelerometer to filter out the noise due to body movements.

Considering the advantages of the technology, this approach might be suitable for the daily life setting. A future application could be the integration of the sensor (or a series of sensors) into a tight-fitting undershirt. In addition to the sensor, a circuit board and battery would be required. Preliminary results show that the sensor has a power draw of about 1.25 mW (as used in this study). This would allow the monitoring of the user's level of talking throughout the day, and furthermore, this measurement could be used as an indicator of social interaction. Such a system might be used in older adults where social isolation and loneliness are common concerns [1,3]. For example, in an institutionalized setting, such a system could provide the staff daily feedback about the level of social interaction of each resident. Once a significant change in behaviour has been detected, targeted interventions could be started. Similarly, this technology could be used in older people living in the community where a low level of social interaction can lead to more frequent home visits by the healthcare professionals.

We acknowledge certain study limitations. Data were collected in the laboratory setting under fairly controlled conditions with young and healthy adults. Participants were asked to read a text out loud, which might be different from conversational speaking. Future studies are warranted to determine whether this approach can be used in a daily life setting and to investigate the accuracy and user acceptance of this system in the older population.

In summary, we have demonstrated that wearable textile-based sensors in combination with a machine learning-based algorithm can be used to detect when the user is talking. In future, this approach may be used to unobtrusively quantify talking as an indicator of social interaction, and consequently may prevent social isolation and loneliness.

Author Contributions: All authors read and approved the manuscript. Conceptualization, A.E. and C.M. Software, A.E. Validation, A.E. Formal analysis, A.E. Investigation, A.E. Resources, A.E. and C.M. Data curation, A.E. and C.M.; Writing—Original Draft Preparation, A.E.; Writing—Review & Editing, A.E. and C.M. Visualization, A.E. Supervision, C.M. Project administration, C.M. Funding acquisition, C.M.

Acknowledgments: The authors would like to thank all participants and individuals who contributed to the data collection.

References

1. Grenade, L.; Boldy, D. Social isolation and loneliness among older people: Issues and future challenges in community and residential settings. *Aust. Health Rev.* **2008**, *32*, 468–478. [CrossRef] [PubMed]
2. Cattan, M.; White, M.; Bond, J.; Learmouth, A. Preventing social isolation and loneliness among older people: A systematic review of health promotion interventions. *Ageing Soc.* **2005**, *25*, 41–67. [CrossRef]
3. Health Quality Ontario. *Social Isolation in Community-Dwelling Seniors: An Evidence-Based Analysis*; Health Quality Ontario: Toronto, ON, Canada, 2008; Volume 8, pp. 1–49.
4. Coughlin, S.S. Recall bias in epidemiologic studies. *J. Clin. Epidemiol.* **1990**, *43*, 87–91. [CrossRef]
5. Choudhury, T.; Pentland, A. Sensing and modeling human networks using the sociometer. In Proceedings of the Seventh IEEE International Symposium on Wearable Computers, White Plains, NY, USA, 21–23 October 2003; pp. 216–222.
6. Wyatt, D.; Choudhury, T.; Bilmes, J.; Kitts, J.A. Inferring colocation and conversation networks from privacy-sensitive audio with implications for computational social science. *ACM Trans. Intell. Syst. Technol.* **2011**, *2*, 1–41. [CrossRef]
7. Cristani, M.; Pesarin, A.; Vinciarelli, A.; Crocco, M.; Murino, V. Look at who's talking: Voice Activity Detection by Automated Gesture Analysis. In Proceedings of the European Conference on Ambient Intelligence, Amsterdam, The Netherlands, 16–18 November 2011; pp. 72–80

8. Rao, R.R. Cross-modal prediction in audio-visual communication. In Proceedings of the 1996 IEEE International Conference on Acoustics, Speech, and Signal Processing, Atlanta, GA, USA, 9 May 1996.
9. Klasnja, P.; Consolvo, S.; Choudhury, T.; Beckwith, R.; Hightower, J. Exploring privacy concerns about personal sensing. *Lect. Notes Comput. Sci.* **2009**, *5538*, 176–183.
10. Rahman, M.; Ahsan, A.; Plarre, K.; al'Absi, M.; Ertin, E.; Kumar, S. mConverse: Inferring Conversation Episodes from Respiratory Measurements Collected in the Field. In Proceedings of the 2nd Conference on Wireless Health, San Diego, CA, USA, 10–13 October 2011.
11. Fuchs, S.; Reichel, U.D.; Rochet-Capellan, A. Changes in speech and breathing rate while speaking and biking. In Proceedings of the 18th International Congress of Phonetic Sciences (ICPhS 2015), Glasgow, UK, 10–14 August 2015.
12. Wilhelm, F.H.; Handke, E.; Roth, W. Detection of speaking with a new respiratory inductive plethysmography system. *Biomed. Sci. Instrum.* **2003**, *39*, 136–141. [PubMed]
13. Haugh, M. Conversational Interaction. In *The Cambridge Handbook of Pragmatics*; Cambridge University Press: Cambridge, UK, 2012; pp. 251–274.
14. Ramos-Garcia, R.I.; Tiffany, S.; Sazonov, E. Using respiratory signals for the recognition of human activities. In Proceedings of the 2016 38th Annual International Conference of the IEEE Engineering in Medicine and Biology Society (EMBC), Orlando, FL, USA, 16–20 August 2016; pp. 173–176.
15. Tognetti, A.; Bartalesi, R.; Lorussi, F.; De Rossi, D. Body segment position reconstruction and posture classification by smart textiles. *Trans. Inst. Meas. Control* **2007**, *29*, 215–253. [CrossRef]
16. Mattmann, C.; Amft, O.; Harms, H.; Troester, G.; Clemens, F. Recognizing upper body postures using textile strain sensors. In Proceedings of the 2007 11th IEEE International Symposium on Wearable Computers (ISWC), Boston, MA, USA, 11–13 October 2007; pp. 29–36.
17. Papi, E.; Spulber, I.; Kotti, M.; Georgiou, P.; McGregor, A.H. Smart sensing system for combined activity classification and estimation of knee range of motion. *IEEE Sens. J.* **2015**, *15*, 5535–5544. [CrossRef]
18. Ferrone, A.; Maita, F.; Maiolo, L.; Arquilla, M.; Castiello, A.; Pecora, A.; Jiang, X.; Menon, C.; Ferrone, A.; Colace, L.; et al. Wearable band for hand gesture recognition based on strain sensors. In Proceedings of the IEEE RAA/EMBS International Conference on Biomedical Robotics and Biomechatronics, Singapore, 26–29 June 2016; pp. 4–7.
19. Adafruit. Available online: https://www.adafruit.com/ (accessed on 10 June 2018).
20. Images SI. Available online: https://www.imagesco.com/ (accessed on 10 June 2018).
21. Ejupi, A.; Ferrone, A.; Menon, C. Quantification of textile-based stretch sensors using machine learning: An exploratory study. In Proceedings of the IEEE International Conference on Biomedical Robotics and Biomechatronics (BioRob), Twente, The Netherlands, 26–29 August 2018.
22. Gholami, M.; Ejupi, A.; Rezaei, A.; Ferrone, A.; Menon, C. Estimation of Knee Joint Angle using a Fabric-based Strain Sensor and Machine Learning: A Preliminary Investigation. In Proceedings of the IEEE International Conference on Biomedical Robotics and Biomechatronics (BioRob), Twente, The Netherlands, 26–29 August 2018.
23. Rezaei, A.; Ejupi, A.; Gholami, M.; Ferrone, A.; Menon, C. Preliminary Investigation of Textile-Based Strain Sensors for the Detection of Human Gait Phases Using Machine Learning. In Proceedings of the IEEE International Conference on Biomedical Robotics and Biomechatronics (BioRob), Twente, The Netherlands, 26–29 August 2018.
24. Gilbert, R.; Auschincloss, J.H.; Peppi, D. Relationship of rib cage and abdomen motion to diaphragm function during quiet breathing. *Chest* **1981**, *80*, 607–612. [CrossRef] [PubMed]
25. Kaneko, H.; Horie, J. Breathing movements of the chest and abdominal wall in healthy subjects. *Respir. Care* **2012**, *57*, 1442–1451. [CrossRef] [PubMed]
26. Grimby, G.; Bunn, J.; Mead, J. Relative contribution of rib cage and abdomen to ventilation during exercise. *J. Appl. Physiol.* **1968**, *24*, 159–166. [CrossRef] [PubMed]
27. McFadden, J.P.; Price, R.; Eastwood, H.D.; Briggs, R. Raised respiratory rate in elderly patients: A valuable physical sign. *Br. Med. J. (Clin. Res. Ed.)* **1982**, *284*, 626–627. [CrossRef]
28. Liaw, A.; Wiener, M. Classification and Regression by randomForest. *R News* **2002**, *2*, 18–22.
29. Specht, D.F. A general regression neural network. *IEEE Trans. Neural Netw.* **1991**, *2*, 568–576. [CrossRef] [PubMed]

30. Drucker, H.; Burges, C.J.C.; Kaufman, L.; Smola, A.; Vapnik, V. Support vector regression machines. *Adv. Neural Inf. Process. Syst.* **1997**, *1*, 155–161.
31. Mika, S.; Ratsch, G.; Weston, J.; Schölkopf, B.; Muller, K.R. Fisher discriminant analysis with kernels. In Proceedings of the 1999 IEEE Signal Processing Society Workshop (Cat. No. 98TH8468), Madison, WI, USA, 25 August 1999; pp. 41–48.
32. tsfresh. Available online: http://tsfresh.readthedocs.io/ (accessed on 10 June 2018).
33. Breiman, L.; Friedman, J.H.; Olshen, R.A.; Stone, C. *Classification and Regression Trees*; Routledge: Abingdon, UK, 1984; Volume 1.
34. Grossmann, A.; Morlet, J. Decomposition of hardy functions into square integrable wavelets of constant shape. *J. Math. Anal.* **1984**, *15*, 723–736. [CrossRef]
35. Cheung, Y.W.; La, K.S. Lag order and critical values of the augmented dickey-fuller test. *J. Bus. Econ. Stat.* **1995**, *13*, 277–280.
36. Cooley, J.W.; Lewis, P.A.W.; Welch, P.D. The fast fourier transform and its applications. *IEEE Trans. Educ.* **1969**, *12*, 27–34. [CrossRef]
37. Welch, P.D. The use of fast fourier transform for the estimation of power spectra: A method based on time averaging over short, modified periodograms. *IEEE Trans. Audio Electroacoust.* **1967**, *15*, 70–73. [CrossRef]
38. Pedregosa, F.; Varoquaux, G. Scikit-Learn: Machine Learning in Python. *J. Mach. Learn. Res.* **2011**, *12*, 2825–2830.
39. Ejupi, A.; Lord, S.R.; Delbaere, K. New methods for fall risk prediction. *Curr. Opin. Clin. Nutr. Metab. Care* **2014**, *17*, 407–411. [CrossRef] [PubMed]
40. Mukhopadhyay, S.C. Wearable sensors for human activity monitoring: A review. *IEEE Sens. J.* **2014**, *15*, 1321–1330. [CrossRef]
41. Zhang, C.; Tian, Y. RGB-D camera-based daily living activity recognition. *J. Comput. Vis. Image Process.* **2012**, *2*, 12.
42. Bari, R.; Adams, R.J.; Rahman, M.; Parsons, M.B.; Buder, E.H.; Kumar, S. rConverse: Moment by moment conversation detection using a mobile respiration sensor. *Proc. ACM Interact. Mob. Wearable Ubiquitous Technol.* **2018**, *2*, 2:1–2:27. [CrossRef]

5

Assessment of Breathing Parameters Using an Inertial Measurement Unit (IMU)-Based System

Ambra Cesareo [1], Ylenia Previtali [1], Emilia Biffi [2,*] and Andrea Aliverti [1]

1 Dipartimento di Elettronica, Informazione e Bioingegneria, Politecnico di Milano, 20133 Milan, Italy; ambra.cesareo@polimi.it (A.C.); ylenia1.previtali@mail.polimi.it (Y.P.); andrea.aliverti@polimi.it (A.A.)

2 Scientific Institute, IRCCS E. Medea, Bioengineering Lab, 23842 Bosisio Parini, Lecco, Italy

* Correspondence: emilia.biffi@lanostrafamiglia.it

Abstract: Breathing frequency (f_B) is an important vital sign that—if appropriately monitored—may help to predict clinical adverse events. Inertial sensors open the door to the development of low-cost, wearable, and easy-to-use breathing-monitoring systems. The present paper proposes a new posture-independent processing algorithm for breath-by-breath extraction of breathing temporal parameters from chest-wall inclination change signals measured using inertial measurement units. An important step of the processing algorithm is dimension reduction (DR) that allows the extraction of a single respiratory signal starting from 4-component quaternion data. Three different DR methods are proposed and compared in terms of accuracy of breathing temporal parameter estimation, in a group of healthy subjects, considering different breathing patterns and different postures; optoelectronic plethysmography was used as reference system. In this study, we found that the method based on PCA-fusion of the four quaternion components provided the best f_B estimation performance in terms of mean absolute errors (<2 breaths/min), correlation ($r > 0.963$) and Bland–Altman Analysis, outperforming the other two methods, based on the selection of a single quaternion component, identified on the basis of spectral analysis; particularly, in supine position, results provided by PCA-based method were even better than those obtained with the ideal quaternion component, determined a posteriori as the one providing the minimum estimation error. The proposed algorithm and system were able to successfully reconstruct the respiration-induced movement, and to accurately determine the respiratory rate in an automatic, position-independent manner.

Keywords: principal component analysis; biomedical signal processing; wearable biomedical sensors; wireless sensor network; respiratory monitoring; optoelectronic plethysmography

---

1. Introduction

Continuous monitoring of respiratory parameters such as breathing frequency (f_B), inspiratory time (T_I) and expiratory time (T_E) could foster early diagnosis of a wide range of respiratory disorders and help to track a patient's condition, discriminating between stable and at-risk patients [1,2]. Conditions of interest could be sleep breathing disorders, sudden infant death syndrome, chronic obstructive pulmonary disease (COPD) and neuromuscular disorders. The current gold standard for measuring f_B is to count the number of breaths in one minute, through auscultation or observation [3,4]. Other methods for breathing function assessment currently used in clinical practice are spirometry or pneumotachograph based on airflow measurement by using mouthpiece or facemask. In overnight polysomnography, breathing activity is assessed both by measuring respiratory flow, through pressure transducer or thermistors near the nostrils, and respiratory efforts (breathing-derived chest-wall movements), by strain-gauge belts. Also, exhaled carbon dioxide sensors, transthoracic inductance and impedance plethysmography and ECG—or PPG—derived f_B have been used to measure breathing signal. Despite their accuracy, these methods are uncomfortable and intrusive, and are not suitable for continuous monitoring in the clinical environment and at home. An emerging area of interest is to use motion sensors to detect the small breathing-derived movements/orientation changes of the chest wall. This method is particularly suitable for long-term breathing monitoring because it is unobtrusive, tolerable, and low-cost. The principle was first presented with a single-axis accelerometer in animal model (dog) using a pressure transducer in the trachea as reference [5]. Starting from this point, a variety of studies demonstrated the feasibility of using one accelerometer placed on the chest wall to derive respiratory signal and/or breathing frequency in different positions [6–14]. Morillo et al. [8] combined a piezoelectric single-axis accelerometer and a polarized capacitive microphone placed on the suprasternal notch to collect information of the cardiac, respiratory, and snoring activities for the screening of patients affected by Sleep Apnea-Hypopnea Syndrome. Measurements were limited to the supine position, that was selected to increase the sensitivity of the single-axis accelerometer, limiting the generality of the findings. The analysis method was based on the estimation of breathing frequency through the identification of the peak of the spectrum or autocorrelation; the main limitation of this approach is that, when the breathing is irregular, a main peak may not exist, and individual breaths must be identified and counted. Hung et al. [7] moved from single-axis to biaxial accelerometers. The aim of their study was to evaluate the reliability of the device in terms of detection of the onsets of expiration and expiration, and to assess the feasibility of differentiating between different breathing patterns (normal breathing, apnea, deep breathing). The signals from both axes (anteroposterior and longitudinal) of the accelerometer were summed, limiting the analysis to the sagittal plane, in sitting and lying positions. An adaptive band-pass filter was applied with a variable passband centered at the detected dominant breathing frequency.

As emerged by these studies, single or dual-axis accelerometers can be used to derive breathing signal when appropriately aligned with the major axis of rotation, which changes when the subject move from a posture to another. Contrarily, the use of a tri-axial accelerometer allows measuring inclination changes due to breathing regardless of orientation. In this case, the problem lies in the identification of the accelerometer axis to consider when posture changes. Bates et al. [13] proposed a method to track the major axis of rotation as it changes, to continuously monitor angular motion due to breathing also when subject change position/orientation. An alternative possibility to the best axis selection is fusing the axes. Jin et al. [12] proposed a posture-independent signal processing method based on three possible algorithms for accelerometer axes fusion. They demonstrated that methods based on Principal Component Analysis (PCA) obtained the highest performance in terms of Signal-to-Noise Ratio (SNR), but no results were provided about breathing rate estimation or validation against a reference method.

With the entry of tri-axial accelerometers new opportunities opened for the monitoring of breathing frequency using inertial sensors, but their use was still confined to static conditions since, when the subject is moving, the degree of the movement-related signal would exceed that due to breathing. One possible approach is to identify non-breathing motion, as proposed by Bates et al [13]. In a successive study, Mann et al. [11] furtherly developed the method proposed by Bates et al. [13], by adding activity tracking, and allowing identification of asymmetric breaths, that was not possible in the original method. An attempt to remove motion artifacts by using signal processing was made by Liu et al. [14]. They proposed an elegant method based on PCA-fusion of the three axes of an accelerometer and on filtering of the first principal component by using an adaptive filter that varied according to the energy expenditure derived by the same accelerometer. To overcome the problems of using a single accelerometer in dynamic conditions, a possibility is to fuse data from accelerometers and from other sensors, such as gyroscopes. Yoon et al. [15] investigated the feasibility of measuring breathing-related motions also during dynamic activities of the subject, by fusing data from a tri-axial accelerometer and a gyroscope and applying Kalman filter. They found that, during dynamic exercises, fusion of accelerometer and gyroscope data provided benefits in terms of reduction of estimation error. Gollee et al. used a more complex system, an inertial measurement unit (IMU) fusing accelerometer, gyroscope and magnetometer but considered only static conditions [16]. Another approach to overcome the problems related to motion artefacts is modularity. Lapi et al. [17] tried to overcome limitations deriving from the use of a single accelerometer by proposing a system based on a couple of 3-axis accelerometers placed bilaterally on the chest. Using two accelerometers permitted to detect respiration-related chest-wall movements regardless of sensor positioning with respect to the gravity vector; secondly, the breathing frequency can be obtained even when one of the two sensors is silenced by postural constraints. Recently, Gaidhani at al. [18] proposed a method that uses two IMUs composed by a 3-axis accelerometer, a 3-axis gyroscope and a 3-axis magnetometer, placed on the anterior and posterior side of the chest to decompose the motions experienced by the two IMUs into trunk movements and breathing actions. This paper presents an automatic processing algorithm to derive breathing frequency and other breathing temporal parameters from quaternion-based orientation signals recorded simultaneously at thoracic and abdominal level by using a modular, wireless, IMU-based device [19]. An important step of the processing algorithm is dimension reduction (DR) that allows the extraction of a single respiratory signal starting from 4-component quaternion data. Three different methods of DR are proposed and compared; two of them are based on the selection of one quaternion component, the third one is based on PCA-fusion of the 4 quaternion components. Results obtained using the IMU-based device, with the three different methods, are validated against optoelectronic plethysmography, an already established method to evaluate ventilation through an external measurement of the chest-wall surface motion [20–25].

2. Materials and Methods

2.1. Device Architecture and Hardware Description

The system used in this study is composed by three IMU-sensor units that communicate via Bluetooth with a smartphone; here data are pre-processed and saved. Two of the three sensor units (peripheral units) are dedicated to the recording of chest-wall respiratory-related movements and are placed on the thorax and on the abdomen to record respiratory information about both the compartments; the third sensor unit (reference central unit) is placed on a body area that is integral with the chest wall, but not involved in respiratory movements (e.g., coccyx or anterior superior iliac crest). The measurement of chest-wall movements, related to both abdominal and thoracic compartments, allows the consideration of the two-degree-of-freedom (DoF) model of chest-wall breathing movements [26], that considers abdomen and rib cage (thorax) as acting independently. Moreover, the compartmental contribution to total chest-wall volume changes according to posture and the breathing strategy adopted by each subject. Thus, the recording of chest-wall movements at different levels provides on the one hand, a more accurate estimation of the breathing signal, and on the other hand allows investigation of asynchronies between compartments, typical of different pathological conditions. The reference central unit, in addition to performing a central role within the Bluetooth piconet, can be used to discriminate between static and dynamic conditions and to map the activity state of the subject. Moreover, it could be used to reduce movement information not linked to breathing by means of frequency domain analysis or by referring orientation change experienced by the peripheral units to the coordinate frame of the reference unit. Each unit is composed by a printed circuit board equipped with a low-power microcontroller, a Bluetooth Low Energy (BLE) module, a 9-DoF IMU (3-axis accelerometer, a 3-axis gyroscope, and a 3-axis magnetometer) and lithium polymer rechargeable battery. A voltage regulator circuit, and Li–Po battery recharge circuit with mini USB port are also included in the design. Differently from the peripheral units, the reference central unit is equipped with a different BLE module, able to support simultaneous central/peripheral role and also brings a Micro Secure Digital (SD) Memory Card Connector for data logging. The dimensions of each peripheral unit, comprehensive of the 3D-printed housing, are 41 mm × 33 mm× 19 mm (LWH), and the weight is 25 g, including the battery, while the reference central unit measures 45 mm × 45 mm × 15 mm (LWH), and weighs 35 g. A prototypal version of this device has been described in [19].

2.2. Quaternion-Based Orientation Estimation and Fusion Algorithm

The final goal is to derive breathing signal by measuring orientation changes during the respiratory movements, both at thoracic and abdominal level. The IMUs provide 3D-acceleration, 3D-magnetic field, and 3D-angular rate. These measures are combined to provide accurate 3D orientation data aboard each unit. The orientation is represented with quaternions [27,28], that even though may suffer from problems of interpretation in terms of meaningfully physical angles, are interesting mathematical entities (four-dimensional complex number ($q = [q_0\ q_1\ q_2\ q_3]$), since they require less computing time and avoid the singularity problems (i.e., "gimbal lock") typical of other orientation descriptors, e.g., Euler angles. The fusion of the data collected from the sensors is done by using the sensor fusion algorithm proposed by Madgwick et al. [29], based on an analytically derived and optimized gradient descent algorithm enabling levels of accuracy exceeding that of the Kalman-based algorithm, with low computational (277 scalar arithmetic operations each filter update) load and low sampling rates (e.g., 10 Hz); this orientation filter also provides an online magnetic distortion compensation algorithm and gyroscope bias drift compensation. The sensors data were collected at 40 Hz and the fusion algorithm was updated with the same rate, but due to limited buffer of the BLE module and to the stricter timings used for the Bluetooth communication, just one quaternion out of 4 computed is considered (10 Hz); nevertheless, the final sampling rate was considered appropriate given the relative low frequency of the respiratory signal [0.1 ÷ 1 Hz]. Thus, the microprocessor of each unit, receives data from accelerometer, gyroscope and magnetometer that are on board and implements Madgwick fusion filter [29] to compute a quaternion representing the change of orientation of each unit relative to the earth frame (${}^{Th}_{Earth}\hat{q}$, ${}^{Ab}_{Earth}\hat{q}$, ${}^{Ref}_{Earth}\hat{q}$), or more correctly the change of orientation of the earth relative to each unit frame [29]. In fact, in quaternion form, an arbitrary orientation of a coordinate frame B relative to coordinate frame A, achieved through a rotation of angle θ around an axis ${}^{A}\mathbf{r}$ (r_x, r_y, r_z) defined in frame A, is univocally represented through the normalized quaternion ${}^{A}_{B}\hat{q}$ defined by Equation (1):

$$ {}^{A}_{B}\hat{q} = [q_0\ q_1\ q_2\ q_3] = \left[\cos\frac{\theta}{2}\ -r_x\sin\frac{\theta}{2}\ -r_y\sin\frac{\theta}{2}\ r_z\sin\frac{\theta}{2}\right] \tag{1} $$

2.3. Quaternion-Derived Breathing Frequency

All the elaborations and computations needed to extract breathing parameters from data collected by the device were performed offline using MATLAB, the processing took on average 1.027 ± 0.129 seconds for the analysis of signals of 1071 ± 270 samples. A signal processing procedure was designed to extract the breathing frequency starting from quaternions representing the change of orientation of each unit relative to the earth frame (${}^{Th}_{Earth}\hat{q}$, ${}^{Ab}_{Earth}\hat{q}$, ${}^{Ref}_{Earth}\hat{q}$). The block diagram of the signal processing part is presented in Figure 1. The algorithm is divided into 4 main blocks: (i) pre-processing, (ii) DR, (iii) spectrum analysis, and (iv) processing.

Pre-processing block includes the preliminary steps that leads to chest-wall respiratory-related orientation change signals. The orientations changes of thoracic and abdominal units were referred to the reference unit frame (that in turn represents orientation changes of trunk) applying Equations (2) and (3) respectively:

$$ {}^{Th}_{Ref}\hat{q} = {}^{Th}_{Earth}\hat{q} \otimes {}^{Ref}_{Earth}\hat{q}^{*} = {}^{Th}_{Earth}\hat{q} \otimes {}^{Earth}_{Ref}\hat{q}, \tag{2} $$

$$ {}^{Ab}_{Ref}\hat{q} = {}^{Ab}_{Earth}\hat{q} \otimes {}^{Ref}_{Earth}\hat{q}^{*} = {}^{Ab}_{Earth}\hat{q} \otimes {}^{Earth}_{Ref}\hat{q}, \tag{3} $$

These two quaternions represent the outputs of the pre-processing block and the input of the DR block.

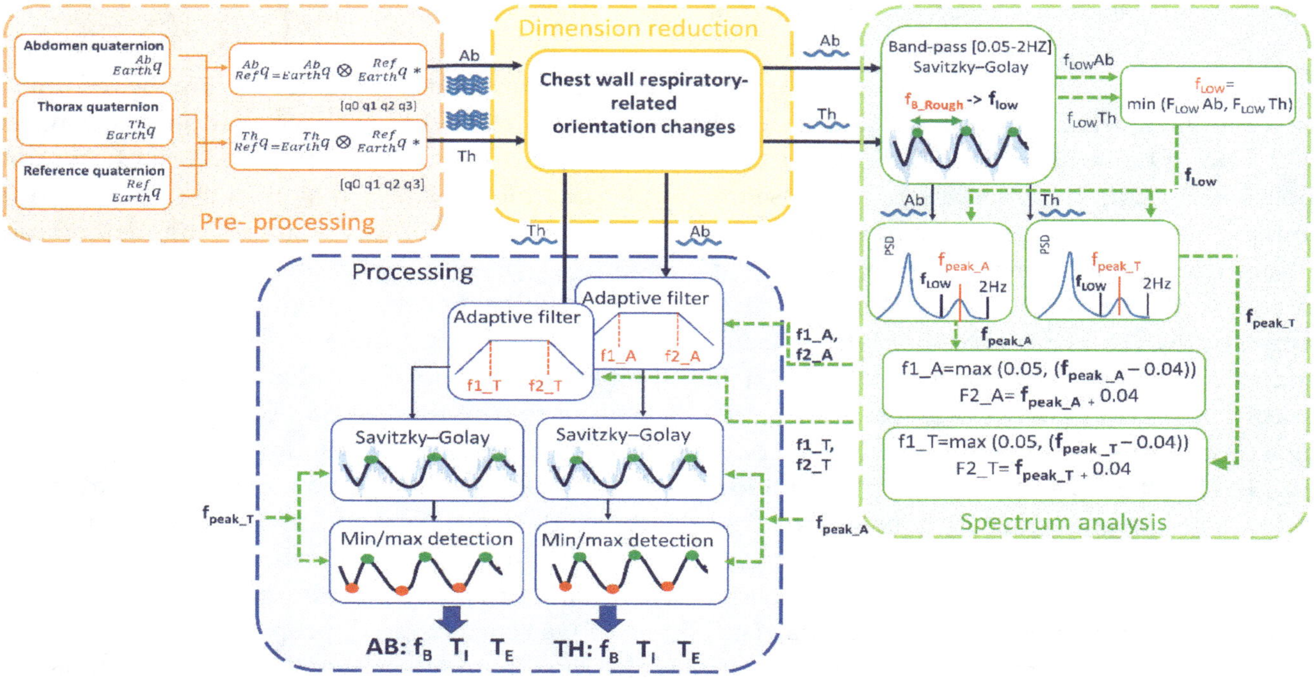

Figure 1. Block Diagram of the Analysis algorithm that allows derivation of breathing temporal parameters (f_B. T_I, T_E) from quaternion-based orientation change signals recorded on Thorax, Abdomen and Reference point.

Dimension-reduction block takes the quaternions obtained from Equations (2) and (3), that are composed by 4 components each, and provides as output 2 single-component signals (1 for the abdomen and 1 for the thorax) representing chest-wall respiratory-related orientation change signals. These two signals represent the input of the power spectrum block and of the processing block. To reduce dimension from 4 components to 1, two possibilities were investigated as shown in Figure 2:

(i). Best quaternion component selection
(ii). PCA-based fusion of the quaternion components

To select the best component among the 4 components representing the orientation quaternion, two different methods were proposed, both based on spectrum analysis. The idea was to choose the component with the highest breathing information, computing the power spectral density estimate (PSD) between 0.5–2 Hz for each component and selecting the component with: (1) maximum PSD peak ("Peak" method) or (2) maximum area under the PSD ("Area" method). To assess the goodness of these two methods in predicting the best quaternion component, the ideal component ("Ideal") was determined a posteriori, case by case, based on minimum breathing frequency estimation error (see Section 2.5).

Since more than one quaternion component is supposed to convey breathing information, the possibility to maximize this information fusing the 4 components of the quaternion by means of PCA was investigated. PCA is a mathematical procedure that transforms an original set of correlated variables into a (smaller) number of uncorrelated variables by determining a set of orthogonal vectors called principal components, which are defined by a linear combination of the original variables [30,31]. To do this, the directions in the data with the most variation, i.e., the eigenvectors corresponding to the largest eigenvalues of the covariance matrix, are computed and the data are projected onto these directions. To compute the eigenvectors, data were arranged into a two-dimensional matrix $\mathbf{X}(m \times n)$, where m was the number of observations of the time series and n the number of variables (quaternion components). Then, the univariate means were subtracted from the n columns, to center the data. Singular Value Decomposition (SVD) was used to compute the eigenvectors ($\mathbf{V} = [v_1, v_2, v_3, v_4]$) and corresponding eigenvalues ($\lambda_1, \lambda_2, \lambda_3, \lambda_4$). Original data were finally projected in the new coordinate system (**Y** = **XV**) and the first principal component, accounting for the largest possible variance, was selected and passed to other blocks [30,31].

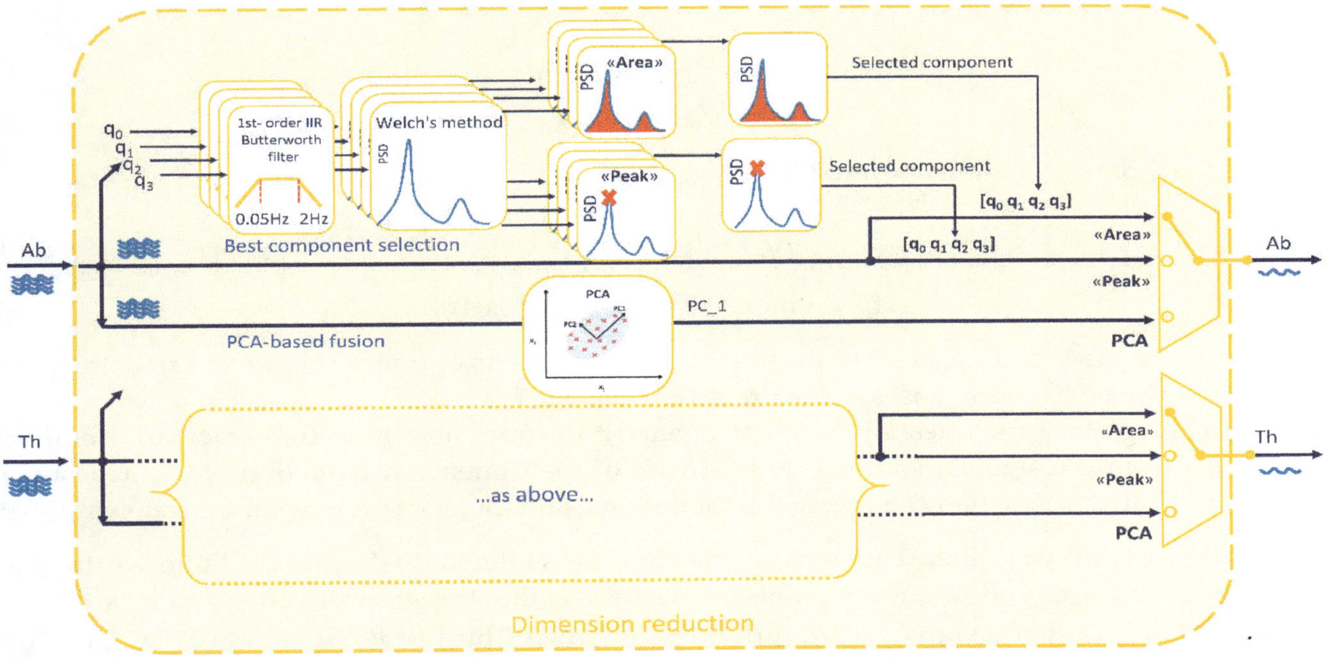

Figure 2. Dimension-reduction block in detail. Starting from the 4 components $[q_0, q_1, q_2, q_3]$ of each quaternion (Abdominal: Ab and Thoracic: Th), three methods are applied to obtain a single-component signal: two methods based on best quaternion component selection ("Area" and "Peak") and one method based on the fusion of the 4 components through Principal Component Analysis (PCA). "Area" method selects the quaternion component with the larger area under the Power Spectral Density (PSD) estimate, while "Peak" method selects the quaternion component with the highest PSD's peak. PCA-fusion method selects the first principal component (PC_1) that accounts for the largest variance in the data.

Spectrum Analysis block include a set of steps needed to optimize the subsequent processing phase. The two signals representing chest-wall (abdominal and thoracic) respiratory-related orientation obtained downstream of the dimension-reduction block underwent the following steps (Figure 1):

(i). A low-frequency threshold (f_{LOW}) was determined based on a first estimate of the breathing frequency (f_B). The rough estimate of f_B was done by identifying maxima points of the signal and computing the f_B, breath by breath, as reciprocal of the temporal distance between consecutive maxima points. Then, the mean (f_{B_Rough}) and the standard deviation ($f_{B\_Rough\_SD}$) of the f_B over the entire trial were computed. To facilitate maxima points identification, signals were at first band-bass filtered using a first-order infinite impulse response (IIR) Butterworth filter [0.05 Hz–2 Hz] and smoothed with a third-order Savitzky–Golay [32] finite impulse response (FIR) filter (fixed window length = 31 samples). Low thresholds f_{LOW}Ab and f_{LOW}Th were determined for the abdominal and thoracic signals respectively as difference $f_{B\_Rough} - f_{B\_Rough\_SD}$. Then the minimum value between f_{LOW}Ab and f_{LOW}Th was chosen as final low-frequency threshold, named f_{LOW}, and it was used in the next step.

(ii). PSD estimate (Welch's method, Hamming window size: 300 samples, overlapping: 50 samples) was computed and the spectrum frequency corresponding to the breathing rate was identified, both for the thorax (f_{peak_T}) and the abdomen (f_{peak_A}), by looking for the local peak of the PSD within the window [$f_{LOW} \div 2$ Hz]. The use of a low threshold, based on a rough estimate of the breathing frequency, supports the selection of the PSD peak linked to breathing rate and avoid selecting wrong peaks, often related to low-frequency oscillation artifacts.

(iii). The breathing frequency derived by the spectrum was used to set an adaptive band-pass filter, as proposed in a previous study [7], centered on f_{peak} frequency. For the abdomen, upper (f_U) and lower (f_L) cut-off frequency points for the band-pass filter were defined, by applying Equations (4) and (5) respectively [7]:

$$f_{U\_A} = f_{peak\_A} + 0.04, \tag{4}$$

$$f_{L\_A} = \max\left(0.05, \left(f_{peak\_A} - 0.04\right)\right), \tag{5}$$

For the thorax, Equations (6) and (7) were applied:

$$f_{U\_T} = f_{peak\_T} + 0.04, \tag{6}$$

$$f_{L\_T} = \max\left(0.05, \left(f_{peak\_T} - 0.04\right)\right), \tag{7}$$

Moreover, based on f_{peak}, a set of parameters was selected to optimize subsequent smoothing and minima/maxima detection phases of the processing block.

Processing block includes all the steps needed to extract breathing frequency and temporal parameters from the signals obtained downstream of the dimension-reduction block. Chest-wall respiratory-related orientation change signals (abdominal and thoracic) underwent the following steps:

(i). Adaptive band-pass filter. The signals were band-pass filtered (first-order IIR Butterworth filter), with f_U and f_L cut-off frequency points determined within the spectrum analysis block.

(ii). Smoothing. Filtered signals were furtherly smoothed (third-order Savitzky–Golay FIR filter) to simplify subsequent identification of maxima and minima points. The level of smoothing (window length) was automatically selected based on f_{peak}, i.e., increasing window length for decreasing f_{peak}. Relation between optimal window length values and f_{peak} values has been determined empirically.

(iii). Minima and maxima points detection. A set of optimized parameters (i.e., minimum peak distance (MPD) and minimum prominence threshold (MPT)) was automatically selected based on f_{peak} to optimize recognition of minima and maxima points of the smoothed signals. Optimal MPD and MPT values depending on f_{peak} were experimentally determined.

(iv). Breathing frequency extraction. Breath by breath, inspiratory time (T_I) was computed as the temporal distance between a minimum point (m_i) and the consecutive maximum point (M_i); Expiratory time (T_E) was computed as the temporal distance between the maximum point (M_i) and the consecutive minimum point ($m_i + 1$); total time (T_{TOT}) was computed as $T_{TOT} = T_I + T_E$ [s], duty cycle (DC) was computed as $\frac{T_I}{T_{TOT}} \times 100$ [%] and breathing frequency was computed as $\frac{60}{(T_{TOT})}$ [breaths/minute]. A mean value for each of the above-mentioned parameter was computed for each trial (~3 min).

2.4. Experimental Setup

To evaluate the capability of the device and of the proposed methods to correctly estimate breathing frequency (and temporal parameters) 8 healthy volunteers (4 males, 4 females) were enrolled. All subjects gave their informed consent for inclusion before they participated in the study. The study was conducted in accordance with the Declaration of Helsinki, and the protocol (Project identification code n° 534) was approved by the Ethics Committee of Scientific Institute IRCCS Medea (date of approval: 25 January 2018). Chest-wall movements during breathing, in seated and supine position, were measured using the proposed device and optoelectronic plethysmography (OEP) simultaneously. OEP [21] is a technique based on a similar functioning principle of the proposed device; in fact, it allows assessment of ventilatory and breathing pattern by measuring chest-wall movements related to breathing, by using motion capture principles. The system is composed of eight infrared video cameras working at a sampling rate of 60 Hz. It can compute the 3D coordinates of retro-reflective markers positioned on the chest wall in specific anatomic points. From the three-dimensional coordinates of the markers, it is possible to obtain the volume enclosed by the chest-wall surface, by applying the Gauss's theorem. The chest wall is modelled by a bicompartmental model, composed of rib cage and abdomen, and thus it is possible to investigate the contribution of both the compartments. This is an advantage for the validation of the proposed device, in fact, using OEP as reference method it is possible to compare the data recorded with the thoracic and abdominal units of the device with those obtained by using OEP for the thoracic and abdominal compartments, respectively. OEP has been widely validated against spirometer, in healthy subjects, in different conditions and positions, also during submaximal and maximal exercise on cycle ergometer, obtaining discrepancies in tidal volume measurements always <5% [22–24,33,34].

The subjects were prepared, placing the reflective markers according to the 89-marker protocol (previously described in [24,35]) used for seated position and the 52-marker protocol (previously described in [36,37]) used for supine position or, more generally, when a back support is present. Then peripheral IMU-units were placed on the thorax and on the abdomen, while reference IMU-unit was placed on the coccyx in seated position, and on the bed in supine position (Figure 3).

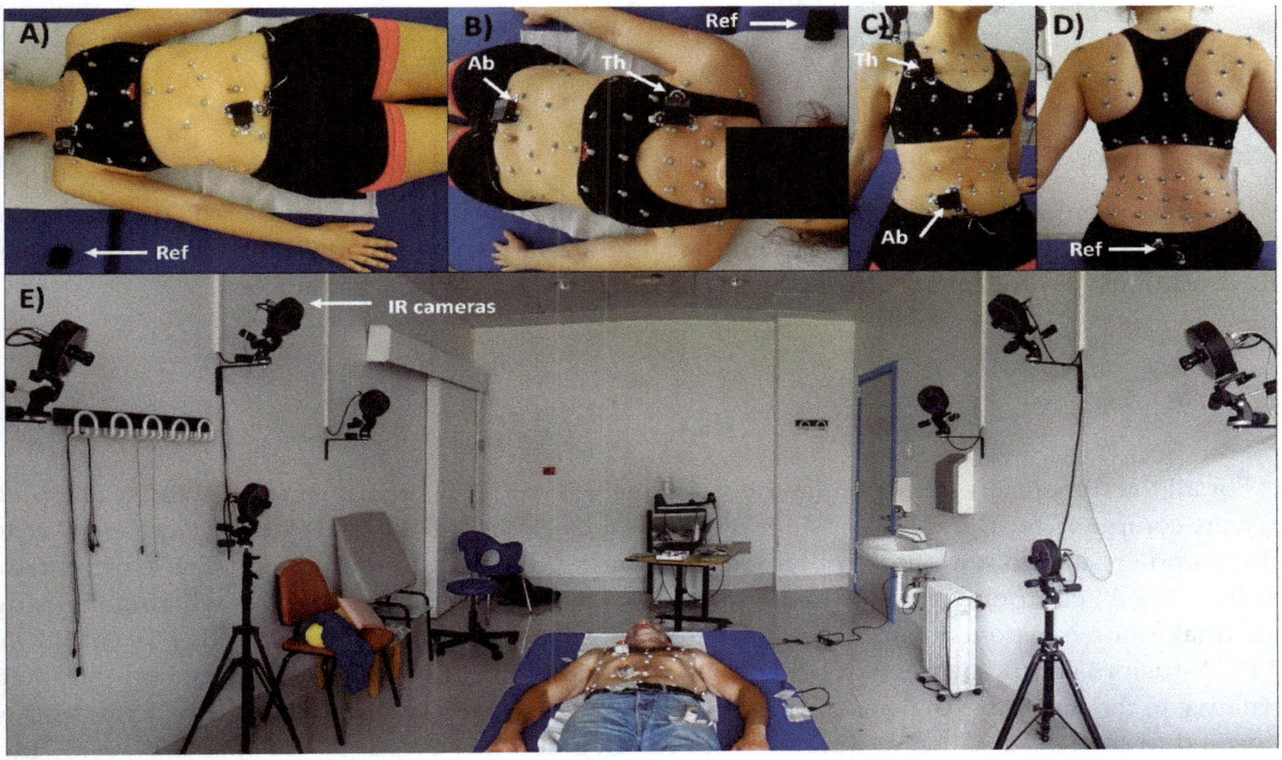

Figure 3. Experimental setup. Retroreflective-marker configuration for optoelectronic plethysmography (OEP) and IMU-unit (Ab: Abdomen, Th: Thorax, Ref: Reference) placement in supine (A and B panels) and seated (C and D panels) positions. Panel E shows the experimental setup and the OEP Lab; Infrared cameras of the motion capture system are also noticeable.

Subjects were then asked to seat or lie on a bed and were invited to perform a slow vital capacity maneuver (SVC) and then to start breathing with the following patterns: (I) quiet breathing (QB), (II) increasing f_B but same tidal volume of QB ($\uparrow f_B$, V_T=), (III) increasing f_B and reducing tidal volume ($\uparrow f_B$, $V_T\downarrow$), (IV) decreasing f_B with the same tidal volume of QB ($\downarrow f_B$, V_T=), (V) decreasing f_B increasing tidal volume of QB ($\downarrow f_B$, $V_T\uparrow$). QB trial was repeated two times, thus, each subject performed 6 trials of the duration of 3 min each. The SVC maneuver was used to align OEP signal and device signals during data analysis, since it is generally recognizable with respect to QB. In fact, SVC requires a maximal inspiration followed by a complete expiration without forced or rapid effort.

The subjects were asked to maintain the same breathing pattern (namely, QB, ↑f_B, V_T=, ↑f_B, V_T↓, ↓f_B, V_T=, ↓f_B, V_T↑) until the end of the trial; in case of fatigue they were asked to perform a second SVC before returning to QB. This procedure was repeated in seated position and in supine position.

2.5. Statistical Analysis

For each trial, mean values of f_B, T_I, T_E and DC were extracted from the best quaternion components identified online by using "Area" and "Peak" methods, and from the signal obtained with the PCA-based fusion method, both for the thoracic and abdominal tracings. Moreover, to evaluate the performance of the selection methods ("Area" and "Peak") and their ability to select the best component, the same parameters were obtained for all the quaternion components (q_0, q_1, q_2, q_3) and compared with those obtained by OEP, on the abdominal and thoracic compartment, respectively. The "Ideal" quaternion component was identified a posteriori, trial by trial, as the one providing the minimum estimation error of the breathing frequency. Obviously, the "Ideal" component cannot be identified during online analysis, or when a reference method is not present. Thus, for each trial, 5 sets of parameters were available:

- f_{B_OEP}, T_{I_OEP}, T_{E_OEP} and $DC_{\_OEP}$
- f_{B_Peak}, T_{I_Peak}, T_{E_Peak} and $DC_{\_Peak}$
- f_{B_Area}, T_{I_Area}, T_{E_Area} and $DC_{\_Area}$
- f_{B_PCA}, T_{I_PCA}, T_{E_PCA} and $DC_{\_PCA}$
- f_{B_Ideal}, T_{I_Ideal}, T_{E_Ideal} and $DC_{\_Ideal}$

Among the entire set of trials, those with $f_{B\_OEP} < 6$ breaths/minute or $f_{B\_OEP} > 60$ breaths/minute were discarded. Then, the absolute (Equation (8)) and relative (Equation (9)) errors of estimation in static conditions (supine and seated position) were computed for each parameter:

$$Absolute\ Error\ (\boldsymbol{E}) = |Device - OEP|, \tag{8}$$

$$Relative\ Error\ (\boldsymbol{E}\%) = \frac{|Device - OEP|}{OEP} \times 100 \tag{9}$$

For all the dimension-reduction methods ("Area", "Peak", "PCA"), mean and standard deviation (SD) were computed for E and E% considering all the subjects and all the trials, for the supine and seated position and compared with those obtained considering the "Ideal" component. The error obtained with the "Ideal" component, identified a posteriori, is thus the minimum error obtainable using a single quaternion component, and represents the performance that the other methods ("Area", "Peak", and PCA-fusion) should achieve or beat. For E% obtained in f_B and DC estimation, non-parametric alternative to the one-way Analysis of variance (ANOVA) with repeated measures (Friedman test) was performed to assess if significant differences between methods ("Area", "Peak", "PCA") and "Ideal" component occurred, "Ideal"); post-hoc analysis was done performing Wilcoxon signed-rank tests on the different combinations of related methods, applying the correction for multiple comparisons using false discovery rate (FDR) method [38,39].

For f_B, T_I, T_E, linear regression analysis and correlation analysis (Pearson's product-moment correlation r_P, or Spearman's rank-order correlation r_S, if data were not normally distributed) were performed between measurements obtained with the device and measurements obtained with the OEP, for the supine and seated position, respectively.

To assess the agreement between measurements obtained with the device and with the OEP, Bland–Altman analysis was performed plotting the difference of the two paired measurements (device–OEP) against the mean of the two measurements [40–42]. Mean of the differences (d) and limits of agreement (LOA: from d − (1.9 × SD) to d + (1.9 × SD)) were calculated. The presence of heteroscedasticity was always examined to assess the presence of proportional biases and/or the correlation between differences and mean values. As proposed by Brehm et al. [43], to determine if data were heteroscedastic a visual inspection of Bland–Altman plots was performed at first. If the errors (y-axes: absolute differences) increased with increasing measured values (x-axes: mean), the data were suspected of being heteroscedastic. Then Kendall's tau (τ) correlation between the absolute differences and the corresponding means was computed to assess the degree of heteroscedasticity. Data were denoted heteroscedastic when a positive, significant correlation ($\tau > 0.1$ and p-value < 0.05) was found, for other cases data were considered homoscedastic [43].

When heteroscedasticity was present the "classical" 95% confidence and tolerance limits cannot be constructed, thus the approach based on the construction of V-shaped limits was applied: the regression line (ordinary least squares (OLS) best fit) was constructed for differences on mean values and the V-shaped confidence limits (upper confidence limit: UCL, lower confidence limit: LCL) were constructed modelling the variability in the SD of the differences directly as a function of the level of the measurement, using a method based on absolute residuals from a fitted regression line [44,45].

3. Results

3.1. Breathing Patterns

Table 1 presents the mean and SD of breathing rate for each breathing pattern (QB_1 e QB_2, $\uparrow f_B$, V_T=, $\uparrow f_B$, $V_T\downarrow$, $\downarrow f_B$, VT=, $\downarrow f_B$, $V_T\uparrow$) estimated with OEP and device, using "PCA", "Area", and "Peak" methods and the "Ideal" component, for all subjects, in supine and seated position. Sample size (n) of each condition is reported in Table 1 for the breathing pattern $\uparrow f_B$, $V_T\downarrow$, just one thoracic tracing was available for seated position (n = 1). It can be noticed that each subject demonstrated a different breathing frequency for each breathing pattern and SD in the forced breathing patterns is higher than those obtained for QB, meaning that subjects interpreted the required speed differently.

Table 1. Breathing frequencies for different breathing patterns.

Supine		QB 1		↑f_B, V_T=		↓f_B, V_T=		↑f_B, V_T↓		↓f_B, V_T↑		QB 2	
		AB (n = 8)	TH (n = 7)	AB (n = 8)	TH (n = 8)	AB (n = 6)	TH (n = 6)	AB (n = 3)	TH (n = 2)	AB (n = 5)	TH (n = 6)	AB (n = 8)	TH (n = 8)
OEP		17.13 ± 2.23	17.62 ± 2.21	39.49 ± 10.26	39.48 ± 10.25	11.17 ± 2.64	11.14 ± 2.63	48.11 ± 13.29	47.66 ± 13.95	8.38 ± 2.40	8.61 ± 2.24	15.29 ± 4.34	15.24 ± 4.48
Device	Area	17.20 ± 2.15	18.53 ± 3.96	39.19 ± 10.84	38.16 ± 14.67	15.52 ± 8.14	19.29 ± 9.42	34.47 ± 34.58	30.01 ± 25.52	10.11 ± 3.91	10.62 ± 4.44	21.28 ± 8.14	16.55 ± 3.62
	Peak	17.20 ± 2.15	16.63 ±2.29	38.92 ± 11.12	38.96 ± 13.01	15.52 ± 8.14	16.97 ± 9.59	34.47 ± 34.58	53.39 ± 7.55	10.11 ± 3.91	9.32 ± 2.12	21.25 ± 8.15	16.55 ± 3.62
	PCA	17.23 ± 2.09	17.03 ± 1.98	40.06 ± 9.22	40.63 ± 8.45	11.51 ± 2.59	11.56 ± 3.04	48.61 ± 12.64	49.93 ± 11.94	8.61 ± 2.19	8.95 ± 2.06	15.11 ± 4.82	15.23 ± 3.79
	Ideal	17.57 ± 2.52	16.34 ± 2.00	39.81 ± 10.50	40.94 ± 9.97	12.11 ± 1.99	13.60 ± 2.61	49.53 ± 12.31	48.12 ± 13.89	9.34 ± 3.33	8.83 ± 2.06	17.74 ± 4.70	15.37 ± 3.82
Seated		**QB 1**		**↑f_B, V_T=**		**↓f_B, V_T=**		**↑f_B, V_T↓**		**↓f_B, V_T↑**		**QB 2**	
		AB (n = 8)	TH (n = 8)	AB (n = 8)	TH (n = 7)	AB (n = 8)	TH (n = 8)	AB (n = 2)	TH (n = 1)	AB (n = 6)	TH (n = 5)	AB (n = 7)	TH (n = 6)
OEP		16.99 ± 2.65	16.94 ± 2.77	42.74 ± 10.97	46.49 ± 7.58	14.57 ± 13.40	14.49 ± 13.41	33.20 ± 16.01	22.01	10.04 ± 3.56	10.05 ± 3.81	18.47 ± 4.32	18.47 ± 4.49
Device	Area	17.15 ± 2.86	15.78 ± 3.62	43.06 ± 11.22	40.71 ± 13.59	15.71 ± 13.52	17.06 ± 13.05	32.63 ± 12.87	27.62	10.83 ± 2.93	12.58 ± 4.08	19.80 ± 5.15	17.04 ± 2.09
	Peak	16.48 ± 3.58	16.27 ± 3.76	43.06 ± 11.22	40.71 ± 13.59	16.53 ± 13.50	17.15 ± 12.99	32.63 ± 12.87	27.62	10.83 ± 2.93	12.58 ± 4.08	17.23 ± 2.19	16.54 ± 1.95
	PCA	16.54 ± 3.01	16.58 ± 2.10	42.26 ± 11.38	45.31 ± 8.56	16.07 ± 13.07	14.91 ± 13.39	33.79 ± 14.50	27.27	10.76 ± 2.90	11.35 ± 3.73	16.59 ± 2.17	15.47 ± 1.69
	Ideal	16.68 ± 2.59	16.61 ± 2.34	42.64 ± 11.21	45.42 ± 7.98	15.29 ± 13.33	11.07 ± 2.36	33.38 ± 13.92	24.53	10.40 ± 3.53	10.29 ± 3.66	19.06 ± 4.89	18.73 ± 5.04

Across subject mean ± SD of the breathing frequency (f_B, [breaths/minute]) measurements with OEP and the device, using best component-selection methods ("Area" and "Peak"), PCA-fusion method and "Ideal" component, for the requested patterns. Data are reported for the supine and seated positions, subdivided in abdominal and thoracic contributions.

3.2. Accuracy Errors

Relative errors of estimation in supine and seated position computed for best component-selection methods ("Peak", "Area"), for PCA-fusion method and for the "Ideal" quaternion component for f_B and DC are presented in Figure 4. For what concerns f_B estimation in supine position, relative errors obtained using PCA were similar or even better than those provided by the "Ideal" component; on the contrary, both component-selection methods, namely "Area" and "Peak", provided errors higher than 10%, both for the abdominal and the thoracic compartments. Errors obtained with PCA resulted significantly lower than those obtained with the "Area" method, both for the abdominal (Wilcoxon post-hoc test FDR-adjusted, $p = 0.038$) and thoracic compartment (Wilcoxon post-hoc test FDR-adjusted, $p = 0.015$); also, PCA was significantly better than "Peak" method considering abdominal compartment (Wilcoxon post-hoc test FDR-adjusted, $p = 0.038$). Errors obtained with "Ideal" component resulted significantly lower than those obtained with the component-selection methods both for the abdominal (Wilcoxon post-hoc test FDR-adjusted, Ideal vs. Area $p = 0.038$, Ideal vs. Peak $p = 0.038$) and thoracic (Wilcoxon post-hoc test FDR-adjusted, Ideal vs. Area $p = 0.000$, Ideal vs. Peak $p = 0.020$) compartments.

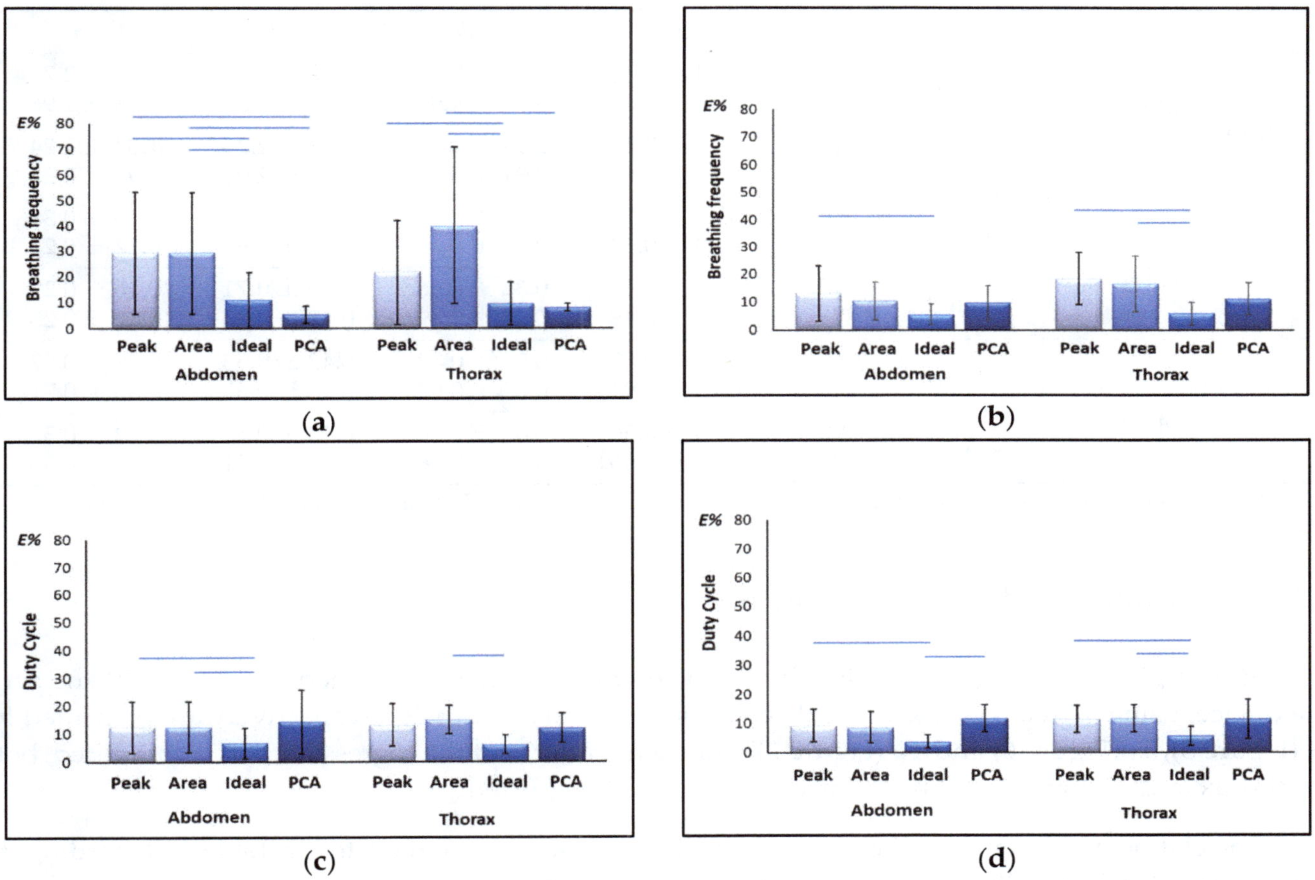

Figure 4. Relative errors (E%) of estimation of breathing frequency (**a**,**b**) and Duty Cycle (**c**,**d**) in supine (**a**,**c**) and seated (**b**,**d**) positions, computed for each method (Peak, Area and PCA) and for the "Ideal" component with respect to the reference (OEP). Errors are computed both for the Thoracic and abdominal compartments. Horizontal blue lines indicate statistical significance of difference (post-hoc analysis, Wilcoxon test FDR corrected).

In seated position, f_B estimation errors obtained with component-selection methods were lower on average than those obtained in supine position, while PCA performances declined. This led to a sort of equalization effect, confirmed also by the statistical analysis: significant differences remained only for comparisons "Ideal" vs. "Area" method (Wilcoxon post-hoc test FDR-adjusted, AB: $p = 0.102$,

TH: p = 0.015) and "Ideal" vs. "Peak" method (Wilcoxon post-hoc test FDR-adjusted, AB: p = 0.006, TH: p = 0.015).

Regarding duty cycle, relative errors of estimation obtained with the different methods are comparable, with exception of those provided by "Ideal" component that are on average lower, both in supine (Wilcoxon post-hoc test FDR-adjusted, AB: Ideal vs. Peak p = 0.042, Ideal vs. Area p = 0.042; TH: Ideal vs. Area p = 0.006) and seated position (Wilcoxon post-hoc test FDR-adjusted, AB: Ideal vs. Peak p = 0.015, Ideal vs. PCA p = 0.006; TH: Ideal vs. Area p = 0.015, Ideal vs. Peak p = 0.015, Ideal vs. PCA p = 0.05).

Absolute estimation errors of f_B, T_I and T_E obtained with the device using different methods (Area, Peak, Ideal, PCA) relative to OEP are reported in Table 2.

Table 2. Absolute errors of breathing frequency (E_f_B), Inspiratory time (E_T_I) and expiratory time (E_T_E) obtained for the device with respect to OEP, using best component-selection methods ("Area" and "Peak"), PCA-fusion method and "Ideal" component.

			Area	**Peak**	**PCA**	**Ideal**
E_f_B [breaths/minute]	supine	AB	3.64 ± 7.46	3.64 ± 7.46	1.00 ± 1.24	1.39 ± 2.76
		TH	5.46 ± 8.89	3.17 ± 4.92	1.55 ± 1.51	1.56 ± 1.96
	seated	AB	2.19 ± 2.49	2.12 ± 2.74	1.71 ± 2.25	1.04 ± 1.24
		TH	3.35 ± 5.68	3.31 ± 5.69	1.79 ± 2.04	0.96 ± 0.22
E_T_I [s]	supine	AB	0.48 ± 0.73	0.48 ± 0.73	0.33 ± 0.51	0.20 ± 0.38
		TH	0.43 ± 0.52	0.41 ± 0.49	0.47 ± 0.67	0.17 ± 0.25
	seated	AB	0.33 ± 0.58	0.36 ± 0.56	0.46 ± 0.71	0.16 ± 0.27
		TH	0.43 ± 0.48	0.44 ± 0.49	0.42 ± 0.35	0.17 ± 0.25
E_T_E [s]	supine	AB	0.58 ± 0.82	0.58 ± 0.82	0.43 ± 0.58	0.29 ± 0.52
		TH	0.79 ± 0.94	0.67 ± 0.92	0.46 ± 0.63	0.36 ± 0.71
	seated	AB	0.43 ± 0.56	0.43 ± 0.56	0.43 ± 0.55	0.22 ± 0.31
		TH	0.56 ± 0.66	0.56 ± 0.66	0.39 ± 0.41	0.24 ± 0.36

Data are reported as mean ± SD, in supine and seated position for thoracic (TH) and abdominal (AB) compartments.

3.3. Linear Regression and Correlation Analysis

Scatter plots showing the relationship between measurements obtained with the OEP and with the device, using "Area", "Peak", "Ideal" components, and PCA-fusion respectively are presented for f_B (Figure 5), T_I (Figure 6) and T_E (Figure 7). For each scatter plot the regression line is computed, both for thorax and abdomen, and the relative equations are reported.

Correlation coefficients for the comparisons Device vs. OEP are reported in Table 3. Regarding the main parameter, f_B, results obtained with correlation analysis confirmed what emerged from estimation error analysis: in supine position, PCA exhibited the best performances in terms of correlation with OEP measurements both in terms of regression line and correlation coefficient. In seated position, "Ideal" component was the one with the highest correlation with OEP measurements, followed by PCA.

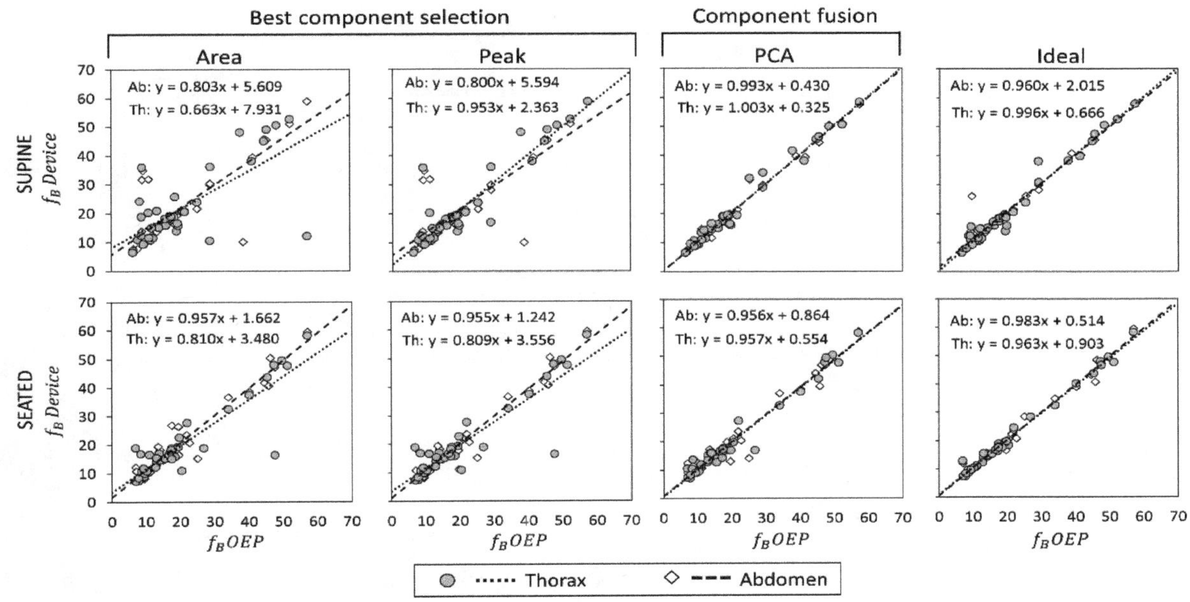

Figure 5. Comparisons of breathing frequency (f_B expressed as breaths/minuteute) measurements by using the proposed device and by using Optoelectronic plethysmography (OEP) presented as regression analysis, in supine (top panels) and seated (bottom panels) positions. For what concerns f_B measurements obtained with the IMU-device, three dimension-reduction methods were considered: Area, Peak and PCA-fusion. The performance obtained by using these three methods is benchmarked against that obtained with the Ideal quaternion component determined a posteriori based on the minimum estimation error. The regression line between measurements done by OEP and the proposed device is plotted, and the relative equation presented, both for the thorax and the abdomen.

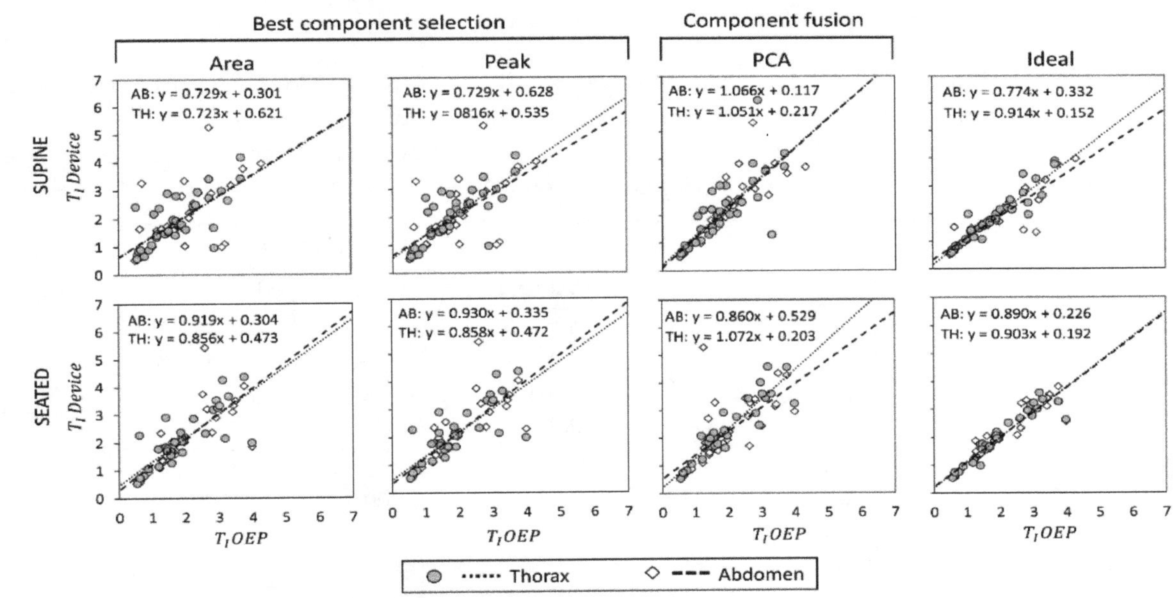

Figure 6. Comparisons of inspiratory time (T_I expressed as seconds) measurements by using the proposed device and by using Optoelectronic plethysmography (OEP) presented as regression analysis, in supine (top panels) and seated (bottom panels) positions. For what concerns T_I measurements obtained with the IMU-device, three dimension-reduction methods were considered: Area, Peak and PCA-fusion. The performance obtained by using these three methods is benchmarked against that obtained with the Ideal quaternion component determined a posteriori based on the minimum estimation error. The regression line between measurements done by OEP and the proposed device is plotted, and the relative equation presented, both for the thorax and the abdomen.

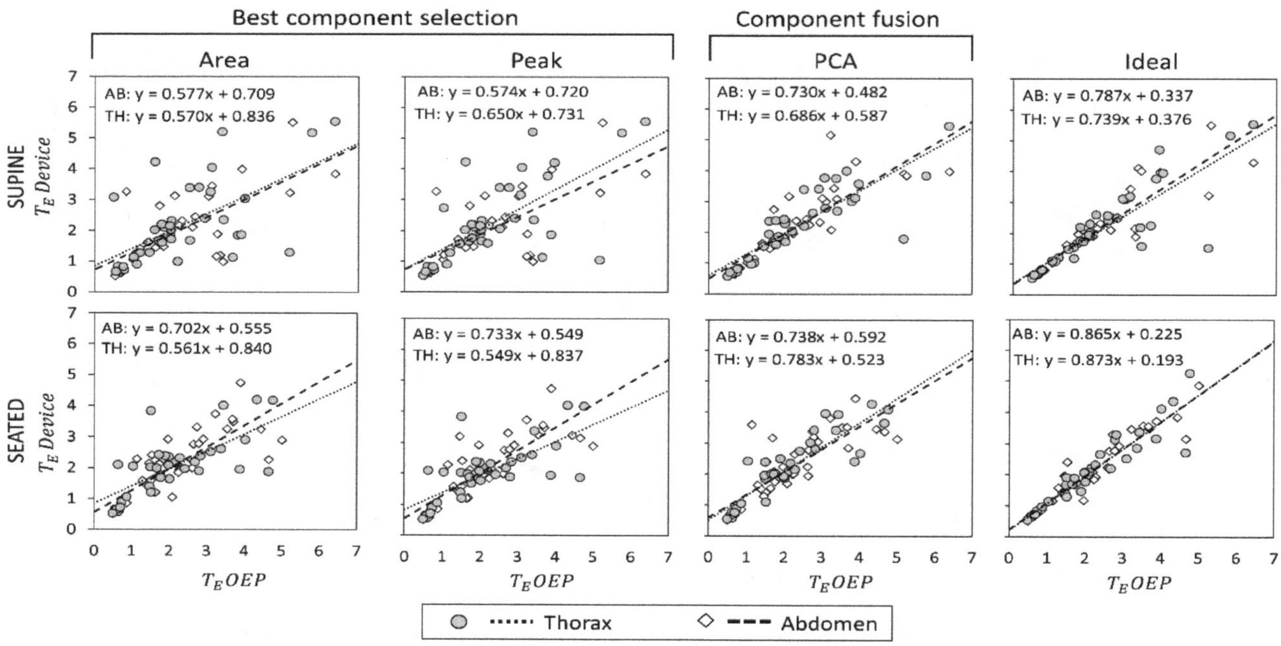

Figure 7. Comparisons of expiratory time (T_E, expressed as seconds) measurements by using the proposed device and by using Optoelectronic plethysmography (OEP) presented as regression analysis, in supine (top panels) and seated (bottom panels) positions. Regarding T_E measurements obtained with the IMU-device, three dimension-reduction methods were considered. Area, Peak and PCA-fusion. The performance obtained by using these three methods is benchmarked against that obtained with the Ideal quaternion component determined a posteriori based on the minimum estimation error. The regression line between measurements done by OEP and the proposed device is plotted, and the relative equation presented, both for the thorax and the abdomen.

Table 3. Correlation outcomes across subjects and breathing patterns. Coefficient of correlation (r) between measurements obtained using Device vs. OEP are reported for f_B. T_I. and T_E using best component-selection methods ("Area" and "Peak"), PCA-fusion method and "Ideal" component, in supine (Thorax: n = 37. Abdomen: n = 37) and seated (Thorax: n = 35. Abdomen: n = 39) position.

		Supine		**Seated**	
		Thorax	**Abdomen**	**Thorax**	**Abdomen**
f_B	**Area**	0.580 $	0.706 $	0.748 $	0.915 $
	Peak	0.833 $	0.706 $	0.759 $	0.861 $
	PCA	**0.963** $	**0.985** $	0.953 $	0.924 $
	Ideal	0.935 $	0.931 $	**0.974** $	**0.977** $
T_I	**Area**	0.727 #	0.665 $	0.812 #	0.812 #
	Peak	0.785 #	0.659 $	0.809 #	0.824 #
	PCA	0.783 #	**0.874** #	0.926 #	0.731 #
	Ideal	**0.943** #	0.862 $	**0.951** #	**0.948** #
T_E	**Area**	0.600 $	0.713 #	0.682 #	0.818 #
	Peak	0.687 $	0.712 #	0.723 #	0.835 #
	PCA	**0.891** #	0.864 #	0.888 #	0.824 #
	Ideal	0.874 #	**0.966** $	**0.938** #	**0.951** #

Correlations are all significant (p-value < 0.001). $ Spearman correlation coefficient; # Pearson correlation coefficient; Bold: best correlation result.

With reference to T_I estimation in supine position, "Ideal" component provided the best performances, followed by PCA method; "Peak" and "Area" methods provided comparable, poor performances. In seated position, measurements of T_I provided by component-selection methods were on average more correlated with OEP measurements than measurements obtained using PCA-fusion method. The "Ideal" component presented the best results, followed by "Area" and "Peak" methods; PCA provided the worst performance considering the abdominal compartment, while correlation between measurements obtained with the thoracic unit and OEP measurements was good.

Estimation of T_E was on average more problematic. In terms of regression lines in fact, slope values were far from the unity for all the considered methods, highlighting a proportional error leading to an overestimation for low values of expiratory time and an underestimation at high expiratory times, as shown in Figure 7. For what concerns supine position, correlation coefficients were good both for "Ideal" component and PCA-fusion method; on the contrary, correlation coefficients were low both for "Area" and "Peak" methods. Also, in seated position correlation coefficients provided by "Ideal" and PCA-fusion method were higher than those provided by "Area" and "Peak" methods, especially with respect to the thoracic compartment.

3.4. Bland–Altman Analysis

Bland–Altman plots representing the agreement between measurements obtained with the OEP and with the device, using "Area", "Peak", "Ideal" components, and PCA-fusion respectively are presented for f_B (Figure 8), T_I (Figure 9) and T_E (Figure 10). In Bland–Altman plots, the difference of the two paired measurements (device–OEP) is plotted against the mean of the two measurements (device+OEP)/2. Results of agreement analysis, including evaluation of heteroscedasticity (Kendall's τ correlation and relative p-value) are reported in Table 4. As shown there, for homoscedastic data, the mean of the differences representing the fixed bias, and LOAs were computed. On the other hand, for heteroscedastic data, OLS line of best fit representing the proportional bias and upper and lower 95% V-shape confidence limits (UCL and LCL) are reported.

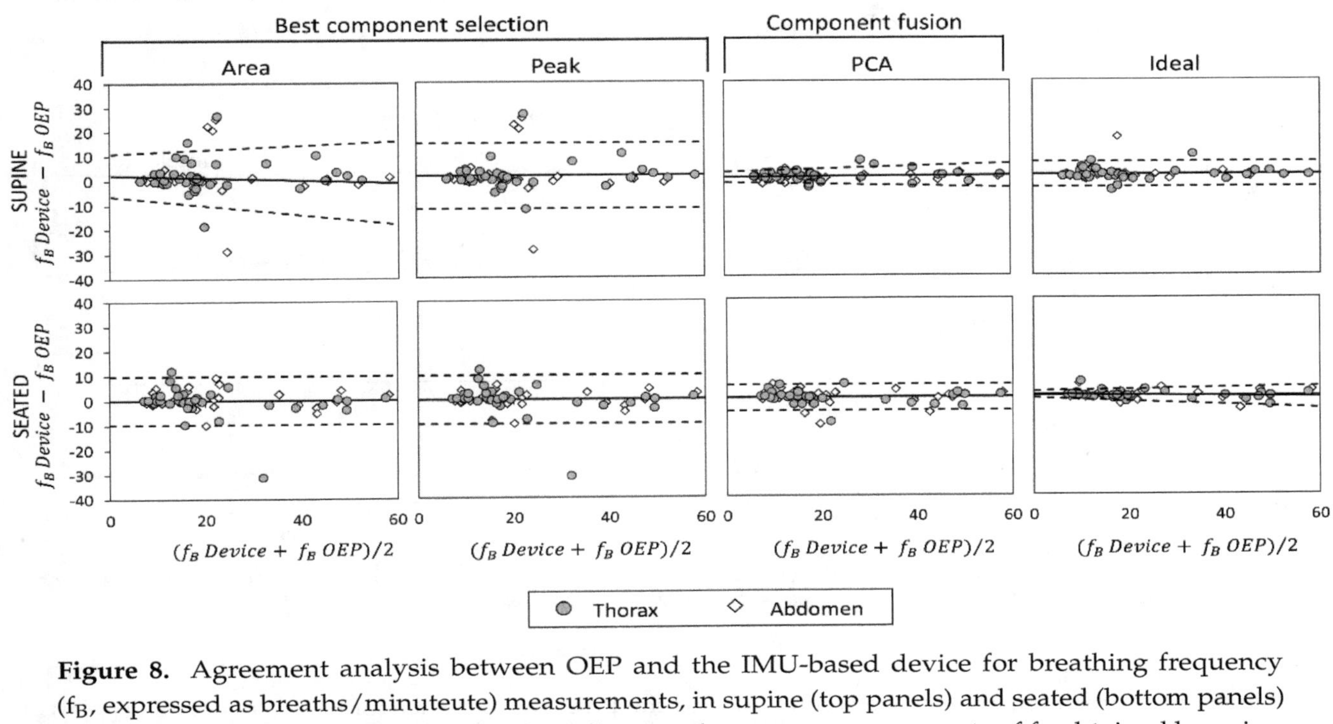

Figure 8. Agreement analysis between OEP and the IMU-based device for breathing frequency (f_B, expressed as breaths/minuteute) measurements, in supine (top panels) and seated (bottom panels) position. In each Bland–Altman plot the differences between measurements of f_B obtained by using the IMU-based device and by using OEP are plotted against the mean of the two measurements. For homoscedastic data, the mean of the differences (bias: —) and limits of agreement (black dotted line) from mean − 1.96 s to mean + 1.96 s are represented by lines parallel to the X axis. For heteroscedastic data, the proportional bias (—) is represented by the ordinary least squares (OLS) line of best fit for the difference on mean values; V-shaped upper and lower 95% confidence limits (- - -) are calculated according to Bland [44].

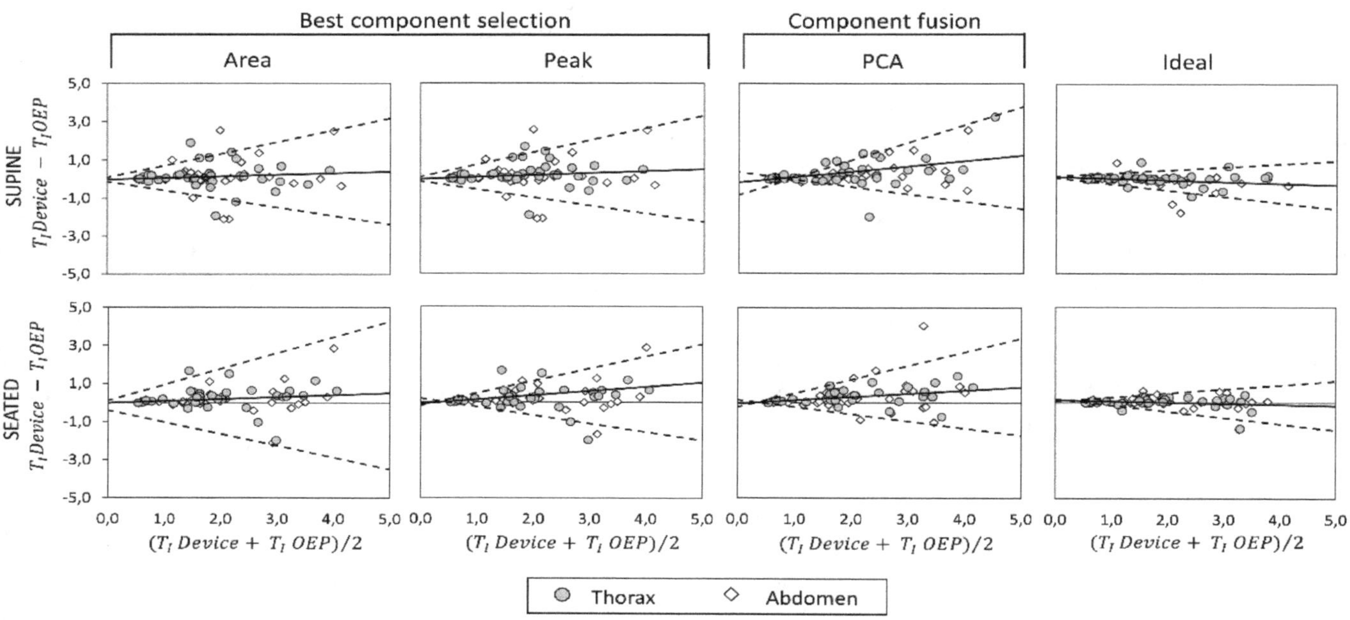

Figure 9. Agreement analysis between OEP and the IMU-based device for inspiratory time (T_I, [s]) measurements, in supine (top panels) and seated (bottom panels) position. In each Bland–Altman plot the differences between measurements of T_I obtained by using the IMU-based device and by using OEP are plotted against the mean of the two measurements. For homoscedastic data, the mean of the differences (bias: —) and limits of agreement (- - -) from mean − 1.96 s to mean + 1.96 s are represented by lines parallel to the X axis. For heteroscedastic data, the proportional bias (—) is represented by the OLS line of best fit for differences on mean values; V-shaped upper and lower 95% confidence limits (- - -) are calculated according to Bland [44].

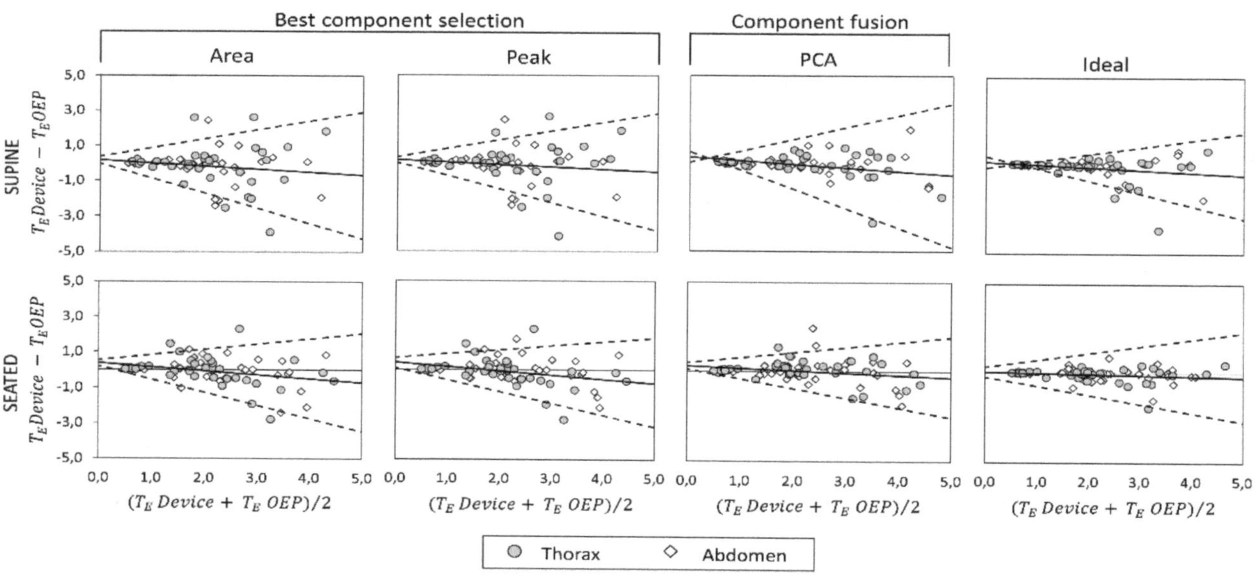

Figure 10. Agreement analysis between OEP and the IMU-based device for expiratory time (T_E, [s]) measurements, in supine (top panels) and seated (bottom panels) position. In each Bland–Altman plot the differences between measurements of T_E obtained by using the IMU-based device and by using OEP are plotted against the mean of the two measurements. For homoscedastic data, the mean of the differences (bias: —) and limits of agreement (- - -) from mean − 1.96 s to mean + 1.96 s are represented by lines parallel to the X axis. For heteroscedastic data, the proportional bias (—) is represented by the OLS line of best fit for differences on mean values; V-shaped upper and lower 95% confidence limits (- - -) are calculated according to Bland [44].

Table 4. Agreement analysis outcomes across subjects and different breathing patterns. Bland and Altman plot statistics for measurements of f_B. T_I. and T_E using best component-selection methods ("Area" and "Peak"), PCA-fusion method and "Ideal" component and, in supine (n = 74) and seated (n = 74) position.

		τ	p-Value	Heteroscedastic?	Fixed Bias [a]/OLS	LOA [c]/V-Shape Limits [d]
f_B supine	**Area**	0.159	0.045	Yes	y = −0.054x + 2.316 [b]	UCL: y = 0.085x + 10.907 [d] LCL: y = −0.192x − 6.275
	Peak	0.142	0.074	No	1.380 [a]	From −11.95 to 14.72 [c]
	PCA	0.211	0.008	Yes	y = 0.008x + 0.130 [b]	UCL: y = 0.054x + 2.299 [d] LCL: y = −0.038x − 2.039
	Ideal	0.038	0.631	No	0.884 [a]	From −4.171 to 5.940 [c]
f_B seated	**Area**	0.142	0.074	No	0.084 [a]	From −9.635 to 9.803 [c]
	Peak	0.132	0.096	No	−0.121 [a]	From −9.931 to 9.688 [c]
	PCA	0.108	0.174	No	−0.23 [a]	From −5.474 to 5.010 [c]
	Ideal	0.196	0.014	Yes	y = −0.021x + 0.597 [b]	UCL: y = 0.028x + 2.057 [d] LCL: y = −0.071x − 0.864
T_I supine	**Area**	0.302	0.000	Yes	y = 0.084x − 0.019 [b]	UCL: y = 0.618x + 0.095 [d] LCL: y = −0.450x − 0.132
	Peak	0.334	0.000	Yes	y = 0.104x − 0.021 [b]	UCL: y = 0.638x + 0.093 [d] LCL: y = −0.430x − 0.135
	PCA	0.375	0.001	Yes	y = 0.283x − 0.175 [b]	UCL: y = 0.926x − 0.840 [d] LCL: y = −0.390x + 0.354
	Ideal	0.292	0.000	Yes	y = −0.090x + 0.121 [b]	UCL: y = 0.158x + 0.163 [d] LCL: y = −0.338x + 0.078
T_I seated	**Area**	0.430	0.000	Yes	y = 0.1022x − 0.0141 [b]	UCL: y = 0.834x + 0.112 [d] LCL: y = −0.618x − 0.409
	Peak	0.422	0.000	Yes	y = 0.220x − 0.075 [b]	UCL: y = 0.642x − 0.173 [d] LCL: y = −0.438x + 0.197
	PCA	0.489	0.000	Yes	y = 0.171x − 0.0332 [b]	UCL: y = 0.7182x − 0.226 [d] LCL: y = −0.377x + 0.160
	Ideal	0.313	0.000	Yes	y = −0.059x + 0.129 [b]	UCL: y = 0.211x + 0.069 [d] LCL: y = −0.329x + 0.189
T_E supine	**Area**	0.421	0.000	Yes	y = −0.170x + 0.166 [b]	UCL: y = 0.508x + 0.358 [d] LCL: y = −0.847x − 0.026
	Peak	0.405	0.000	Yes	y = −0.138x + 0.144 [b]	UCL: y = 0.496x + 0.306 [d] LCL: y = −0.771x − 0.017
	PCA	0.522	0.000	Yes	y = −0.209x + 0.328 [b]	UCL: y = 0.667x + 0.037 [d] LCL: y = −1.084x + 0.620
	Ideal	0.484	0.000	Yes	y = −0.153x + 0.148 [b]	UCL: y = 0.3987x − 0.185 [d] LCL: y = −0.705x + 0.481
T_E seated	**Area**	0.384	0.000	Yes	y = −0.216x + 0.364 [b]	UCL: y = 0.303x + 0.532 [d] LCL: y = −0.735x + 0.197
	Peak	0.396	0.000	Yes	y = −0.231x + 0.413 [b]	UCL: y = 0.226x + 0.666 [d] LCL: y = −0.657x + 0.101
	PCA	0.422	0.000	Yes	y = −0.127x + 0.320 [b]	UCL: y = 0.284x + 0.498 [d] LCL: y = −0.538x + 0.142
	Ideal	0.316	0.000	Yes	y = −0.058x + 0.054 [b]	UCL: y = 0.383x + 0.337 [d] LCL: y = −0.500x − 0.228

τ: Kendall's τ correlation coefficient and relative p-value (heteroscedasticity test). [a] Fixed Bias. obtained as the mean of differences (device – OEP). for homoscedastic data. [b] OLS: ordinary least squares line of best fit (proportional bias) for heteroscedastic data. [c] LOA: limits of agreement. computed as mean difference ± 1.96SD (for homoscedastic data). [d] V-shape limits: UCL and LCL 95% confidence limits. calculated according to Bland [44].

With respect to the main parameter (f_B), agreement between OEP and the device is very strong when the "Ideal" component or the PCA-fusion are used, both in supine and seated position. In relation to time estimation, the agreement decreases for all the methods considered. In particular, for what concerns inspiratory times, a significant relationship between errors and mean value emerged, with a general increase of the difference (device–OEP) at higher time values (overestimation of the device), both in supine and seated position. Also, for expiratory times absolute errors increased with increasing time values, but in this case the device underestimated at high time values (negative slope of the OLS).

3.5. Quaternion Component Selection

Considering the quaternion components selected by the "Area" and "Peak" methods as best component or identified as "Ideal" component, a clear rule did not emerge. In fact, there was not a quaternion component that was selected as best component with a considerable frequency. Relative frequencies of quaternion component selection with the different methods are presented in Figure 11. It is interesting to notice that quaternion component q_0 was never selected by "Area" and "Peak" methods, while the "Ideal" component was q_0 in 14.86 % of cases (n = 74) in supine position and 6.76% of cases (n = 74) in seated position. In seated position, the component q_1 was selected more frequently as best component both by using "Area" (44.59) and "Peak" (39.19%) methods. In contrast, in supine position, the components q_2 ("Area" 51.35%, "Peak": 41.89) and q_3 ("Area": 39.19% and "Peak": 40.54%) were selected more frequently.

Excluding q_0 component, that was clearly less selected, the other quaternion components were almost equally selected as "Ideal" component considering all the trials, both in supine position (q_0: 14.86%, q_1: 22.97%, q_2: 32.43%, q_3: 29.73%), and seated position (q_0: 6.76%, q_1: 33.78, q_2: 22.97%, q_3: 36.49%).

In regard to the ability of the two component-selection methods ("Area" and "Peak") to identify the "Ideal" component, i.e., the component providing the minimum f_B estimation error, in supine position, the "Area" method was able to identify the "Ideal" component in 45.94% of the cases (relative frequency for the event "the component selected by "Area" method and the "Ideal" component corresponded"), the "Peak" method identified the "Ideal" component in 52.70% of the cases, while for the 45.94% of the cases neither the "Area" method nor the "Peak" method were able to identify the "Ideal" component. In 44.59% of cases, "Area" method and "Peak" method selected the same quaternion component, that was also identified as "Ideal" component.

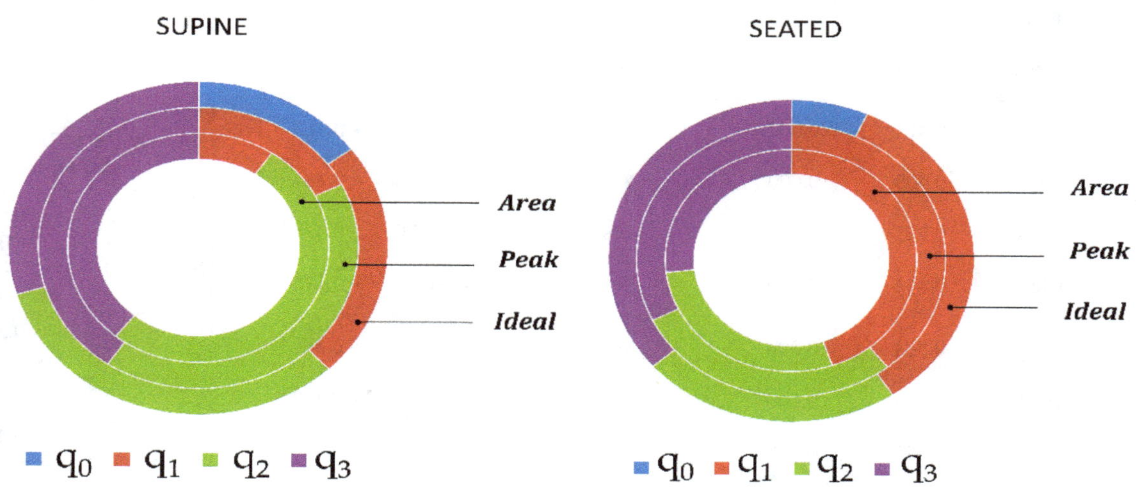

Figure 11. Relative frequencies of quaternion component (q_0, q_1, q_2, q_3) selection using Area and Peak methods and of quaternion component selection as Ideal component, in supine and seated position. Each portion of the rings represents the ratio between the number of times that each quaternion component has been selected (by Area and Peak methods or as Ideal component respectively) and the total number of trials (n = 74).

4. Discussion

In this study, we presented an automatic, position-independent processing algorithm to derive breathing signal, and subsequently breathing temporal parameters, from chest-wall orientation changes acquired using an IMU-based device previously developed by our group [19], composed of three sensor units. Even if the modular configuration of the device was designed to reduce non-breathing movements, the aim of this work was neither to demonstrate the effectiveness of this approach nor to support the presence of the reference unit. On the contrary the focus is on the analysis algorithm, which uses quaternion form to represent orientation, avoiding singularity problem that affects Euler representation; thus, thoracic and abdominal orientation change signals are 4-dimensional entities. The proposed algorithm includes therefore a dimension-reduction block to obtain a 1-dimension signal representing chest-wall orientation changes due to breathing activity.

Another aim of this study was, therefore, to compare three different dimension-reduction methods. The first two methods ("Peak" and "Area") are based on the selection of the quaternion component with the highest breathing information. The third method is based on the fusion of the 4 components of the quaternion using PCA.

The PCA-fusion method performed better than the best component-selection methods ("Peak" and "Area") as regards breathing frequency estimation, both in supine and seated position. In supine position, it provided better results than "Ideal" component, while in seated position it provided closer performances to those obtained by using the "Ideal" component with respect to "Area" and "Peak" methods.

About estimation of other temporal parameters (T_I, T_E and duty cycle), "Ideal" component provided the best results, while PCA-fusion method gave results comparable to the best component-selection methods. Thus, a quaternion component providing the best performance exists, the problem lies in its a priori identification. In fact, both "Area" and "Peak" methods failed to identify it on the basis of spectral analysis (in 45.94% of the cases neither the "Area" method nor the "Peak" method were able to identify the "Ideal" component), and no quaternion component emerged as the most selected as "Ideal" component (supine q_0:14.86%, q_1: 22.97%, q_2: 32.43%, q_3: 29.73%; seated q_0: 6.76%, q_1: 33.78, q_2: 22.97%, q_3: 36.49%).

Geometrical or morphological considerations to determine which quaternion component is more involved in breathing movement are problematic when considering quaternions, and are position- and IMU-placement dependent, thus not suitable in dynamic conditions. On the contrary, PCA-fusion method represents an interesting solution to this problem because it fuses the information of the four quaternion components regardless the position of the subject or the IMUs placement, avoiding the necessity to select a best component/axes, as reported in previous studies [7,11,13].

In this study, we found that PCA-fusion method provided the best f_B estimation performance in terms of mean absolute errors (<2 breaths/minute), correlation (r > 0.963) and agreement (see Table 4) with the reference method. Comparing our results in terms of accuracy errors with those obtained by previous studies is difficult because in most cases only relative errors were reported, but these errors depend on the breathing frequency adopted. Liu et al. [14] reported a mean absolute error of 15.45 breaths/minute (thus about 7 times higher than the error obtained in this study) during quiet sitting. Bates et al. [13] obtained an RMS error of 0.38 breaths/minute and a peak error of 3 breaths/minute in a postoperative patient during sleep. Considering comparable conditions (abdominal compartment in supine position) we obtained an RMS error of 1.51 breaths/minute, using PCA-fusion method, but in our study different, forced, breathing patterns were included, leading to higher mean error.

Regarding correlation between f_B measurements obtained with the proposed method and OEP, our results are comparable to those obtained by Bates et al. [13] that reported a correlation coefficient equal to 0.985 between measurements of f_B obtained with the accelerometer and nasal cannula. Mann et al. [11] obtained a correlation coefficient of 0.97 between measurements of f_B obtained with a tri-axial accelerometer and with a system based on oxygen consumption measurement (Oxycon Mobile). In both cases [11,13], breath-by-breath analysis was not possible. Liu et al. [14] reported correlation coefficients lower than 0.6 between f_B computed with a 3-axis accelerometer and with the reference (Airflow CO_2 analysis).

There are few studies in the literature that performs Bland–Altman analysis to assess the agreement between breathing frequency measurements obtained by using inertial sensors and other validated methods. In the study from Morillo et al. [8] agreement analysis using Bland Altman plots was done against PSG thermistor. The authors reported a mean difference (fixed bias) of 0.02 (SD = 1.09) breaths/minute and LOAs from −3.05 to +2.11 breaths/minute in the range ~12 ÷ 35 breaths/minute. In that case, the use of a single-axis accelerometer, prevent the use of that method during postural changes. Dehkrodi et al. [9] used a tri-axial accelerometer placed on the suprasternal notch extending the validation presented in [8] to different sleeping positions and breathing conditions (Deep: 13.5 ± 4.3, Normal: 16.5 ± 5.2 and Shallow: 39.7 ± 30.3 breath/minute). They reported a mean difference (fixed bias) of 0.042 breaths/minute and LOAs from –0.65 to 0.74 breaths/minute. Lapi et al. [17] performed agreement analysis with Bland Altman plots for measurements of breathing frequency (range 12 ÷ 26 breaths/minute) obtained with the accelerometer and with the standard method (counting breaths by visual inspection), in supine position. They reported a mean difference (fixed bias) of 0.33 breaths/minute and LOA from −1.92 to 2.60 with 3.2% of data outside that range. For all the above-mentioned studies heteroscedasticity of data was not considered or reported making it difficult compare them directly with our results. In fact, taking into account heteroscedasticity of data, for f_B in supine position, we built Bland–Altman plot with proportional bias (OLS: y = 0.008x + 0.130, thus going from 0.18 (at x = 6 breaths/minute) to 0.61 (at x = 60 breaths/minute) breaths/minute) and V-shaped limits (LCL: y = −0.038x − 2.039 thus the lower limit goes from −2.26 (at x = 6 breaths/minute) to −4.32 (at x = 60 breaths/minute) breath/minute; UCL: y = 0.054x + 2.299; thus the upper limit goes form 2.62 (at x = 6 breaths/minute) to 5.539 (at x = 60 breaths/minute) breaths/minute)). Thus, considering comparable breathing frequency ranges our results are closer to those obtained by Morillo et al. [8] and Lapi et al. [17]. On the contrary, Dehkrodi et al. [9] obtained better results; unfortunately, the steps to obtain the acceleration derived respiratory (ADR) signal are not described in detail.

For the best of our knowledge, this is the first study that provides a detailed analysis of respiratory timing measurements obtained by using inertial sensor systems, validating them against an established method.

5. Conclusions

PCA-fusion method provided overall best performances with respect to selecting the best quaternion component identified based on spectrum analysis. In supine position results obtained fusing the 4 quaternion components were even better than those obtained with the "Ideal" component, identified a posteriori considering the minimum breathing frequency estimation error. Performance in seated position were worse than those obtained in supine position, probably because subjects were seated without the back support and some oscillations of the trunk were more likely to occur. This could particularly affect PCA-based method where the first principal component selected for further analysis is the one with the largest variance, and thus more subject to larger body motions. This must be taken into account in dynamic conditions; signal baseline removal prior to PCA-fusion should be considered in this case.

The analysis algorithm proposed in this work, applying PCA-fusion as dimension-reduction method, can be used to analyze further data. In fact, an extended validation of the proposed device and method is needed also in dynamic conditions, during daily activities, considering not only healthy subjects but also patients that could particularly take advantage of this system (e.g., COPD, neuromuscular patients, sleep apnea, etc.). This would also allow study of asynchronies of thoraco-abdominal compartments taking advantage of the modular configuration of the device. Another key step will be the adaptation of our method, currently implemented as an offline analysis, to online monitoring, moving the computation process aboard the smartphone. This enhancement could allow immediate computation of an average breathing frequency over a certain period (e.g., 60 s) directly aboard the smartphone, fostering the use of the device in other applications such as sport and fitness, exercise testing, breathing training to use different respiratory muscles, rehabilitation protocols and treatment evaluation where respiratory assessment could be of great interest.

6. Patents

The present work is partially described in the International Patent application n° PCT/IB2018/054956, priority date 11 July 2017, title "A wearable device for the continuous monitoring of the respiratory rate". Inventors: Ambra Cesareo, Andrea Aliverti, Assignee: Politecnico di Milano.

Author Contributions: A.C. and A.A. contributed IMU circuit design and fabrication; A.C. conceived and designed the experiments; A.C. and Y.P. performed the experiments and analyzed the data; A.C. and E.B. prepared the original draft; E.B. and A.A. reviewed the paper; E.B. and A.A. supervised the project and contributed to funding acquisition.

Acknowledgments: This work was supported by "FoRST -Fondazione per la Ricerca Scientifica Termale".

References

1. Subbe, C.; Davies, R.; Williams, E.; Rutherford, P.; Gemmell, L. Effect of Introducing the Modified Early Warning Score on Clinical Outcomes, cardio-pulmonary Arrests and Intensive Care Utilisation in Acute Medical Admissions. *Anaesthesia* **2003**, *58*, 797–802. [CrossRef] [PubMed]
2. Cretikos, M.A.; Bellomo, R.; Hillman, K.; Chen, J.; Finfer, S.; Flabouris, A. Respiratory Rate: The Neglected Vital Sign. *Med. J. Aust.* **2008**, *188*, 657.
3. World Health Organization. *Acute Respiratory Infections in Children: Case Management in Small Hospitals in Developing Countries, a Manual for Doctors and Other Senior Health Workers*; World Health Organization: Geneva, Switzerland, 1990.
4. Karlen, W.; Gan, H.; Chiu, M.; Dunsmuir, D.; Zhou, G.; Dumont, G.A.; Ansermino, J.M. Improving the Accuracy and Efficiency of Respiratory Rate Measurements in Children using Mobile Devices. *PLoS ONE* **2014**, *9*, e99266. [CrossRef] [PubMed]
5. Torres, A.; Fiz, J.; Galdiz, B.; Gea, J.; Morera, J.; Jané, R. Assessment of Respiratory Muscle Effort Studying Diaphragm Movement Registered with Surface Sensors. Animal Model (Dogs). In Proceedings of the 26th Annual International Conference of the IEEE Engineering in Medicine and Biology Society (IEMBS'04), San Francisco, CA, USA, 1–4 September 2004; pp. 3917–3920.
6. Reinvuo, T.; Hannula, M.; Sorvoja, H.; Alasaarela, E.; Myllyla, R. Measurement of Respiratory Rate with High-Resolution Accelerometer and EMFit Pressure Sensor. In Proceedings of the 2006 IEEE Sensors Applications Symposium, Houston, TX, USA, 7–9 February 2006; pp. 192–195.
7. Hung, P.; Bonnet, S.; Guillemaud, R.; Castelli, E.; Yen, P.T.N. Estimation of Respiratory Waveform using an Accelerometer. In Proceedings of the 5th IEEE International Symposium on Biomedical Imaging: From Nano to Macro (ISBI 2008), Paris, France, 14–17 May 2008; pp. 1493–1496.
8. Morillo, D.S.; Ojeda, J.L.R.; Foix, L.F.C.; Jiménez, A.L. An Accelerometer-Based Device for Sleep Apnea Screening. *IEEE Trans. Inf. Technol. Biomed.* **2010**, *14*, 491–499. [CrossRef] [PubMed]
9. Dehkordi, P.K.; Marzencki, M.; Tavakolian, K.; Kaminska, M.; Kaminska, B. Validation of Respiratory Signal Derived from Suprasternal Notch Acceleration for Sleep Apnea Detection. In Proceedings of the 2011 Annual International Conference of the IEEE Engineering in Medicine and Biology Society (EMBC), Boston, MA, USA, 30 August–3 September 2011; pp. 3824–3827.
10. Fekr, A.R.; Janidarmian, M.; Radecka, K.; Zilic, Z. A Medical Cloud-Based Platform for Respiration Rate Measurement and Hierarchical Classification of Breath Disorders. *Sensors* **2014**, *14*, 11204–11224. [CrossRef] [PubMed]
11. Mann, J.; Rabinovich, R.; Bates, A.; Giavedoni, S.; MacNee, W.; Arvind, D. Simultaneous Activity and Respiratory Monitoring using an Accelerometer. In Proceedings of the 2011 International Conference Body Sensor Networks (BSN), Dallas, TX, USA, 23–25 May 2011; pp. 139–143.
12. Jin, A.; Yin, B.; Morren, G.; Duric, H.; Aarts, R.M. Performance Evaluation of a Tri-Axial Accelerometry-Based Respiration Monitoring for Ambient Assisted Living. In Proceedings of the Annual International Conference of the IEEE Engineering in Medicine and Biology Society (EMBC 2009), Minneapolis, MN, USA, 2–6 September 2009; pp. 5677–5680.

13. Bates, A.; Ling, M.J.; Mann, J.; Arvind, D. Respiratory Rate and Flow Waveform Estimation from Tri-Axial Accelerometer Data. In Proceedings of the 2010 International Conference on Body Sensor Networks (BSN), Singapore, 7–9 June 2010; pp. 144–150.
14. Liu, G.; Guo, Y.; Zhu, Q.; Huang, B.; Wang, L. Estimation of Respiration Rate from Three-Dimensional Acceleration Data Based on Body Sensor Network. *Telemed. e-Health* **2011**, *17*, 705–711. [CrossRef] [PubMed]
15. Yoon, J.; Noh, Y.; Kwon, Y.; Kim, W.; Yoon, H. Improvement of Dynamic Respiration Monitoring through Sensor Fusion of Accelerometer and Gyro-Sensor. *J. Electr. Eng. Technol.* **2014**, *9*, 334–343. [CrossRef]
16. Gollee, H.; Chen, W. Real-Time Detection of Respiratory Activity using an Inertial Measurement Unit. In Proceedings of the 29th Annual International Conference of the IEEE Engineering in Medicine and Biology Society (EMBS 2007), Lyon, France, 23–26 August 2007; pp. 2230–2233.
17. Lapi, S.; Lavorini, F.; Borgioli, G.; Calzolai, M.; Masotti, L.; Pistolesi, M.; Fontana, G.A. Respiratory Rate Assessments using a Dual-Accelerometer Device. *Respir. Physiol. Neurobiol.* **2014**, *191*, 60–66. [CrossRef]
18. Gaidhani, A.; Moon, K.S.; Ozturk, Y.; Lee, S.Q.; Youm, W. Extraction and Analysis of Respiratory Motion using Wearable Inertial Sensor System during Trunk Motion. *Sensors* **2017**, *17*, 2932. [CrossRef]
19. Cesareo, A.; Gandolfi, S.; Pini, I.; Biffi, E.; Reni, G.; Aliverti, A. A Novel, Low Cost, Wearable Contact-Based Device for Breathing Frequency Monitoring. In Proceedings of the 2017 39th Annual International Conference of the IEEE Engineering in Medicine and Biology Society (EMBC), Seogwipo, Korea, 11–15 July 2017; pp. 2402–2405.
20. Romei, M.; Mauro, A.L.; D'angelo, M.; Turconi, A.; Bresolin, N.; Pedotti, A.; Aliverti, A. Effects of Gender and Posture on Thoraco-Abdominal Kinematics during Quiet Breathing in Healthy Adults. *Respir. Physiol. Neurobiol.* **2010**, *172*, 184–191. [CrossRef]
21. Aliverti, A.; Pedotti, A. Opto-electronic plethysmography. In *Mechanics of Breathing*; Springer: Milano, Italy, 2002; pp. 47–59.
22. Aliverti, A.; Dellacà, R.; Pelosi, P.; Chiumello, D.; Gattinoni, L.; Pedotti, A. Compartmental Analysis of Breathing in the Supine and Prone Positions by Optoelectronic Plethysmography. *Ann. Biomed. Eng.* **2001**, *29*, 60–70. [CrossRef] [PubMed]
23. Aliverti, A.; Dellaca, R.; Pelosi, P.; Chiumello, D.; Pedotti, A.; Gattinoni, L. Optoelectronic Plethysmography in Intensive Care Patients. *Am. J. Respir. Crit. Care Med.* **2000**, *161*, 1546–1552. [CrossRef] [PubMed]
24. Cala, S.; Kenyon, C.; Ferrigno, G.; Carnevali, P.; Aliverti, A.; Pedotti, A.; Macklem, P.; Rochester, D. Chest Wall and Lung Volume Estimation by Optical Reflectance Motion Analysis. *J. Appl. Physiol.* **1996**, *81*, 2680–2689. [CrossRef] [PubMed]
25. Ferrigno, G.; Carnevali, P.; Aliverti, A.; Molteni, F.; Beulcke, G.; Pedotti, A. Three-Dimensional Optical Analysis of Chest Wall Motion. *J. Appl. Physiol.* **1994**, *77*, 1224–1231. [CrossRef] [PubMed]
26. Konno, K.; Mead, J. Measurement of the separate volume changes of rib cage and abdomen during breathing. *J. Appl. Physiol.* **1967**, *22*, 407–422. [CrossRef] [PubMed]
27. Hamilton, W.R. XI. On Quaternions; Or on a New System of Imaginaries in Algebra. *Lond. Edinb. Dublin Philos. Mag. J. Sci.* **1848**, *33*, 58–60. [CrossRef]
28. Rosenfeld, B. *The History of Non-Euclidean Geometry: Evolution of the Concept of a Geometrical Space*; Springer-Verlag: Berlin, Germany, 1988.
29. Madgwick, S.O.; Harrison, A.J.; Vaidyanathan, R. Estimation of IMU and MARG Orientation using a Gradient Descent Algorithm. In Proceedings of the 2011 IEEE International Conference on Rehabilitation Robotics (ICORR), Zurich, Switzerland, 29 June–1 July 2011; pp. 1–7.
30. Pearson, K. LIII. On Lines and Planes of Closest Fit to Systems of Points in Space. *Lond. Edinb. Dublin Philos. Mag. J. Sci.* **1901**, *2*, 559–572. [CrossRef]
31. Hotelling, H. Analysis of a Complex of Statistical Variables into Principal Components. *J. Educ. Psychol.* **1933**, *24*, 417. [CrossRef]
32. Savitzky, A.; Golay, M.J. Smoothing and Differentiation of Data by Simplified Least Squares Procedures. *Anal. Chem.* **1964**, *36*, 1627–1639. [CrossRef]
33. Kenyon, C.M.; Cala, S.J.; Yan, S.; Aliverti, A.; Scano, G.; Duranti, R.; Pedotti, A.; Macklem, P.T. Rib cage mechanics during quiet breathing and exercise in humans. *J. Appl. Physiol.* **1997**, *83*, 1242–1255. [CrossRef]
34. Layton, A.M.; Moran, S.L.; Garber, C.E.; Armstrong, H.F.; Basner, R.C.; Thomashow, B.M.; Bartels, M.N. Optoelectronic plethysmography compared to spirometry during maximal exercise. *Respir. Physiol. Neurobiol.* **2013**, *185*, 362–368. [CrossRef] [PubMed]

35. LoMauro, A.; Cesareo, A.; Agosti, F.; Tringali, G.; Salvadego, D.; Grassi, B.; Sartorio, A.; Aliverti, A. Effects of a Multidisciplinary Body Weight Reduction Program on Static and Dynamic Thoraco-Abdominal Volumes in Obese Adolescents. *Appl. Physiol. Nutr. Metab.* **2016**, *41*, 649–658. [CrossRef] [PubMed]
36. Lo Mauro, A.; D'Angelo, M.G.; Romei, M.; Motta, F.; Colombo, D.; Comi, G.P.; Pedotti, A.; Marchi, E.; Turconi, A.C.; Bresolin, N.; et al. Abdominal Volume Contribution to Tidal Volume as an Early Indicator of Respiratory Impairment in Duchenne Muscular Dystrophy. *Eur. Respir. J.* **2010**, *35*, 1118–1125. [CrossRef] [PubMed]
37. Cesareo, A.; LoMauro, A.; Santi, M.; Biffi, E.; D'Angelo, M.G.; Aliverti, A. Acute Effects of Mechanical Insufflation-Exsufflation on the Breathing Pattern in Stable Subjects with Duchenne Muscular Dystrophy. *Respir. Care* **2018**. [CrossRef] [PubMed]
38. Benjamini, Y.; Hochberg, Y. Controlling the False Discovery Rate: A Practical and Powerful Approach to Multiple Testing. *J. R. Stat. Soc. Ser. B Methodol.* **1995**, *57*, 289–300. [CrossRef]
39. Benjamini, Y.; Yekutieli, D. The Control of the False Discovery Rate in Multiple Testing Under Dependency. *Ann. Stat.* **2001**, 1165–1188.
40. Altman, D.G.; Bland, J.M. Measurement in Medicine: The Analysis of Method Comparison Studies. *Statistician* **1983**, 307–317. [CrossRef]
41. Bland, J.M.; Altman, D. Statistical Methods for Assessing Agreement between Two Methods of Clinical Measurement. *Lancet* **1986**, *327*, 307–310. [CrossRef]
42. Bland, J.M.; Altman, D.G. Measuring Agreement in Method Comparison Studies. *Stat. Methods Med. Res.* **1999**, *8*, 135–160. [CrossRef]
43. BREHM, M.; Scholtes, V.A.; Dallmeijer, A.J.; Twisk, J.W.; Harlaar, J. The Importance of Addressing Heteroscedasticity in the Reliability Analysis of ratio-scaled Variables: An Example Based on Walking energy-cost Measurements. *Dev. Med. Child Neurol.* **2012**, *54*, 267–273. [CrossRef]
44. Bland, J. How Do I Estimate Limits of Agreement When the Mean or SD of Differences Is Not Constant? Available online: https://www-users.york.ac.uk/~{}mb55/meas/glucose.htm (accessed on 4 October 2018).
45. Ludbrook, J. Confidence in Altman–Bland Plots: A Critical Review of the Method of Differences. *Clin. Exp. Pharmacol. Physiol.* **2010**, *37*, 143–149. [CrossRef] [PubMed]

6

Inertial Measurement Unit Based Upper Extremity Motion Characterization for Action Research Arm Test and Activities of Daily Living

Hyung Seok Nam [1,2], Woo Hyung Lee [1], Han Gil Seo [2], Yoon Jae Kim [3], Moon Suk Bang [2,4,*] and Sungwan Kim [1,5,*]

1 Department of Biomedical Engineering, Seoul National University College of Medicine, Seoul 03080, Korea; ignite31@snu.ac.kr (H.S.N.); v3night9@snu.ac.kr (W.H.L.)
2 Department of Rehabilitation Medicine, Seoul National University Hospital, Seoul 03080, Korea; hangilseo@snu.ac.kr
3 Interdisciplinary Program for Bioengineering, Seoul National University Graduate School, Seoul 08826, Korea; kyj182731@naver.com
4 Department of Rehabilitation Medicine, Seoul National University College of Medicine, Seoul 03080, Korea
5 Institute of Medical and Biological Engineering, Seoul National University, Seoul 03080, Korea
* Correspondence: msbang@snu.ac.kr (M.S.B.); sungwan@snu.ac.kr (S.K.)

Abstract: In practical rehabilitation robot development, it is imperative to pre-specify the critical workspace to prevent redundant structure. This study aimed to characterize the upper extremity motion during essential activities in daily living. An IMU-based wearable motion capture system was used to access arm movements. Ten healthy subjects performed the Action Research Arm Test (ARAT) and six pre-selected essential daily activities. The Euler angles of the major joints, and acceleration from wrist and hand sensors were acquired and analyzed. The size of the workspace for the ARAT was 0.53 (left-right) × 0.92 (front-back) × 0.89 (up-down) m for the dominant hand. For the daily activities, the workspace size was 0.71 × 0.70 × 0.86 m for the dominant hand, significantly larger than the non-dominant hand ($p \leq 0.011$). The average range of motion (RoM) during ARAT was 109.15 ± 18.82° for elbow flexion/extension, 105.23 ± 5.38° for forearm supination/pronation, 91.99 ± 0.98° for shoulder internal/external rotation, and 82.90 ± 22.52° for wrist dorsiflexion/volarflexion, whereas the corresponding range for daily activities were 120.61 ± 23.64°, 128.09 ± 22.04°, 111.56 ± 31.88°, and 113.70 ± 18.26°. The shoulder joint was more abducted and extended during pinching compared to grasping posture ($p < 0.001$). Reaching from a grasping posture required approximately 70° elbow extension and 36° forearm supination from the initial position. The study results provide an important database for the workspace and RoM for essential arm movements.

Keywords: inertial measurement unit; upper extremity; motion; action research arm test; activities of daily living

1. Introduction

In the last decade, there have been dramatic improvements in rehabilitation robots and kinematic analyses of the upper extremities. Many types of multi-axis exoskeletons have been developed, as well as relatively simple end-effector type robots [1–5]. Exoskeletons are commonly defined as having a structure in which the robot joints correspond to human joints, whereas end-effector type robot structures do not correspond to human anatomical structures [1,6]. However, even in exoskeletons, the angular movements of human and robot joints do not exactly match. This discrepancy comes from the fundamental difference in that exoskeleton joints have mechanical joint axes with their corresponding motors, whereas human joints consist of bones, muscle and tendons, and soft tissues [7]. Therefore, the goal of exoskeleton rehabilitation robot development should not focus on perfectly resembling the human arm joint and structure, but rather on designing a modified structure based on a better understanding of human kinematics.

Many types of sensors are used for a motion analysis of the upper extremities including electromagnetic sensors, mechanical sensors, optical sensors, and inertial sensors. Aizawa et al. [8] reported the range of motions (RoM) of the major upper extremity joints during selected activities of daily living (ADL), using a commercial electromagnetic sensor system. Gates et al. [9] also quantified the RoM of the upper extremities during eight ADLs using reflective sensors. Kim et al. [10] conducted a kinematic analysis of drinking movements using reflective markers. Chen and Lum [11] used a spring-operated exoskeleton to compare the RoM with and without robotic assistance during the given tasks, where the angles were evaluated using mechanical sensors within the robot. Perez et al. [12] introduced a portable motion analysis for the upper limbs using inertial measurement unit (IMU) sensors. A recent review showed that accelerometers and IMUs are most frequently used devices for an analysis of upper limb motion [13]. Although many of these reports present quantitative angular values during specific ADL tasks, assessments focusing on clinically relevant applications of the motion data remain scarce.

To minimize the size and complexity of neurorehabilitation robots, the number of axes and the workspace of a robotic hand or end-effector should be minimized; at the same time, however, essential tasks need to be performable during daily activities. From the viewpoint of performing a specific task, although the human performance using an arm may seem similar to the actuation of a robot, when considering the mechanism of the performance, they are significantly different. Moreover, it is possible to state that biological and engineering mechanisms are in significant opposition [7]. It is important to have a database on the position and joint angles while performing essential daily activities; however, the movement patterns in healthy subjects and stroke patients differ significantly, and the exoskeleton cannot be actuated in exactly the same manner as a human limb. It is necessary to create a design that patients may not only wear but also actuate in an appropriate manner to help the movement of a paralyzed limb and induce neuroplasticity.

The purpose of this study was to provide a database on the dimensions of the essential workspace and the RoM of the major upper extremity joints during the normal motion of healthy subjects from clinical and practical perspectives.

2. Materials and Methods

In this section, we present the IMU-based motion capture system used in this study with validation protocol, followed by participants information and task protocols. Detailed information on extracted parameters and statistical methods are also provided.

2.1. Upper Extremity Motion Capture System and Its Validation

For motion capture of the upper extremities, Perception Neuron® (Noitom Ltd., Beijing, China), a wearable multi-IMU based modular motion capture system was used. In this study, we utilized 25 IMU sensors for the upper body assessment; three sensors for the body axis, four sensors for each arm, and seven sensors for each hand including the fingers (Figure 1). User-interface software, Axis Neuron (Noitom Ltd., Beijing, China), was applied for motion recording and data extraction. The sampling rate of the data was set to 60 Hz.

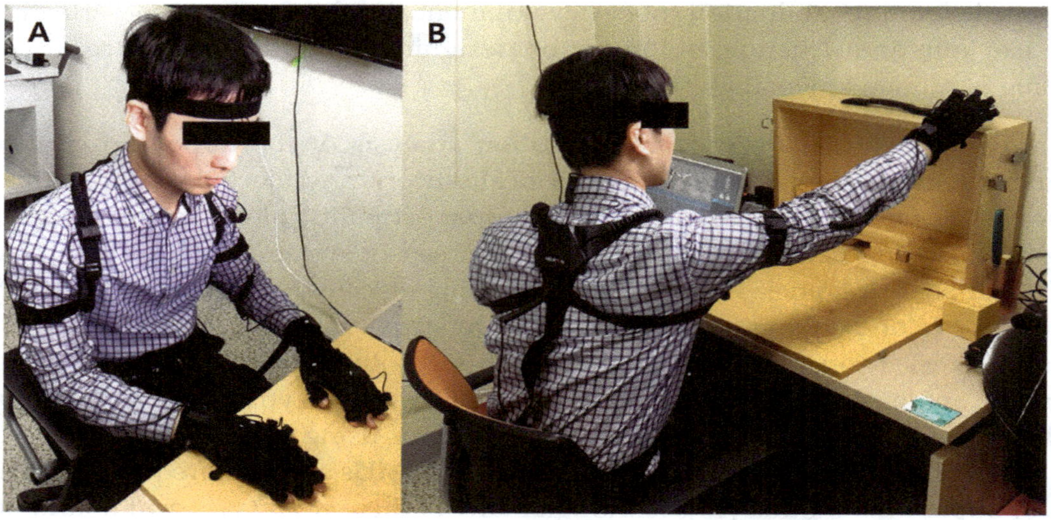

Figure 1. (**A**) A volunteer subject is wearing the IMU-based upper extremity motion capture system. (**B**) The subject is performing a task in the Action Research Arm Test.

To validate the accuracy and consistency of the system, root mean square error (RMSE) analyses for the elbow flexion/extension and wrist dorsiflexion/volarflexion axes were performed using an electro-goniometer as a reference. During real motion with the system worn on the body, it is not possible to isolate single joint movements in a single plane with all other joint being fixed. Therefore, coefficient of variation (CoV) analyses for forearm supination/pronation and elbow flexion/extension for the angles from a gyrosensor, and the z-axis (up-down) and y-axis (front-back) distances from accelerometers in the forearm and hand sensors were conducted using the data collected during the tasks.

2.2. *Participants*

Ten healthy volunteers (six males, four females) were recruited for this study, and participated after providing written informed consent. Their mean age was 29.3 ± 4.7 years (age range: 23–35).

2.3. *Tasks and Procedure*

All subjects wore the IMU sensor based motion capture system on both upper extremities. After sensor calibration, they performed all 19 test items of the Action Research Arm Test (ARAT) with using both their right and left hands alternatively [14]. ARAT consists of four domains: domain 1 includes six grasp and reaching tasks with various size of wooden blocks, ball, or a stone; domain 2 consists of four grip activities such as pouring water from glass to glass or putting a hollow tube through a stick; domain 3 includes six pinch and reaching tasks using various size of marbles using different fingers; and domain 4 consists of four gross movements placing the hand on three different parts of the head [14]. They also performed six pre-specified ADL tasks: (1) opening a water bottle and drinking, (2) peeling off a banana, (3) buttoning and unbuttoning a shirt, (4) combing their hair, (5) squeezing toothpaste from a tube and brushing their teeth, and (6) turning a door knob. These pre-specified ADL tasks were selected from the survey results from our previous study which evaluated the practical needs of stroke patients owing to their hemiplegia [15]. During the ADL tasks, the subjects were instructed to perform the task in the most natural way possible, without specifying which hand to use to hold or manipulate the object.

2.4. *Extracted Parameters*

Using Axis Neuron (Noitom Ltd., Beijing, China) software, acceleration and position data of the wrist and hand sensors from the accelerometer, and the Euler angles for the sensors of all major joints with reference to their proximal segment sensors during the ARAT and ADL tasks, were extracted. For each ARAT domain and ADL task, the size of the workspace in three orthogonal coordinates and the angular position and RoM for each upper extremity joint were calculated. For a sub-analysis, grasping/pinching and reaching movements when conducting the tasks in ARAT domains 1 and 3 were additionally analyzed regarding the initial grasping/pinching position and RoM during a reaching movement.

2.5. Statistical Analysis

For validation purposes, the intra-subject covariance and inter-subject covariance were both calculated for repetitive grasping/pinching and reaching tasks. Paired *t* tests were conducted to compare the workspace dimensions and RoM between dominant and non-dominant arms. Paired *t* tests were also conducted for a comparison of the major joint angles in the grasping/pinching position and reaching position, the initial position between grasping and pinching, and the reaching position from grasping and pinching. The statistical program SPSS ver. 25 (SPSS Inc., Chicago, IL, USA) was used for analysis. A p value of less than 0.05 was considered statistically significant.

3. Results

The validation results followed by data analysis on movement characteristics are provided in this section.

3.1. Validation of Upper Extremity Motion Capture System

The range of RMSE for the elbow flexion/extension angle ranged from 2.11° to 4.75° (3.61 ± 1.32°), and 0.42° to 1.22° (0.85 ± 0.40°) for wrist dorsiflexion/volarflexion angle. During the reaching task, the mean change in forearm supination/pronation was 36.65 ± 6.98°, with an intra-subject CoV of 17.29% and inter-subject CoV of 19.05%. The change in elbow flexion/extension was 69.96 ± 16.89°, and intra-subject and inter-subject CoV was 11.67% and 24.14%, respectively. Distance data extracted from the sensors during the reaching tasks were evaluated and then compared with the real movement distance. Regarding the accelerometer on the forearm sensor, the average of calculated movement distance was 34.14 ± 4.15 cm in the z-axis, and 33.54 ± 4.79 cm in the y-axis, where the measured distance in each direction was 34.0 cm and 33.5 cm, respectively. Data calculated from hand sensors were 36.78 ± 3.09 cm and 32.35 ± 4.64 cm), respectively. The intra-subject CoV ranged from 5.5% to 9.5%, whereas the inter-subject CoV ranged from 8.4% to 14.3%. The complete results are shown in Table 1.

Table 1. Coefficient of variation (CoV) for major movements [a].

Sensor Type	Axis	Average Change during Task (Across Subjects)	Intra-Subject CoV Average	Inter-Subject CoV	Estimated Real Distance *
Gyrosensor	Forearm supination/pronation	36.65 ± 6.98°	17.29%	19.05%	-
	Elbow flexion/extension	69.96 ± 16.89°	11.67%	24.14%	-
Accelerometer (forearm sensor)	z-axis distance (up/down)	34.14 ± 4.15 cm	6.18%	12.17%	34.0 cm
	y-axis distance (front/back)	33.54 ± 4.79 cm	7.16%	14.28%	33.5 cm
Accelerometer (hand sensor)	z-axis distance (up/down)	36.78 ± 3.09 cm	5.56%	8.41%	34.0 cm
	y-axis distance (front/back)	32.35 ± 4.64 cm	9.49%	14.33%	33.5 cm

[a] Tasks performed by 10 normal subjects, six trials per reaching. * Estimated distance between initial object position and target position is approximately 33.5 cm for y-axis and 34.0 cm for z-axis. Note that this is the distance regarding common position of the forearm and hand sensors during the task and it varies by trials and subjects.

3.2. Workspace and RoM in Basic Upper Extremity Movements

All ten subjects were right-handed. For an orthogonal coordination, the axes were defined as follows: left-right direction for the x-axis, front-right direction for the y-axis, and up-down direction for the z-axis. For ARAT tasks, the size of the workspace for the right hand with reference to the sensor on the dorsum of the hand was 0.53 ± 0.11 m for the x-axis, 0.92 ± 0.08 m for the y-axis, and 0.89 ± 0.10 m for the z-axis. For the left side, the average workspace size was 0.62 × 0.80 × 0.86 m (in x, y, z-axis order). For pre-specified ADL tasks, the workspace for the dominant hand was 0.71 ± 0.22 m, 0.70 ± 0.17 m, and 0.86 ± 0.11 m (in x, y, z-axis order). The workspace of the non-dominant hand was significantly smaller, with an average size of 0.52 × 0.53 × 0.65 m ($p = 0.001$, 0.011, and 0.001 for the x-, y-, and z-axes, respectively). For the RoM in the major upper extremity joints, the angular ranges were similar between the right and left sides. The elbow flexion/extension and forearm supination/pronation showed the highest RoM in both ARAT and ADL for the dominant arm. The mean RoM values were 109.15 ± 18.82° and 105.23 ± 15.38° (elbow flexion/extension and forearm supination/pronation, respectively) for ARAT tasks, and 120.61 ± 23.64° and 128.09 ± 22.04° for ADL tasks. The RoM of the dominant side was significantly greater than on the non-dominant side for all joint directions except for the wrist dorsiflexion/volarflexion, which showed similar values (mean 113.70 ± 18.26° versus 110.08 ± 12.16°; right versus left, $p = 0.526$). All workspaces and RoM data during the ARAT and ADL tasks are shown in Table 2.

Table 2. Range of motion angle between right and left upper extremities during ARAT and ADL tasks.

	Axis	Right	Left	p [a]
ARAT	x-axis (left-right, hand sensor)	0.53 ± 0.11 m	0.62 ± 0.07 m	0.082
	y-axis (front-back, hand sensor)	0.92 ± 0.08 m	0.80 ± 0.11 m	0.049 *
	z-axis (hand sensor)	0.89 ± 0.10 m	0.86 ± 0.08 m	0.224
	Shoulder abduction/adduction	50.16 ± 11.14°	55.34 ± 13.48°	0.249
	Shoulder flexion/extension	79.52 ± 19.34°	75.71 ± 21.56°	0.478
	Elbow flexion/extension	109.15 ± 18.82°	106.89 ± 12.83°	0.705
	Forearm supination/pronation	105.23 ± 15.38°	108.64 ± 12.64°	0.426
	Shoulder IR/ER	91.99 ± 20.98°	84.44 ± 44.75°	0.584
	Wrist dorsiflexion/volarflexion	82.90 ± 22.52°	81.26 ± 11.16°	0.833
ADL tasks	x-axis (left-right, hand sensor)	0.71 ± 0.22 m	0.52 ± 0.13 m	0.001 *
	y-axis (front-back, hand sensor)	0.70 ± 0.17 m	0.53 ± 0.15 m	0.011 *
	z-axis (hand sensor)	0.86 ± 0.11 m	0.65 ± 0.13 m	0.001 *
	Shoulder abduction/adduction	58.84 ± 14.53°	35.43 ± 10.09°	<0.001 *
	Shoulder flexion/extension	68.41 ± 17.56°	40.49 ± 18.54°	0.002 *
	Elbow flexion/extension	120.61 ± 23.64°	102.53 ± 19.51°	0.044 *
	Forearm supination/pronation	128.09 ± 22.04°	108.00 ± 16.23°	0.027 *
	Shoulder IR/ER	111.56 ± 31.88°	77.04 ± 21.28°	0.030 *
	Wrist dorsiflexion/volarflexion	113.70 ± 18.26°	110.08 ± 12.16°	0.526

[a] p value for paired t test between right and left side; * p value less than 0.05 considered statistically significant.

3.3. Characteristics of Grasping/Pinching and Reaching

The upper extremity postures during grasping/pinching and reaching were analyzed as a subset analysis of the motion data extracted from grasping/pinching and reaching tasks in ARAT domains 1 and 3. Comparing grasping and pinching postures, the shoulder was more significantly abducted during pinching (19.39 ± 7.84°) compared to grasping (15.33 ± 6.91°, $p = 0.040$) and more extended during pinching (29.12 ± 12.33°) than grasping (22.99 ± 10.63°, $p = 0.038$). Elbow flexion/extension, forearm supination/pronation, and shoulder internal/external rotation did not significantly differ between the two postures. While reaching after grasping, the elbow was extended for an average of 87.87 ± 25.18° from the initial flexed posture, and pronated for an average of 36.65 ± 6.98° from the initial posture. The degrees of elbow extension and forearm pronation while reaching after pinching were similar ($p = 0.849$ and 0.294, respectively). The full results are shown in Table 3.

Table 3. Major joint angle position and change during grasping/pinching and reaching.

Axis	Grasping Initial Position	ROM during Reaching	*p*	Pinching Initial Position	ROM during Reaching	*p*	Grasp-Pinch *p* [a]	Reaching Difference *p* [b]
Shoulder abduction/adduction	15.33 ± 6.91° (abduction)	22.48 ± 19.81° (toward abduction)	0.006 *	19.39 ± 7.84° (abduction)	23.67 ± 13.35° (toward abduction)	<0.001 *	0.040 *	0.015 *
Shouler flexion/extension	22.99 ± 10.63° (extension)	47.80 ± 17.70° (toward flexion)	<0.001 *	29.12 ± 12.33° (extension)	41.83 ± 13.69° (toward flexion)	<0.001 *	0.038 *	0.948
Elbow flexion/extension	87.87 ± 25.18° (near fully flexed)	69.96 ± 16.89° (toward extension)	<0.001 *	84.82 ± 20.25° (near fully flexed)	67.91 ± 14.16° (toward extension)	<0.001 *	0.543	0.849
Forearm supination/pronation [c]	34.37 ± 11.07° (supinated)	36.65 ± 6.98° (toward pronation)	<0.001 *	30.98 ± 13.71° (supinated)	36.02 ± 12.44° (toward pronation)	<0.001 *	0.181	0.294
Shoulder IR/ER	0.68 ± 23.56° (inward direction)	16.55 ± 23.02° (toward external rotation)	0.049 *	2.01 ± 13.74° (inward direction)	18.10 ± 13.02° (toward external rotation)	0.002 *	0.794	0.860
Wrist deviation	8.94 ± 12.12° (to thumb side)	−1.76 ± 10.21° (to finger side)	0.599	1.05 ± 8.19° (to thumb side)	4.81 ± 8.85° (to thumb side)	0.120	0.004 *	0.522
Wrist rotation	4.59 ± 7.35° (toward palm down)	7.12 ± 4.59° (toward palm up)	0.001 *	0.80 ± 5.25° (toward palm down)	4.75 ± 4.05° (toward palm up)	0.005 *	0.023 *	0.385
Wrist dorsiflexion/volarflexion	18.79 ± 16.35° (dorsiflexed)	6.79 ± 6.00° (toward volarflexion)	0.006 *	11.30 ± 13.90° (dorsiflexed)	7.28 ± 11.22° (toward volarflexion)	0.070	0.166	0.123

[a] Comparison between grasping and pinching posture by paired *t* test; [b] Comparison between RoM change during reaching after grasping and pinching by paired *t* test; [c] Full pronation: 0°, full supination: 180°; * *p* value less than 0.05 considered statistically significant.

4. Discussion

The purpose of this study was to provide clinically relevant information regarding the workspace and major joint angle range while performing essential ADLs or important movements. By identifying these factors, it is possible to limit the extent of exoskeleton movements and, therefore, modify the design of the robot such that it can move within the designated workspace with a relatively simpler structure. In this study, we evaluated the RoM and workspace while conducting ARAT tasks, which is a common functional evaluation tool used in the clinics, because it is well known to significantly correlate with the patients' functional status or recovery state [16–18]. ARAT consists of four domains: domain 1 and 3 tasks consist of the grasping and pinching of various sized objects and reaching afterwards. Domain 2 mainly involves moving items on a table focusing on the grip function, and domain four items are gross movement tasks that require lifting the arm to the head or face [19].

Validation of the IMU-based motion analysis system used in this study showed that the accuracy and reliability of the sensors themselves are very high regarding angles. However, in the form of wearable multi-sensor system, it is impossible to isolate a single joint movement, because all joints systemically move in three dimensions, including body trunk and contralateral upper extremity. Intra-subject covariance and inter-subject covariance were calculated for the forearm supination/pronation and elbow flexion/extension angles to evaluate the system reliability, and the range was deemed acceptable when considering that the reaching tasks were not completely identical. For the position data from the accelerometers, we compared the calculated data in the y and z directions using the estimated real movement distance. The calculated distance data were similar to the measured data, and the variability was considered acceptable. In addition, the calculated workspace and RoM during ARAT tasks were similar between the two extremities with no significant difference (Table 2). This may also support the reliability of the system-derived parameter values. Although it is difficult to state that the system provides a completely accurate measurement, it seems to provide consistent and meaningful data.

The workspaces of the right and left hands were mostly similar, because ARAT repeats the same tasks with both hands alternatively. The slight difference between both sides is likely due to the difference in posture and orientation based on the limb dominance. During the ADL tasks, the workspace of the dominant hand, right hand for all subjects, was significantly larger than that of the non-dominant side by up to nearly 20 cm for all directions. In the view of stroke rehabilitation, most of the patients demonstrated hemiplegia of up to 80% or more [20], which means that their intact limb should be able to perform all normal functions. Patients with hemiplegia will use their intact hand as their dominant hand and, therefore, in certain occasions, the exoskeleton may only need to cover a smaller workspace than the dominant side.

The RoMs of the major upper extremity joints during essential daily activities are presented in Table 2. The forearm supination/pronation and elbow flexion/extension showed the highest values for the dominant side. The RoM for the forearm supination/pronation was 128.09° and 108.00° on average for the right and left sides, respectively, during all ADL tasks. In a study using a reflective marker-based motion capture system, the whole RoM calculated by overlapping all 95% confidential interval range during various ADL tasks was approximately 92° [9]. Another study applied using an electromagnetic sensor system reported that the maximal supination angle from full pronation was 110° while glass drinking and 75° while combing their hair [8]. In a study by van Andel et al. [21], four selected ADL tasks were evaluated using an optic marker-based system, and their reported RoM for forearm supination/pronation was approximately 130°. Regarding elbow flexion/extension RoM, other studies also showed similar results. Aizawa et al. [8] reported a RoM of approximately 120° to 130° during various tasks, and Gates et al. [9] showed that the peak flexion angle of the elbow joint was 121° on average when drinking from a cup, which was the highest value among the evaluated tasks. Another study reported a RoM of around 140° from full extension [21]. Wrist dorsiflexion/volarflexion RoM was also similar with other studies, which ranged from 90° to 130°, whereas it was 113.70° and 110.08° for right and left side, respectively, in our study. It is important to ensure a sufficient

RoM for elbow flexion/extension, forearm supination/pronation, and wrist dorsiflexion/volarflexion movements during rehabilitation, because such joint movements are essential for conducting ADL tasks, while recovery for distal joints are relatively slow and insufficient for a large portion of stroke patients [22–24].

The angular changes in the major joints when reaching after a grasping/pinching motion are evaluated because such actions are the fundamental movements for conducting any kind of tasks [25,26], and most of the activities are performed within the spatial range of these actions. Pinching was performed at a slightly but significantly more abducted and flexed posture of the shoulder joint, and showed a significant difference in fine tuning movements of the wrist joint.

In contrast to a simple pure reaching movement, a reaching movement associated with a task may differ significantly regarding the arm postures, grasping position, and orientation [27,28]. The human motor system has high redundancy in terms of a multi-degree-of-freedom control system, and while task-relevant factors are specifically controlled, task-irrelevant variables are given relatively high variability [27]. In this study, the shoulder joint angles showed significantly different postures between grasping and pinching, which reflects different positions of the elbow joint while conducting a task. The wrist deviation and rotation angles also showed a significant difference, reflecting the difference in the fine motor posture and movements. Given the difference in posture, the main components of the reaching movement, elbow flexion/extension and forearm supination/pronation, did not differ significantly between the two types of tasks. This result may be applied to the swivel angle model suggested by Li et al. [27], where the shoulder joint angles can be simplified to a swivel angle regarding the orientation and posture, and the other distal joint angles account for essential reaching movements. In regular stroke rehabilitation, proximal muscle power recovery occurs in the early stage and more sufficiently compared to distal muscles [22–24] and, thus, it will be reasonable to motivate the patient to practice taking an appropriate posture for providing the right orientation of the upper extremity using the proximal muscles voluntarily, with the help of a gravity support system if applicable, whereas the individual robot joint actuation should focus on the essential distal joint movements such as elbow, forearm, and wrist movements.

Based on the current study dataset and the analysis, the workspace of the end-effector and its corresponding elbow or forearm position workspace, along with the essential elbow flexion/extension and forearm supination/pronation, may provide minimal structural requirements for the rehabilitation robot to maintain basic grasping, pinching, and reaching movements which are necessary to perform daily activities. This may be applied in both neurorehabilitation exoskeletons and assistive exoskeletons. These results may have helpful applications in virtual reality rehabilitation systems, especially in developing games or tasks which are clinically relevant.

This study has several limitations. To generalize the findings of the motion analysis, the number of subjects was relatively small. However, the statistical analyses provided minimal requirements regarding the validity and reliability and the data pattern for each subject was nearly identical especially during the structured movements (ARAT). Still, further studies with advanced protocol are necessary to verify and generalize the study results. In addition, gender and age factors could not be investigated sufficiently due to small number of subjects. Nevertheless, we have performed non-parametric tests to compare the major sensor-based parameters between men and women, and because the age range for this study was relatively in the young age, they were compared with additional dataset of the intact limb of the older people with hemiplegia. Most of the parameters did not show statistically significant difference according to the gender or age, except that older people tend to perform tasks within a smaller workspace during free ADL tasks and that women tend to abduct the shoulder more than men during pinching. IMU-based sensors basically have their own inevitable limitations, which include drift phenomenon in both the position and angular values, which may affect the values of the outcome measures [29]. In addition, a gimbal-lock phenomenon regarding the shoulder joint angles in particular may have occurred during the data measurements [8]. In this regard, the data may not be accurate in terms of the absolute values; however, because the data are sufficiently consistent, it seems that the general pattern of the data is reliable.

5. Conclusions

These study results provide the essential workspace and RoM of the major upper extremity joints during ARAT and ADL tasks in healthy subjects, which will serve as a basis in designing a practical and simple upper extremity exoskeleton robot. Further motion analyses on stroke patients are necessary to characterize upper extremity movements in neurological disorders and determine the key features in the stroke recovery process, which will be important in extracting the clinically relevant movement characteristics for designing new exoskeletons for neurorehabilitation purposes.

Author Contributions: Conceptualization: H.S.N., H.G.S., M.S.B. and S.K.; data curation: H.S.N. and W.H.L.; formal analysis: H.S.N.; funding acquisition: M.S.B. and S.K.; investigation: H.S.N., M.S.B. and S.K.; methodology: H.G.S.; software: Y.J.K.; supervision: S.K.; validation: W.H.L. and Y.J.K.; writing—original draft, H.S.N.; writing—review and editing: H.S.N., W.H.L., H.G.S., Y.J.K., M.S.B. and S.K.

Acknowledgments: This study was approved by the Institutional Review Board of Seoul National University Hospital (IRB No. 1505-017-668).

Declaration: This manuscript is a revision of part of the first author's (Nam HS) Ph. D. thesis from Seoul National University.

References

1. Bertani, R.; Melegari, C.; De Cola, M.C.; Bramanti, A.; Bramanti, P.; Calabro, R.S. Effects of robot-assisted upper limb rehabilitation in stroke patients: A systematic review with meta-analysis. *Neurol. Sci.* **2017**, *38*, 1561–1569. [CrossRef]
2. Mehrholz, J.; Pohl, M.; Platz, T.; Kugler, J.; Elsner, B. Electromechanical and robot-assisted arm training for improving activities of daily living, arm function, and arm muscle strength after stroke. *Cochrane Database Syst. Rev.* **2015**. [CrossRef] [PubMed]
3. Ren, Y.; Kang, S.H.; Park, H.S.; Wu, Y.N.; Zhang, L.Q. Developing a multi-joint upper limb exoskeleton robot for diagnosis, therapy, and outcome evaluation in neurorehabilitation. *IEEE Trans. Neural Syst. Rehabil. Eng.* **2013**, *21*, 490–499. [CrossRef] [PubMed]
4. Klamroth-Marganska, V.; Blanco, J.; Campen, K.; Curt, A.; Dietz, V.; Ettlin, T.; Felder, M.; Fellinghauer, B.; Guidali, M.; Kollmar, A.; et al. Three-dimensional, task-specific robot therapy of the arm after stroke: A multicentre, parallel-group randomised trial. *Lancet Neurol.* **2014**, *13*, 159–166. [CrossRef]
5. Fasoli, S.E.; Krebs, H.I.; Stein, J.; Frontera, W.R.; Hogan, N. Effects of robotic therapy on motor impairment and recovery in chronic stroke. *Arch. Phys. Med. Rehabil.* **2003**, *84*, 477–482. [CrossRef] [PubMed]
6. Lo, H.S.; Xie, S.Q. Exoskeleton robots for upper-limb rehabilitation: State of the art and future prospects. *Med. Eng. Phys.* **2012**, *34*, 261–268. [CrossRef] [PubMed]
7. Valero-Cuevas, F.J.; Santello, M. On neuromechanical approaches for the study of biological and robotic grasp and manipulation. *J. Neuroeng Rehabil.* **2017**, *14*, 101. [CrossRef]
8. Aizawa, J.; Masuda, T.; Koyama, T.; Nakamaru, K.; Isozaki, K.; Okawa, A.; Morita, S. Three-dimensional motion of the upper extremity joints during various activities of daily living. *J. Biomech.* **2010**, *43*, 2915–2922. [CrossRef]
9. Gates, D.H.; Walters, L.S.; Cowley, J.; Wilken, J.M.; Resnik, L. Range of Motion Requirements for Upper-Limb Activities of Daily Living. *Am. J. Occup. Ther.* **2016**, *70*, 7001350010p1–7001350010p10. [CrossRef]
10. Kim, K.; Song, W.K.; Lee, J.; Lee, H.Y.; Park, D.S.; Ko, B.W.; Kim, J. Kinematic analysis of upper extremity movement during drinking in hemiplegic subjects. *Clin. Biomech. (Bristol, Avon)* **2014**, *29*, 248–256. [CrossRef] [PubMed]
11. Chen, J.; Lum, P.S. Pilot testing of the spring operated wearable enhancer for arm rehabilitation (SpringWear). *J. Neuroeng Rehabil.* **2018**, *15*, 13. [CrossRef] [PubMed]

12. Perez, R.; Costa, U.; Torrent, M.; Solana, J.; Opisso, E.; Caceres, C.; Tormos, J.M.; Medina, J.; Gomez, E.J. Upper limb portable motion analysis system based on inertial technology for neurorehabilitation purposes. *Sensors* **2010**, *10*, 10733–10751. [CrossRef] [PubMed]
13. Wang, Q.; Markopoulos, P.; Yu, B.; Chen, W.; Timmermans, A. Interactive wearable systems for upper body rehabilitation: A systematic review. *J. Neuroeng Rehabil.* **2017**, *14*, 20. [CrossRef] [PubMed]
14. Lyle, R.C. A performance test for assessment of upper limb function in physical rehabilitation treatment and research. *Int. J. Rehabil. Res.* **1981**, *4*, 483–492. [CrossRef] [PubMed]
15. Nam, H.S.; Seo, H.G.; Leigh, J.H.; Kim, Y.J.; Kim, S.; Bang, M.S. External Robotic Arm vs Upper Limb Exoskeleton: What Do the Potential Users Need? Unpublished.
16. Hsieh, C.L.; Hsueh, I.P.; Chiang, F.M.; Lin, P.H. Inter-rater reliability and validity of the action research arm test in stroke patients. *Age Ageing* **1998**, *27*, 107–113. [CrossRef] [PubMed]
17. Koh, C.L.; Hsueh, I.P.; Wang, W.C.; Sheu, C.F.; Yu, T.Y.; Wang, C.H.; Hsieh, C.L. Validation of the action research arm test using item response theory in patients after stroke. *J. Rehabil. Med.* **2006**, *38*, 375–380. [CrossRef]
18. Chen, H.F.; Lin, K.C.; Wu, C.Y.; Chen, C.L. Rasch validation and predictive validity of the action research arm test in patients receiving stroke rehabilitation. *Arch. Phys. Med. Rehabil.* **2012**, *93*, 1039–1045. [CrossRef]
19. Yozbatiran, N.; Der-Yeghiaian, L.; Cramer, S.C. A standardized approach to performing the action research arm test. *Neurorehabil. Neural Repair* **2008**, *22*, 78–90. [CrossRef]
20. Parker, V.M.; Wade, D.T.; Langton Hewer, R. Loss of arm function after stroke: Measurement, frequency, and recovery. *Int. Rehabil. Med.* **1986**, *8*, 69–73. [CrossRef]
21. Van Andel, C.J.; Wolterbeek, N.; Doorenbosch, C.A.; Veeger, D.H.; Harlaar, J. Complete 3D kinematics of upper extremity functional tasks. *Gait Posture* **2008**, *27*, 120–127. [CrossRef]
22. Krakauer, J.W. Arm function after stroke: From physiology to recovery. *Semin. Neurol.* **2005**, *25*, 384–395. [CrossRef] [PubMed]
23. Shelton, F.N.; Reding, M.J. Effect of lesion location on upper limb motor recovery after stroke. *Stroke* **2001**, *32*, 107–112. [CrossRef] [PubMed]
24. Brunnstrom, S. Motor testing procedures in hemiplegia: Based on sequential recovery stages. *Phys. Ther.* **1966**, *46*, 357–375. [CrossRef] [PubMed]
25. Shumway-Cook, A.; Woollacott, M.H. *Motor Control: Translating Research into Clinical Practice*, 5th ed.; Wolters Kluwer: Philadelphia, PA, USA, 2017; pp. 465–489.
26. Guccione, A.A.; Wong, R.; Avers, D. *Geriatric Physical Therapy*, 3rd ed.; Elsevier: Louis, MO, USA, 2012.
27. Li, Z.; Milutinovic, D.; Rosen, J. From reaching to reach-to-grasp: The arm posture difference and its implications on human motion control strategy. *Exp. Brain Res.* **2017**, *235*, 1627–1642. [CrossRef] [PubMed]
28. Scharoun, S.M.; Scanlan, K.A.; Bryden, P.J. Hand and Grasp Selection in a Preferential Reaching Task: The Effects of Object Location, Orientation, and Task Intention. *Front. Psychol.* **2016**, *7*, 360. [CrossRef] [PubMed]
29. Luinge, H.J.; Veltink, P.H. Measuring orientation of human body segments using miniature gyroscopes and accelerometers. *Med. Biol. Eng. Comput.* **2005**, *43*, 273–282. [CrossRef]

7

Complexity of Daily Physical Activity is More Sensitive than Conventional Metrics to Assess Functional Change in Younger Older Adults

Wei Zhang [1,*], Michael Schwenk [2,3], Sabato Mellone [4], Anisoara Paraschiv-Ionescu [1], Beatrix Vereijken [5], Mirjam Pijnappels [6], A. Stefanie Mikolaizak [2], Elisabeth Boulton [7], Nini H. Jonkman [6], Andrea B. Maier [6,8], Jochen Klenk [2,9], Jorunn Helbostad [5], Kristin Taraldsen [5] and Kamiar Aminian [1]

1 Laboratory of Movement Analysis and Measurement, Ecole Polytechnique Federale de Lausanne, 1015 Lausanne, Switzerland; anisoara.ionescu@epfl.ch (A.P.-I.); kamiar.aminian@epfl.ch (K.A.)
2 Robert Bosch Foundation for Medical Research, 70376 Stuttgart, Germany; michael.schwenk@rbk.de (M.S.); stefanie.mikolaizak@rbk.de (A.S.M.); jochen.klenk@rbk.de (J.K.)
3 Network Aging Research, Heidelberg University, 69115 Heidelberg, Germany
4 Department of Electrical, Electronic and Information Engineering, University of Bologna, 40136 Bologna, Italy; sabato.mellone@unibo.it
5 Department of Neuromedicine and Movement Science, Norwegian University of Science and Technology, 7491 Trondheim, Norway; beatrix.vereijken@ntnu.no (B.V.); jorunn.helbostad@ntnu.no (J.H.); kristin.taraldsen@ntnu.no (K.T.)
6 Department of Human Movement Sciences, Vrije Universiteit Amsterdam, Amsterdam Movement Sciences, 1081BT Amsterdam, The Netherlands; m.pijnappels@vu.nl (M.P.); n.h.jonkman@vu.nl (N.H.J.); andrea.maier@mh.org.au (A.B.M.)
7 School of Health Sciences, Faculty of Medicine, Biology and Health, University of Manchester, and Manchester Academic Health Science Centre, Manchester M13 9PL, UK; elisabeth.boulton@manchester.ac.uk
8 Department of Medicine and Aged Care, @AgeMelbourne, Royal Melbourne Hospital, University of Melbourne, Melbourne 3050, Australia
9 Institute of Epidemiology and Medical Biometry, Ulm University, 89081 Ulm, Germany
* Correspondence: w zhang@epfl ch

Abstract: The emerging mHealth applications, incorporating wearable sensors, enables continuous monitoring of physical activity (PA). This study aimed at analyzing the relevance of a multivariate complexity metric in assessment of functional change in younger older adults. Thirty individuals (60–70 years old) participated in a 4-week home-based exercise intervention. The Community Balance and Mobility Scale (CBMS) was used for clinical assessment of the participants' functional balance and mobility performance pre- and post- intervention. Accelerometers worn on the low back were used to register PA of one week before and in the third week of the intervention. Changes in conventional univariate PA metrics (percentage of walking and sedentary time, step counts, mean cadence) and complexity were compared to the change as measured by the CBMS. Statistical analyses (21 participants) showed significant rank correlation between the change as measured by complexity and CBMS ($\rho = 0.47$, $p = 0.03$). Smoothing the activity output improved the correlation ($\rho = 0.58$, $p = 0.01$). In contrast, change in univariate PA metrics did not show correlations. These findings demonstrate the high potential of the complexity metric being useful and more sensitive than conventional PA metrics for assessing functional changes in younger older adults.

Keywords: wearable sensors; multivariate analysis; longitudinal study; functional decline; exercise intervention

1. Introduction

The aging process is often accompanied by functional decline and increased risk of chronic diseases [1]. However, functional ability varies between older adults, depending on individual health condition and lifestyles. Physical inactivity is one of the known risk factors that can lead to morbidity and mortality [2]. The transition from work to retirement, which often occurs between 60 and 70 years of age, can involve a significant change in structured daily activities, with physical activity declining. A study on the Dutch population found that retirement introduces a reduction in physical activity from work-related transportation that is not compensated for by an increase in sports participation or an increase in non-sports leisure-time physical activity [3]. Thus, this population is of particular importance for addressing maintenance of their functional status.

In recent years, mobile health (mHealth) applications, incorporating wearable sensing technologies with modern mobile communication devices, are emerging. From the early adoption in younger populations for fitness tracking in particular, mHealth has been continuously developing and diversifying its applications for different populations [1,4]. The scalability of mHealth technologies enables data collection in diverse geographic locations over prolonged time periods [5]. This provides a new perspective in studying physical activities in real life and allows new analytical tools to be developed to analyze and present the data.

An earlier systematic review on body-worn, accelerometer-based physical activity monitoring revealed the challenge of achieving consensus on the reporting and the interpretation of the measurements provided by various mHealth applications [6]. Furthermore, the review pointed out that energy expenditure, walking time, and total activity are most frequently reported and are comparable variables across studies. In addition, several variables, such as walking time, number of steps, and cadence are the most widely adopted variables in research [5,7,8] to characterize walking pattern, the most common daily physical activity across all age groups. Descriptive statistics (e.g., mean, maximum values) are applied to the above walking parameters for analysis. Detrended fluctuation analysis proposed by Hausdorff et al. is used to quantify the stride-to-stride variability in supervised walking tasks [9]. However, physical activity involves multiple components and has more than one dimension. Different types of activities in daily life, as well as the quantity and the quality (performance) of each activity jointly determine a person's functional status. Thus, a variable that models a person's physical activity behaviour based on these aspects is warranted.

Complexity analysis as introduced by Paraschiv-Ionescu et al. [10] aims at combining both the quantity and quality dimensions of multiple, commonly performed daily activities into one metric to describe physical activity behaviour. This complexity metric has demonstrated discriminative power to distinguish groups of patients suffering from chronic pain [11,12]. Besides analyzing accelerometry-derived activities, the metric has been validated also for analyzing activity behaviour of older adults using an application based on wearable pressure insoles [13].

While several cross-sectional studies exist for clinical validation of complexity metrics, the sensitivity of those metrics for detecting changes in physical function over time has not yet been determined. Therefore, we aimed to examine the ability of the aforementioned complexity metric to detect change in a longitudinal intervention study conducted in younger older adults in comparison to conventionally applied univariate physical activity metrics. Within this context, we further explored the impact of smoothing sensor-based physical activity data on the complexity metric.

2. Materials and Methods

2.1. Study Protocol

The study is part of the larger PreventIT project [1], developing and testing an ICT-based mHealth system that enables early identification of risk for age-related functional decline, and engenders behavioural change in younger older adults (aged 60–70 years) in order to adopt a healthy, active lifestyle.

Thirty participants, aged between 60 and 70 years, were recruited at three different sites, Trondheim (Norway), Amsterdam (the Netherlands), and Stuttgart (Germany), to participate in a 4-week pre-post pilot intervention study. All participants were instructed by an experienced physical therapist or exercise therapist to follow an adapted Lifestyle-integrated Functional Exercise (aLiFE) programme specifically developed for improving balance and strength and increasing physical activity in younger older adults [14]. aLiFE was taught during four weekly home visits, and the participants were asked to integrate the aLiFE activities into everyday routines. Pre and post intervention, the participants completed a balance and mobility assessment using the Community Balance and Mobility Scale (CBMS). The scale has been validated to capture high-level balance, gait, and mobility performances in healthy active younger older adults based on the quality of performing the tasks [15]. CBMS assessments were performed in the research hospital or university by trained assessors. In addition, daily physical activity (PA) of each participant was measured twice for one week with wearable sensors. The participants were instructed to wear an inertial sensor (DynaPort, MoveMonitor, McRoberts, The Hague, The Netherlands) at their lower back at the level of L5 using an elastic belt during the day and night. The sensor needed to be removed when showering or during any water activity and needed to be put back on afterwards. The sensor did not need to be recharged during the one week measurement. All sensors were collected at the end of the measurement and raw sensor data was downloaded for offline data analysis. The first measurement was prior to the start of the intervention period. The measurement was repeated during the third week of the pilot study to capture the change of daily activity patterns during the intervention.

2.2. Sensor Data Processing

The sensor consists of a 3D accelerometer with sampling frequency of 100 Hz. The recording start time of each sensor was registered on the device by manual insertion of a timestamp. A non-commercial activity classification software was used to extract quantitative as well as qualitative features of PA from raw sensor data. The software is an outcome of the FARSEEING EU project (FP7/2007–2013, grant agreement 288940). It has been applied in studies with dementia patients [16] and older people residing in independent-living retirement homes [17]. The software has been further developed based on two datasets of elderly subjects. The first one is the ADAPT dataset [18], where video recording was performed using ceiling-mounted cameras in lab settings and an action camera in free-living conditions. The second dataset is from the University of Auckland [17], where subjects performed both scripted and unscripted activities of daily living collected in a free-living environment. First, the algorithm estimates Metabolic Equivalents (METs); signals are filtered and processed as described in [19]. An interval is labelled as 'sedentary', if associated energy expenditure is below or equal to 1.5 MET [20]. Otherwise, the interval is labelled as 'active'. 'Sedentary' intervals with a mean angle between the vertical axis and the medio-lateral or the anterior–posterior direction of the trunk below 30° are labelled as 'lying'. The 'active' intervals, where steps are detected are labelled as 'walking'. Step detection is based on [21]. Each interval is then characterized by the category (label), the duration, and the activity counts (counts/minute) from which METs are estimated [19]. In addition, number of steps and the cadence (steps/minute) are extracted for each 'walking' bout. Data is labelled as 'non-wearing', if the sensor is detected lying flat with very low variance in acceleration signals for longer than half an hour.

The classified activities were sorted into natural days based on the registered timestamp. Days with less than 16 h of measurements (i.e., the first and the last day of the measurement) were excluded from further processing and analysis. Given the high resolution (1 s) of the PA output data, bouts of one activity may be interspersed with short episodes of other activities. For example, short breaks of a few seconds are often present during one walking bout due to environmental factors (e.g., walking episodes whiles shopping in a supermarket), which may lead to a string of several walking episodes rather than one continuous walking bout. Such short breaks during an activity introduce artificial changes in the dynamics of the PA time series, which are not relevant to one's physical behaviour. Therefore, a smoothing technique was devised to filter such artefacts and to aggregate bouts in the original PA output belonging to the same PA category based on the following steps, as illustrated in Figure 1. First, we applied a moving forward sliding window of 30 s without overlap to smooth the PA time series [22]. The activity category of these 30 s was replaced by the activity with the highest density (counts) within the window. Second, the process was repeated for K folds. At each fold, the smoothing starts with a random shift between 1 and 30 s at the beginning of the time series. Third, the activity category of each second in the aggregated time series was determined by the majority vote of the K-fold smoothing. The sliding window length was chosen according to the 'barcode' design (explained in the later section Complexity analysis), where 30-s is the threshold of activity duration corresponding to indoor walking.

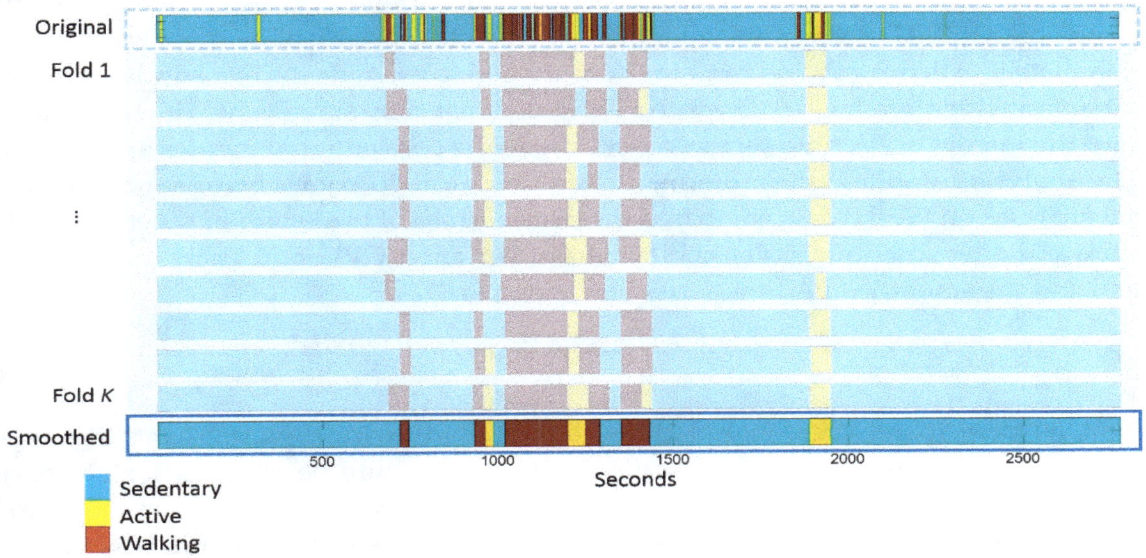

Figure 1. Smoothing activity classification output to aggregate activity bouts in a measurement time series of 45 min. The top bar shows the original PA sequence and the bottom bar shows the smoothed sequence.

2.3. *Univariate Analysis*

For each activity bout, its duration and activity counts per minute ('ActiCount') were estimated. In addition, the total number of steps and the average cadence (steps/min) were provided for each classified walking bout. PA was characterized by various univariate metrics including the percentage of time being sedentary, the percentage of time spent walking, the number of steps normalized to the measurement duration (in hours), and the mean cadence of walking bouts of each day. The univariate metrics were computed based on the original and the smoothed PA time series.

2.4. *Complexity Analysis*

Complexity was introduced in order to analyze the variability of biological and physiological time series data [23,24]. The technique was subsequently adapted and applied to analyze ambulatory activity patterns [25]. Paraschiv-Ionescu et al. proposed complexity analysis on a multivariate PA pattern ('barcode') derived from wearable sensor data [10]. The 'barcode' is constructed for the analyzed period based on the classified activity category, the duration and the intensity. The entropy rate of the resulting multi-state 'barcode' represents complexity. In the analysis of the pilot data, an adapted 'barcode' was used, where the 'ActiCount' was modeled according to a validation study presented in [19]. Entropy rate of the 'barcode' was computed in terms of Lempel-Ziv complexity based on the method described in [26]. (Additional materials are presented in Appendix A.1). Complexity of the 'barcode' generated from both the original and the smoothed time series of PA were computed to analyze the influence of activity classification on the calculated complexity.

2.5. Statistical Analysis

For each participant, the univariate metrics and the complexity metric of PA were analyzed for each day. The average value of each metric over the one-week measurement before (Week0) and during (Week3) the pilot study was calculated. According to study [27], participants having more than two days' sensor data during the one-week measurement, in both Week0 and Week3, were included for statistical analysis. The changes in PA metrics between Week0 and Week3 were computed. The change in CBMS score pre and post the pilot study was calculated. The primary analysis was to examine the correlations between the change in PA metrics and the change in CBMS score. Given the small sample size and ordinal data type (CBMS scores), spearman coefficient (ρ) was used to analyse the strength of correlation. In addition, a non-parametric effect size calculator, Cliff's Delta, was applied to measure the degree of overlap between the distribution of various variables extracted pre- and during/post interventions [28]. Cliff's Delta approaching 1 or −1 indicates absence of overlap, whereas 0 indicates overlap completely. Wilcoxon signed rank test was applied to examine the statistical significance of the change. Changes with a p value < 0.05 was considered statistically significant. The secondary analysis consisted of the impact of PA time series smoothing on the conventional metrics and the complexity metric. The analysis compared the aforementioned statistical outcomes before and after smoothing. Additional analyses on Week0 data compared the distributions of the length of sedentary and walking bouts before and after smoothing. The coefficients of variance (CV) of the daily complexity value of the original and the smoothed PA time series were compared.

3. Results

In total, 30 participants were included in the pilot study with 10 participants at each trial site. Due to technical problems with the sensor devices (no data could be retrieved), eight participants were excluded from further data processing and analysis (n = 5 in Week0 and n = 3 in Week3). One participant's CBMS score was not available at the baseline assessment and was excluded from further data analysis leaving 21 participants for statistical analyses. All participants in statistical analysis had minimum 3 days of data in Week0 and Week3. Table 1 summarizes the descriptive statistics of PA metrics and CBMS score for the included participants (n = 21, except the CV of complexity, where n = 25 from Week0 were analyzed) in the pilot study. The included participants were not significantly different from the excluded participants in CMBS scores at the pre- (Willcoxon ranksum test, p = 0.14) or the post- (p = 0.23) intervention assessment. To illustrate, Figure 2 shows one participant's barcode (based on smoothed PA time series) in Week0 (left) and Week3 (right). The barcode in Week3 shows richer colours filled in throughout several days of measurements, which was reflected by the higher mean complexity score of 0.120 compared to 0.111 in Week0.

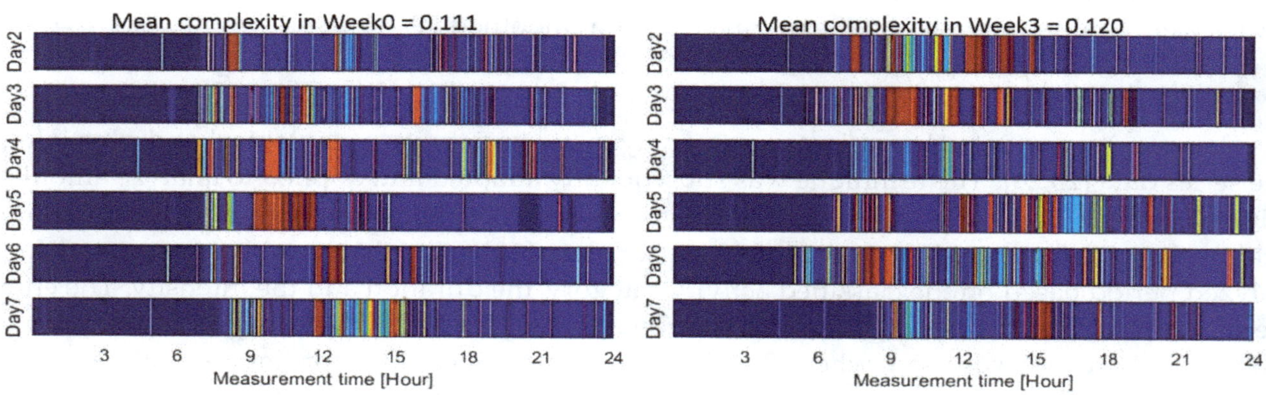

Figure 2. Barcode and mean complexity of one-week PA time series of Week0 (**left**) and Week3 (**right**) in one participant.

Table 1. Descriptive statistics of PA metrics, complexity, and CBMS scores in pre- and post- intervention assessments. PA metrics and complexity based on original and smoothed PA time series are compared with CMBS scores.

	Week0 or Pre Pilot (Mean ± SD) Original/Smoothed	Week3 or Post Pilot (Mean ± SD) Original/Smoothed	Association (ρ) with CBMS Original/Smoothed	Effect Size (Cliff's Delta) Original/Smoothed
Percentage of sedentary time (%)	44.9 ± 6.0/47.7 ± 6.5	44.4 ± 5.6/47.5 ± 6.0	−0.35/−0.28	−0.12/−0.08
Percentage of walking time (%)	9.1 ± 2.0/9.1 ± 2.2	9.9 ± 3.0/10.0 ± 3.3	0.05/−0.01	0.13/0.15 [a]
Normalised nr. of steps (steps/hour)	489 ± 123/361 ± 111	532 ± 182/395 ± 160	0.02/−0.17	0.11/0.08
Mean cadence (steps/minute)	78 ± 5/52 ± 8	78 ± 6/51 ± 7	−0.25/−0.33	0/−0.13
Complexity	0.178 ± 0.024/0.101 ± 0.006	0.185 ± 0.024/0.103 ± 0.007	0.47 [a]/0.58 [a]	0.18/0.15
CV of complexity [b]	0.11 ± 0.05/0.07 ± 0.02			
CBMS score	66.4 ± 12.8	70.2 ± 12.9		0.20 [a]

[a] Statistically significant ($p < 0.05$), [b] based on 25 participants' data at Week0.

For the primary analysis, scatter plots in Figure 3 show the correlations. Spearman correlations between changes in PA metrics (based on original PA time series) and CBMS score (between the change in CBMS score and the changes measured by various conventional univariate metrics and the complexity metric) are based on original PA time series. Changes in univariate metrics had no significant association with the change as measured by the CBMS score. In contrast, complexity had a significant positive correlation (ρ = 0.47, p = 0.03) with the change in CBMS. Complexity was higher after intervention with an effect size of 0.18, which was comparable to the effect size as measured by the CBMS score (0.20). Despite an increase in complexity post intervention, the change was not statistically significant. Changes in univariate metrics had smaller effect size and were not statistically significant (see Table 1).

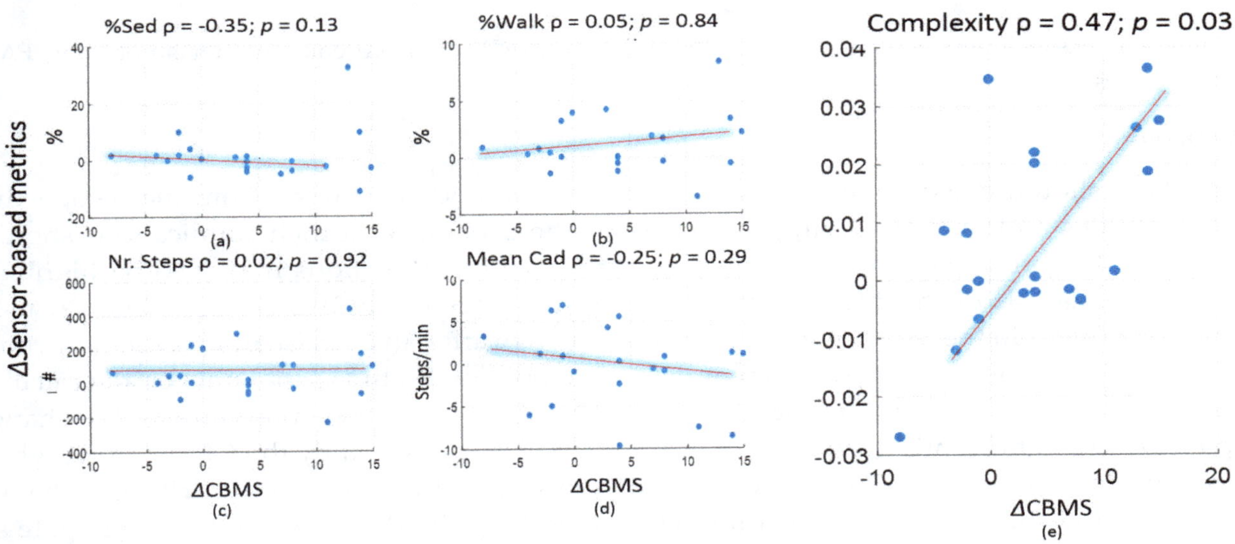

Figure 3. Spearman correlations between changes in PA metrics (based on original PA time series) and CBMS score. (**a**) Change in percentage of sedentary time vs. change in CBMS. (**b**) Change in percentage of walking time vs. change in CBMS. (**c**) Change in normalized number of steps vs. change in CBMS. (**d**) Change in mean cadence vs. change in CBMS. (**e**) Change in complexity vs. change in CBMS.

For the secondary analysis, after smoothing the PA time series, multiple very short sedentary bouts were merged into one longer bout. Similarly, multiple walking bouts with short interruptions were concatenated to form a continuous walking bout (see Appendix A.2). Comparison of mean values of various univariate metrics presented in Table 1 indicated that smoothing had little impact on the percentage of sedentary time and the percentage of walking time, whereas the total number of steps and mean cadence were reduced. The value of complexity for the smoothed PA time series was smaller, compared to the original complexity. The change in complexity for the smoothed PA time series resulted in a stronger association with the change in CBMS score (ρ = 0.58, $p = 0.01$ as shown in Figure 4. Association between complexity change and CBMS score change after smoothing PA time series.). Moreover, the mean CV of complexity of the participants in Week0 decreased from 0.11 to 0.07 after smoothing the PA time series (see Appendix A.2).

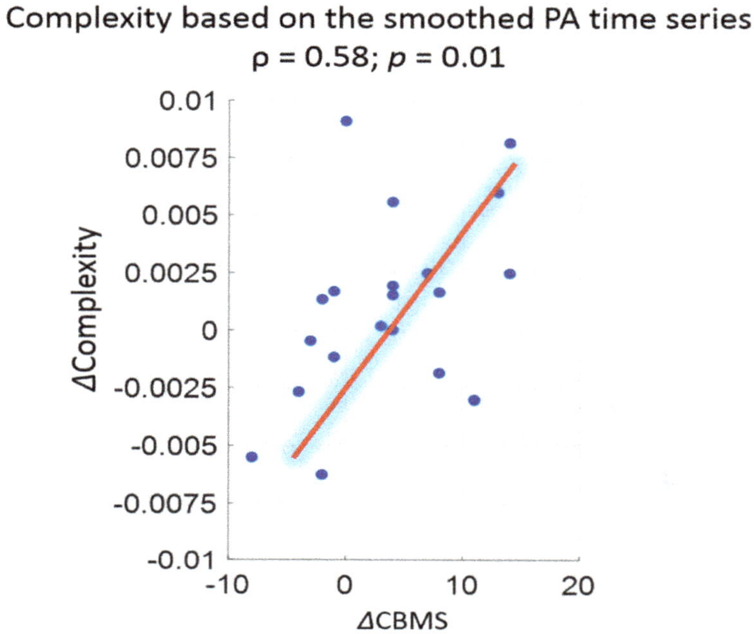

Figure 4. Association between complexity change and CBMS score change after smoothing PA time series.

4. Discussion

Authors should discuss the results and how they can be interpreted from the perspective of previous studies and of the working hypotheses. The findings and their implications should be discussed in the broadest context possible. Future research directions may also be highlighted. The primary analysis of this study focused on the relevance of various conventional PA metrics and the complexity in the assessment of functional change after an exercise intervention in younger older adults. In addition, we analyzed the impact of smoothing PA time series data on the calculation of various PA metrics and the complexity metric. Despite a very short intervention, the change in complexity was significantly correlated with the change as measured by the CBMS score, whereas, the changes in conventional PA metrics did not show significant correlation with the change as measured by the clinical assessment. Moreover, smoothing the PA time series, to aggregate short activity bouts, improved the complexity metric in terms of stronger correlation with functional change as measured by a clinical assessment and higher measurement reproducibility as quantified by the CV of one-week measurements.

These results revealed that complexity is a useful and a more sensitive metric than conventionally applied univariate PA metrics in the assessment of functional change in younger older adults. Conventional PA metrics derived from wearable sensors, step counts, or cadence, might not be sensitive enough to capture the functional change after short interventions. Metrics characterizing one aspect of daily physical activity, such as the time spent walking or being sedentary, do not provide a comprehensive picture of the determinants of functional status. The complexity metric of physical behaviour, on the other hand, characterizes the quantity, the quality, and the dynamic changes between different activities and different performances while doing the same activity (such as a change in cadence) in the 'barcode'. Further, the entropy rate increases while the number of sub-patterns in the 'barcode' increases as illustrated in Figure 2. Since it captures more aspects of physical behaviour simultaneously, the complexity metric has the potential to capture the underlined important aspect in the aging process that the variety and dimension of activities decreases due to functional decline [29,30].

The 'barcode', as defined in Table A1 and illustrated in Figure 2, is constructed with generic activity features derived from the wearable sensors. This makes complexity a generic metric for PA data analysis in principle without constraints in specific sensor configuration or wearing position. The activity features required by the 'barcode', such as walking time and number of steps, are universally recognized by the state-of-the-art wearable sensors [10,12,25]. Selection of activity features to be included in barcode construction is a topic worth separate investigation. For example, efficacy and sensitivity to wearing position of a 'barcode' that states sensor-derived activity levels (sedentary, light, and moderate-to-vigorous) can be analyzed [31].

The complexity metric analyses the entropy rate of the 'barcode'. Changes in 'barcode' states depend on the richness of the activity performed but is also influenced by the resolution of the activity features. The higher the resolution, the more detailed the features in the activity performed can be described; however, the resolution becomes less resistant to noise in the activity data. As demonstrated in Figure 1, the original PA time series (the top bar) has second-by-second feature resolution, which shows frequent fast changes between sedentary and walking activities (for example, see between 1000 and 1250 s). In the original PA time series, almost all sedentary bouts were shorter than five minutes, and less than 5% of walking continued for more than one minute in all participants (see distribution of PA activity data before and after smoothing in Figure A1). It is plausible that very short bouts were artifacts of the activity features due to the noise in the accelerometry signal acquired at the waist. The complexity metric aims to capture the dynamic change of real activity patterns that are encoded in the 'barcode' rather than the signal noise. Thus, a pre-processing method to remove the noise, or smooth the activity features before barcoding for complexity analysis is necessary and important. We proposed a smoothing method in this study to remove the noise. As shown in the secondary analysis, the resulting complexity value was lower than the complexity of the original PA time series, indicating that there was less frequent change in the activities after smoothing. The smoothing method improved the reproducibility of the complexity metric, which implies that the smoothing removed irrelevant noise existing in the original PA time series. However, it preserved the clinically relevant activity patterns as shown in the significant correlation with the clinical outcome. We observed a decrease in step counts and mean cadence after smoothing, which was likely due to the procedure, where steps in very short walking bouts were removed, but no step was inserted in the concatenated walking bouts.

There are some limitations in the study presented in this manuscript. First, the sample size was relatively small. Due to missing data, only 21 participants were included in the statistical analyses. Even though, there was no significant difference in functional status as measured by the CBMS score between the included and the excluded subject, the strength of association and effect size of change measured in this pilot study will need to be confirmed in a larger cohort of comparable participants. Secondly, the assessment of daily activity with wearable sensors during the intervention (Week3) was collected one week prior to the post-intervention assessment of CBMS. For the short intervention pilot, this time discrepancy might have introduced bias. This bias likely has made our estimates of pre- or post-intervention change in PA metrics to be more conservative. Lastly, the window of 30 s chosen for the smoothing method is based on the lowest threshold for walk analysis in the 'barcode' design. Conceptually, this threshold corresponds to most indoor walking activities [7,10]. However, future research should conduct a systematic evaluation to confirm the optimized activity feature resolution for complexity analysis.

In the context of PreventIT project, the on-going multi-national randomized controlled trial (RCT) study will provide a larger cohort data of 180 participants with comparable demographic and health profile as studied in this pilot. The RCT will assess the participant's CBMSs and monitor their PAs using a similar sensor configuration at baseline, 6-month, and 12-month follow-up. Correlation between the change in complexity and the change in CBMS will be validated after the longer intervention. Analyses on the association between complexity and CBMS at baseline will be conducted. In addition, relationship between complexity and each individual balance and mobility components assessed in CBMS will be analyzed.

5. Conclusions

This study demonstrated the clinical relevance of using a multivariate metric for physical behavioural complexity to capture change in functional status in a longitudinal study in younger older adults. The complexity metric showed higher sensitivity to functional change than conventionally applied univariate PA metrics such as sedentary time and step count. Complexity can be applied as a generic metric to analyze the daily life activity patterns derived from wearable sensors. A meaningful resolution of sensor-derived activity features is important for reliable complexity analysis. The complexity metric is a useful metric to be further developed for the outcome measure of the feasibility and the effectiveness of PreventIT interventions.

Author Contributions: Conceptualization, B.V., M.P., A.B.M., J.H. and K.A.; Methodology, W.Z., M.S., A.P.-I. and K.A.; Software, W.Z., S.M. and A.P.I.; Data Analysis, W.Z. and M.S.; Data Curation, A.S.M., N.H.J. and K.T.; Writing-Original Draft Preparation, W.Z.; Writing-Review & Editing, all authors.

Acknowledgments: We thank ADAPT project for providing dataset for technical development of the activity classification algorithm. We thank all PreventIT consortium partners for the inspiring discussions in project meetings. We are grateful to all participants, therapists and trainers in the aLiFE study.

Appendix

Appendix A.1 Adapted Barcode Design and Complexity Computation

A 'barcode' state was assigned to each second of the time series according to Table A1. The definition was modified for the type 'active' from the original design presented in [10] that applied the absolute value of acceleration. As acceleration is sensitive to the sensor wearing location, the acceleration based threshold was replaced by the 'ActiCount' in this study. The 'ActiCount' thresholds are determined based on a validation study presented in [19]. Complexity computation was according to Equation (A1), where 'nrPattern' is the total number of sub-patterns found in the 'barcode'. 'nBC' is the total number of 'barcode' states. In our analysis, nBC = 18. N is the total length of PA time series in seconds.

$$\text{Complexity} = \frac{\text{nrPattern} * (\frac{\log_{10}(\text{nrPattern})}{\log_{10}(\text{nBC})} + 1)}{\text{N}} \tag{A1}$$

Table A1. Definition of barcode state according to PA category, intensity and duration.

Category	Intensity	Duration	State
Lying			1
Sedentary			2
Active	ActiCounts $\leq$ 3500 (counts/minute)		3
	3500 < ActiCounts $\leq$ 7000		4
	7000 < ActiCounts $\leq$ 10000		5
	ActiCounts > 10000		6
Walking	Cadence $\leq$ 60 (steps/minute)	Duration $\leq$ 30 s	7
	60 < Cadence $\leq$ 90		8
	90 < Cadence $\leq$ 140		9
	Cadence > 140		10
	Cadence $\leq$ 60	30 < Duration $\leq$ 120	11
	60 < Cadence $\leq$ 90		12
	90 < Cadence $\leq$ 140		13
	Cadence > 140		14
	Cadence $\leq$ 60	Duration > 120	15
	60 < Cadence $\leq$ 90		16
	90 < Cadence $\leq$ 140		17
	Cadence > 140		18

Appendix A.2 Effect of Smoothing on the Duration of Activity Bouts and Reliability of Complexity

Figure A1 shows that, after smoothing, 90% of the sedentary bouts lasted up to 15 min, whereas only 10% of the walking bouts were longer than two and half minutes before a stop. Figure A2 compares the mean and standard deviation of daily complexity in one-week measurement before and after smoothing. Smoothing lowered the mean values and the CV of the complexity.

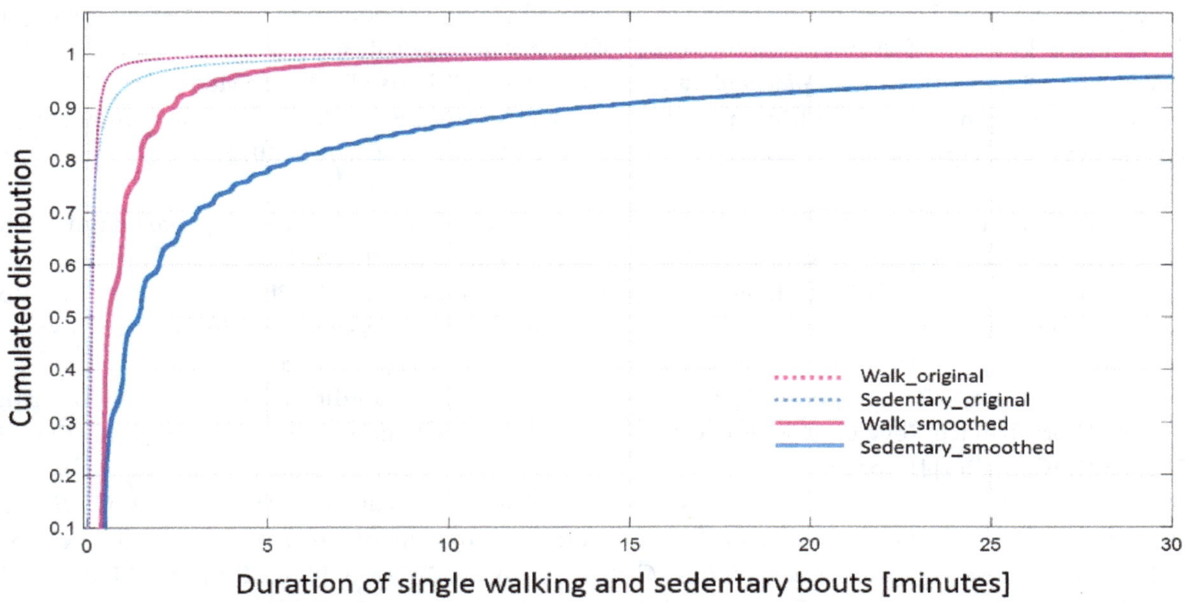

Figure A1. Comparison of cumulated distribution of walking and sedentary bouts before and after smoothing of activity classification output.

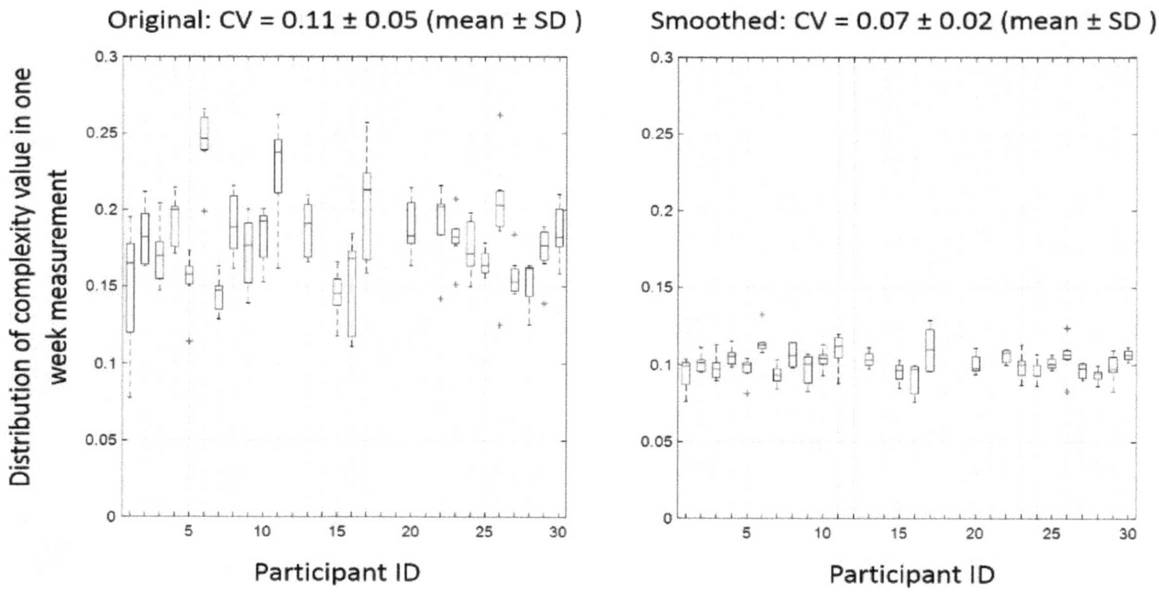

Figure A2. CV before and after smoothing PA time series.

References

1. Helbostad, J.L.; Vereijken, B.; Becker, C.; Todd, C.; Taraldsen, K.; Pijnappels, M.; Aminian, K.; Mellone, S. Mobile Health Applications to Promote Active and Healthy Ageing. *Sensors* **2017**, *17*, 622. [CrossRef] [PubMed]
2. World Health Organization. *Global Health Risks: Mortality and Burden of Disease Attributable to Selected Major Risks*; World Health Organization: Geneva, Switzerland, 2009.
3. Slingerland, A.S.; van Lenthe, F.J.; Jukema, J.W.; Kamphuis, C.B.M.; Looman, C.; Huisman, M.; Narayan, K.M.; Mackenbach, J.P.; Brug, J. Aging, Retirement, and Changes in Physical Activity: Prospective Cohort Findings from the GLOBE Study. *Am. J. Epidemiol.* **2007**, *165*, 1356–1363. [CrossRef] [PubMed]
4. Bort-Roig, J.; Gilson, N.D.; Puig-Ribera, A.; Contreras, R.S.; Trost, S.G. Measuring and influencing physical activity with smartphone technology: A systematic review. *Sports Med.* **2014**, *44*, 671–686. [CrossRef] [PubMed]
5. Althoff, T.; Sosič, R.; Hicks, J.L.; King, A.C.; Delp, S.L.; Leskovec, J. Large-scale physical activity data reveal worldwide activity inequality. *Nature* **2017**, *547*, 336–339. [CrossRef] [PubMed]
6. Taraldsen, K.; Chastin, S.F.M.; Riphagen, I.I.; Vereijken, B.; Helbostad, J.L. Physical activity monitoring by use of accelerometer-based body-worn sensors in older adults: A systematic literature review of current knowledge and applications. *Maturitas* **2012**, *71*, 13–19. [CrossRef] [PubMed]
7. Brodie, M.A.; Lord, S.R.; Coppens, M.J.; Annegarn, J.; Delbaere, K. Eight-Week Remote Monitoring Using a Freely Worn Device Reveals Unstable Gait Patterns in Older Fallers. *IEEE Trans. Biomed. Eng.* **2015**, *62*, 2588–2594. [CrossRef] [PubMed]
8. Ahlrichs, C.; Samà, A.; Lawo, M.; Cabestany, J.; Rodríguez-Martín, D.; Pérez-López, C.; Sweeney, D.; Quinlan, L.R.; Laighin, G.Ò.; Counihan, T.; et al. Detecting freezing of gait with a tri-axial accelerometer in Parkinson's disease patients. *Med. Biol. Eng. Comput.* **2016**, *54*, 223–233. [CrossRef] [PubMed]
9. Hausdorff, J.M. Gait Dynamics, Fractals and Falls: Finding Meaning in the Stride-To-Stride Fluctuations of Human Walking. *Hum. Mov. Sci.* **2007**, *26*, 555–589. [CrossRef] [PubMed]
10. Paraschiv-Ionescu, A.; Perruchoud, C.; Buchser, E.; Aminian, K. Barcoding Human Physical Activity to Assess Chronic Pain Conditions. *PLoS ONE* **2012**, *7*, e32239. [CrossRef] [PubMed]
11. Paraschiv-Ionescu, A.; Perruchoud, C.; Rutschmann, B.; Buchser, E.; Aminian, K. Quantifying dimensions of physical behavior in chronic pain conditions. *J. Neuroeng. Rehabil.* **2016**, *13*, 85. [CrossRef] [PubMed]
12. Paraschiv-Ionescu, A.; Buchser, E.; Aminian, K. Unraveling dynamics of human physical activity patterns in chronic pain conditions. *Sci. Rep.* **2013**, *3*, 2019. [CrossRef] [PubMed]

13. Moufawad el Achkar, C.; Lenoble-Hoskovec, C.; Paraschiv-Ionescu, A.; Major, K.; Büla, C.; Aminian, K. Physical Behavior in Older Persons during Daily Life: Insights from Instrumented Shoes. *Sensors* **2016**, *16*, 1225. [CrossRef] [PubMed]
14. ISRCTN—ISRCTN37750605: Feasibility of the Adapted LiFE (aLiFE) Intervention—A pilot Study. Available online: http://www.isrctn.com/ISRCTN37750605 (accessed on 16 February 2017).
15. Balasubramanian, C.K. The community balance and mobility scale alleviates the ceiling effects observed in the currently used gait and balance assessments for the community-dwelling older adults. *J. Geriatr. Phys. Ther.* **2015**, *38*, 78–89. [CrossRef] [PubMed]
16. Fleiner, T.; Haussermann, P.; Mellone, S.; Zijlstra, W. Sensor-based assessment of mobility-related behavior in dementia: Feasibility and relevance in a hospital context. *Int. Psychogeriatr.* **2016**, *28*, 1687–1694. [CrossRef] [PubMed]
17. Chigateri, N.; Kerse, N.; MacDonald, B.; Klenk, J. Validation of Walking Episode Recognition in Supervised and Free-living Conditions Using Triaxial Accelerometers. In Proceedings of the 2017 World Congress of International Society for Posture & Gait Research, Fort Lauderdale, FL, USA, 25–29 June 2017; pp. 289–290.
18. Bourke, A.K.; Ihlen, E.A.F.; Bergquist, R.; Wik, P.B.; Vereijken, B.; Helbostad, J.L. A Physical Activity Reference Data-Set Recorded from Older Adults Using Body-Worn Inertial Sensors and Video Technology—The ADAPT Study Data-Set. *Sensors* **2017**, *17*, 559. [CrossRef] [PubMed]
19. Sasaki, J.E.; John, D.; Freedson, P.S. Validation and comparison of ActiGraph activity monitors. *J. Sci. Med. Sport* **2011**, *14*, 411–416. [CrossRef] [PubMed]
20. Mansoubi, M.; Pearson, N.; Clemes, S.A.; Biddle, S.J.; Bodicoat, D.H.; Tolfrey, K.; Edwardson, L.; Yates, T. Energy expenditure during common sitting and standing tasks: Examining the 1.5 MET definition of sedentary behaviour. *BMC Public Health* **2015**, *15*, 516. [CrossRef] [PubMed]
21. Ryu, U.; Ahn, K.; Kim, E.; Kim, M.; Kim, B.; Woo, S.; Chang, Y. Adaptive Step Detection Algorithm for Wireless Smart Step Counter. In Proceedings of the 2013 International Conference on Information Science and Applications (ICISA), Suwon, Korea, 24–26 June 2013; pp. 1–4.
22. Razjouyan, J.; Grewal, G.S.; Rishel, C.; Parthasarathy, S.; Mohler, J.; Najafi, B. Activity Monitoring and Heart Rate Variability as Indicators of Fall Risk: Proof-of-Concept for Application of Wearable Sensors in the Acute Care Setting. *J. Gerontol. Nurs.* **2017**, *43*, 53–62. [CrossRef] [PubMed]
23. Orlov, Y.L.; Potapov, V.N. Complexity: An internet resource for analysis of DNA sequence complexity. *Nucleic Acids Res.* **2004**, *32*, W628–W633. [CrossRef] [PubMed]
24. Seely, A.J.; Macklem, P.T. Complex systems and the technology of variability analysis. *Crit. Care* **2004**, *8*, R367. [CrossRef] [PubMed]
25. Cavanaugh, J.T.; Kochi, N.; Stergiou, N. Nonlinear Analysis of Ambulatory Activity Patterns in Community-Dwelling Older Adults. *J. Gerontol. Ser. A* **2010**, *65A*, 197–203. [CrossRef] [PubMed]
26. Lempel, A.; Ziv, J. On the Complexity of Finite Sequences. *IEEE Trans. Inf. Theory.* **1976**, *22*, 75–81. [CrossRef]
27. De Bruin, E.D.; Najafi, B.; Murer, K.; Uebelhart, D.; Aminian, K. Quantification of everyday motor function in a geriatric population. *J. Rehabil. Res. Dev.* **2007**, *44*, 417–428. [CrossRef] [PubMed]
28. Macbeth, G.; Razumiejczyk, E.; Ledesma, R.D. Cliff's Delta Calculator: A non-parametric effect size program for two groups of observations. *Univ. Psychol.* **2011**, *10*, 545–555.
29. Lipsitz, L.A. Physiological Complexity, Aging, and the Path to Frailty. *Sci. Aging Knowl. Environ.* **2004**, *2004*, pe16. [CrossRef] [PubMed]
30. Vaillancourt, D.E.; Newell, K.M. Changing complexity in human behavior and physiology through aging and disease. *Neurobiol. Aging.* **2002**, *23*, 1–11. [CrossRef]
31. Razjouyan, J.; Naik, A.D.; Horstman, M.J.; Kunik, M.E.; Amirmazaheri, M.; Zhou, H.; Sharafkhaneh, A.; Najafi, B. Wearable Sensors and the Assessment of Frailty among Vulnerable Older Adults: An Observational Cohort Study. *Sensors* **2018**, *18*, 1336. [CrossRef] [PubMed]

8

Design of a Wearable 12-Lead Noncontact Electrocardiogram Monitoring System

Chien-Chin Hsu [1,2], Bor-Shing Lin [3], Ke-Yi He [4] and Bor-Shyh Lin [4,*]

1 Department of Emergency Medicine, Chi Mei Medical Center, Tainan 710, Taiwan; nych2525@gmail.com
2 Department of Biotechnology, Southern Taiwan University of Science and Technology, Tainan 71005, Taiwan
3 Department of Computer Science and Information Engineering, National Taipei University, New Taipei 23741, Taiwan; bslin@mail.ntpu.edu.tw
4 Institute of Imaging and Biomedical Photonics, National Chiao Tung University, Tainan 711, Taiwan; nctukeyiho@gmail.com
* Correspondence: borshyhlin@gmail.com

Abstract: A standard 12-lead electrocardiogram (ECG) is an important tool in the diagnosis of heart diseases. Here, Ag/AgCl electrodes with conductive gels are usually used in a 12-lead ECG system to access biopotentials. However, using Ag/AgCl electrodes with conductive gels might be inconvenient in a prehospital setting. In previous studies, several dry electrodes have been developed to improve this issue. However, these dry electrodes have contact with the skin directly, and they might be still unsuitable for patients with wounds. In this study, a wearable 12-lead electrocardiogram monitoring system was proposed to improve the above issue. Here, novel noncontact electrodes were also designed to access biopotentials without contact with the skin directly. Moreover, by using the mechanical design, this system allows the user to easily wear and take off the device and to adjust the locations of the noncontact electrodes. The experimental results showed that the proposed system could exactly provide a good ECG signal quality even while walking and could detect the ECG features of the patients with myocardial ischemia, installation pacemaker, and ventricular premature contraction.

Keywords: electrocardiogram; conductive gels; noncontact electrode; myocardial ischemia; pacemaker; ventricular premature contraction

---

1. Introduction

The standard 12-lead electrocardiogram (ECG) is an important tool to assist the diagnosis of myocardial ischemia and arrhythmia. In particular, for the diagnosis of myocardial infarction, 12-lead ECG provides important and meaningful information. The timely treatment of occluded coronary artery is critical to reduce myocardial injury and mortality. In order to save the ischemia myocardium, a 12-lead ECG of the patient must be obtained in emergency or prehospital settings. Myocardial infarction must be identified as early as possible and the patient must be taken to a hospital with a cardiac cath lab. In general, the conventional Ag/AgCl ECG electrodes with conductive gels are used to measure ECG signals. The use of conductive gels can effectively improve the conductivity of the skin electrode interface to acquire a better ECG signal quality [1]. However, the use of conductive gels usually encounters the dying issue of long-time measurement or the dislodgement of electrodes due to wet skin.

In order to improve the above issue of the conventional ECG electrodes, several novel dry electrodes have been proposed in previous studies. Some studies applied the technique of microelectromechanical systems (MEMS) in the development of novel dry electrodes [2]. However, the manufacturing cost and process of these MEMS-based dry electrodes is relatively expensive and complex. Moreover, the measuring method of these MEMS-based dry electrodes are semi-invasive, and this also increases the risk of a skin allergy. Several conductive fabrics, conductive materials, or metals are also used for the development of dry electrodes [3–15]. In 2013, Zhou et al. proposed microstructure-array metal dry electrodes [16]. In 2012, Jung et al. developed carbon nanotube (CNT)/polydimethylsiloxane (PDMS) composite flexible dry electrodes for ECG measurement [17]. The above dry electrodes are also semi-invasive and could provide a good signal quality in a hairless site. In 2011, Lin et al. proposed a novel foam dry electrode [18,19] to acquire biopotentials without conductive gels. However, the abovementioned dry electrodes have to contact the skin directly and may be unsuitable for measuring biopotentials in a hairy site due to the fact that the hair layer might increase the impedance of the skin-electrode interface.

Different from the above dry electrodes which have to contact with the skin directly, the noncontact dry electrode was developed in recent years. In general, the design of dry electrodes has to minimize the impedance of the skin-electrode interface. Different from other skin-electrode models of other dry electrodes, the skin-electrode interface model of a noncontact dry electrode can be viewed as a coupling capacitance. In 2013, Lin et al. successfully applied the technique of noncontact electrode to acquire a lead I ECG signal [20,21]. Based on our experience of the noncontact electrode design, a wearable 12-lead ECG monitoring system with noncontact electrodes was proposed in this study. By using the properties of the noncontact electrode technique, ECG signal can be measured across thin clothes to avoid contacting a wound of the subject. Moreover, by using the wearable mechanical design, the proposed system can be easily worn and taken off, and the locations of noncontact electrodes can be quickly and easily adjusted. Finally, the performance of the proposed noncontact electrode has also be validated and applied in the detection of myocardial ischemia, installation pacemaker, and ventricular premature contraction.

2. Materials and Methods

2.1. Fundamental Theory of Noncontact Electrode

The electrode-skin interface models of conventional Ag/AgCl electrode and noncontact electrode are shown in Figure 1a,b. In general, conductive gel has to be applied in the conventional Ag/AgCl electrode to form a conductive layer between the electrode and skin and to reduce the impedance of the electrode-skin interface. Therefore, the equivalent circuit of the conductive gel layer can be simply viewed as a resistor. The skin layer can be viewed as a plate, and its equivalent circuit can be presented as a resistance and a capacitor in parallel. Therefore, the measurement of a biopotential by using the conventional Ag/AgCl electrode has to pass through these equivalent impedances, such as the skin layer, the conductive gel layer, and the metal electrode.

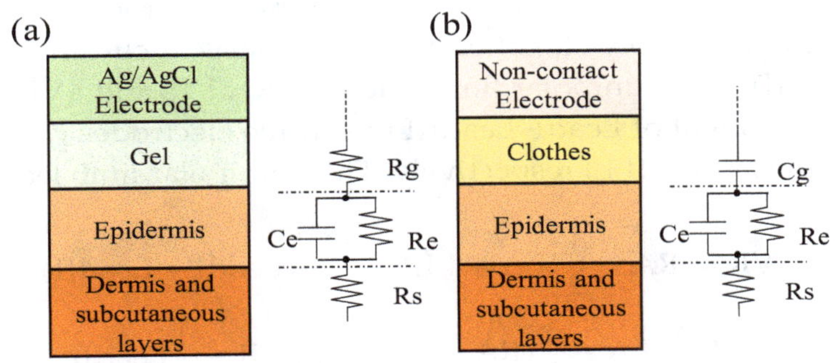

Figure 1. The skin-electrode interface models of (**a**) an Ag–AgCl electrode and (**b**) a noncontact dry electrode.

In the electrode-skin interface model of a noncontact electrode, the skin layer and the metal electrode can be viewed as two parallel plates, and the clothes can be viewed as an isolation layer. Therefore, the electrode-skin interface model of a noncontact electrode can be viewed as a capacitor.

Figure 2a shows the basic scheme of the designed noncontact electrode. Its major parts contain a metal electrode; an impedance converter, which is used to provide an ultrahigh input impedance to reduce the influence of the variation of the skin-electrode interface impedance; and a high-impedance pathway, which is used to reduce the influence of the bias variation of the unit buffer to ensure it works within the active region. Here, the metal electrode was coated with an isolated layer of solder mask. Figure 2b shows the equivalent electrical model of the used noncontact electrodes. Let V_i and V_o denote the ECG signal source of the human body and the output of the noncontact electrode, respectively, C_g denote the coupling capacitance formed by the skin and the metal electrode plate, R_g be the equivalent impedance of the bias pathway, and R_i and C_i denote the equivalent resistance and the equivalent capacitance of the used operational amplifier, respectively. Therefore, the transfer function of the used noncontact electrode can be expressed as followings.

$$\frac{V_o(S)}{V_i(S)} = \frac{R_g//R_i//\frac{1}{SC_i}}{\frac{1}{SC_g} + R_g//R_i//\frac{1}{SC_i}} = \frac{SC_gR_gR_i}{SC_gR_gR_i + SC_iR_gR_i + R_g + R_i} \tag{1}$$

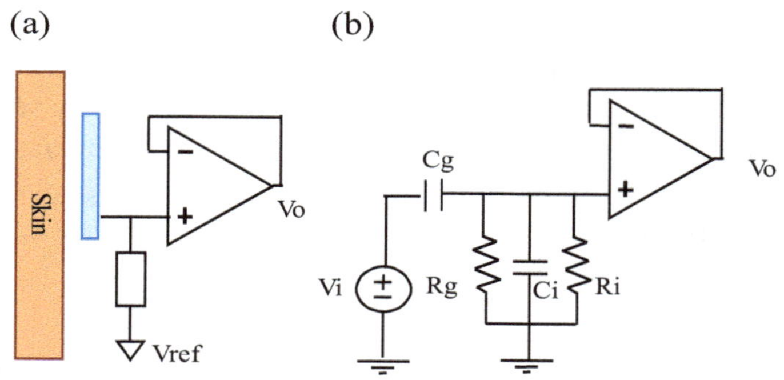

Figure 2. (**a**) A basic scheme and (**b**) the equivalent electrical model of a used noncontact electrode.

From the above formula, it showed that decreasing C_i could provide the larger amplitude response when C_g, R_g, and R_i are large enough. In the design of the noncontact electrode, R_i and C_i are decided by the selection of the used operational amplifier. C_g is a coupling capacitor, formed by the metal plate of the noncontact electrode and the skin. In order to increase the value of C_g, the electrode surface area has to be increased or the distance between the skin and the electrode has to be decreased.

2.2. Measurement of Standard 12-Lead Electrocardiogram

The standard 12-lead ECG system is used to collect 12 different ECG signals from different locations simultaneously to completely estimate the vector of electrocardiogram. The measurement of 12-lead ECG system can be simply classified into three parts, including three bipolar limb leads (LeadI, LeadII, and LeadIII), three unipolar limb leads (aVR, aVL, and aVF), and six unipolar chest leads (V1–V6). The measurement of LeadI–LeadIII uses three electrodes placed on the left arm (LA), the right arm (RA), and the left leg (LL) respectively. These unipolar limb leads can be represented as Equations (2)–(4).

$$\text{aVR} = \text{RA} - \frac{1}{2}(\text{LA} + \text{LL}) = -\frac{1}{2}(\text{LeadI} + \text{LeadII}) \tag{2}$$

$$\text{aVL} = \text{LA} - \frac{1}{2}(\text{RA} + \text{LL}) = \text{LeadI} - \frac{1}{2}\text{LeadII} \tag{3}$$

$$\text{aVF} = \text{LL} - \frac{1}{2}(\text{RA} + \text{LA}) = \text{LeadII} - \frac{1}{2}\text{LeadI} \tag{4}$$

The six unipolar chest leads (V1 to V6) represent the voltage difference between the chest voltage and the average voltages of LA, RA, and LL, and they can be expressed by

$$V_k = \text{Chest}_k - \frac{1}{3}(\text{RA} + \text{LL} + \text{LA}) \quad (5)$$

where V_k and Chest_k denote the *k*th chest leads and the voltage of the *k*th chest electrode, respectively.

3. Design and Implementation of Wearable 12-Lead ECG Monitoring System

The system architecture and photograph of the proposed system is shown in Figure 3, and it mainly contains a wearable mechanical design, a wireless 12-lead ECG acquisition module, and a back-end host system. The wireless 12-lead ECG acquisition module is designed to measure ECG signals and can be embedded into the wearable mechanical design. The wearable mechanical design is designed to be worn easily in daily life and can provide a suitable pressure to avoid the sliding of the wireless 12-lead ECG acquisition module to acquire a good ECG signal quality. Finally, the acquired ECG signal will be transmitted to the back-end host system wirelessly via Bluetooth.

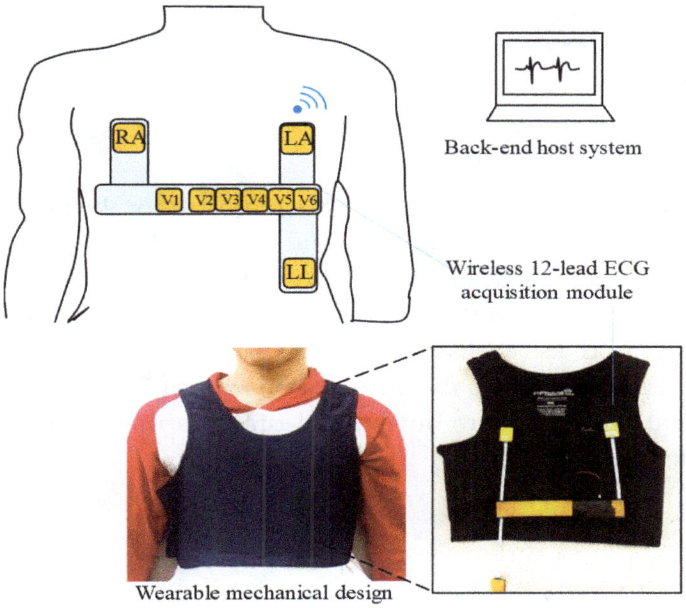

Figure 3. A basic scheme and photograph of the wearable 12-Lead electrocardiogram (ECG) monitoring system.

The block diagram of the wireless 12-lead ECG acquisition module is shown in Figure 4, and it mainly consists of several parts: noncontact dry electrodes, multiplexers, a summing amplifier, a front-end amplifier, a microprocessor, and a wireless transmission circuit. First, the biopotentials would be acquired by these noncontact dry electrodes. In order to measure the six unipolar chest leads, the reference signal, combined from the voltages of RA, LL, and LA, has to be obtained. Here, the summing amplifier is used to obtain the combination of the RA, LL, and LA voltages. According to the definition of the 12-lead ECG system, nine dry electrodes would be switched by two multiplexers and, then, would be inputted into the front-end amplifier to obtain the 12-lead ECG signals. The front-end amplifier contains an instrumentation amplifier (AD620, Analog Devices, Norwood, MA, USA; gain = 20), a band-pass filter (gain = 20, and frequency band = 0.1 Hz–150 Hz), and a notch filter of 60 Hz. Then, the preprocessed ECG signals would be digitized by an analog-to-digital converter built into the microprocessor with the sampling rate of 500 Hz and, then, would be sent to the wireless transmission circuit to transmit to the back-end host system. The wearable mechanical design mainly consists of an elastic chest vest and Velcros. By using these Velcros, the designed wireless 12-lead ECG acquisition module could be easily embedded on the elastic chest vest, and it also allows the adjustment of the positions of the noncontact electrodes to reduce the influence of the individual body size difference.

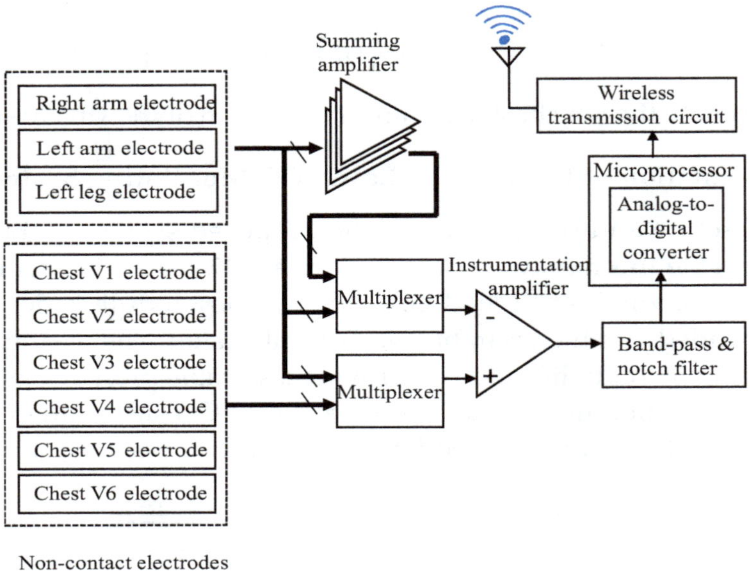

Figure 4. A block diagram of the wearable 12-Lead ECG acquisition module.

In this system, a commercial tablet was used as the platform for the host system, and a 12-lead ECG monitoring program was also designed to continuously monitor the 12-lead ECG signals. This program would first build the graphical user interface to allow the user operating and setting the program parameters. When clicking the start button, it would call the Bluetooth application programming interface (API) to search the wireless 12-lead ECG acquisition module and to make a connection with this module. After connecting with this module, the thread of DataREC would receive the 12-lead ECG signals, store them into the program buffer, real-time display them on the screen, and store the raw data into the local files.

4. Results

4.1. Electrical Specifications of Noncontact Electrodes

In this section, the electrical specifications of the designed noncontact electrodes were first investigated. Figure 5a,b shows the magnitude response and phase response of the designed noncontact electrodes. Here, a function generator was used to generate a 1 voltage p-p sine wave with varying frequency (from 0.1 Hz to 1000 Hz), and it was connected to a copper plate coated with an insulation tape as the input of the noncontact electrode. From the experimental results, the magnitude response of the noncontact electrode at the frequency range between 1 Hz and 1000 Hz is stable and flat, and its phase response is also almost linear. Figure 5c shows the referred noise spectrum of the noncontact electrode. In this test, the input of the noncontact electrode was connected to the ground. It showed that the referred noise spectrum of the noncontact electrode in higher frequency would be slightly decayed, and the whole referred noise is almost below 10^{-5} V/Hz.

Next, the ECG signal quality obtained by the proposed noncontact electrode was compared with that of the conventional ECG electrode with conductive gels. In this experiment, the noncontact electrodes were placed across the chest through a thin T-shirt, and their locations were close to that of these conventional ECG electrodes. Figure 6a–c shows the comparisons between the lead II, aVL, and V6 ECG signals randomly selected from 12-lead ECG signals of different ECG electrodes and their spectra. Here, the ECG machine (PageWriter TC30, Philips, Amsterdam, Netherlands) with Ag/AgCl electrodes in Chi Mei Medical Center, Taiwan was used, and the function of the linear correlation coefficient in the Matlab software was used to estimate the difference between the ECG signal qualities obtained by different ECG electrodes. It showed that the correlation between ECG signals obtained by different electrodes was over 0.95 and that the correlation for the ECG spectra was over 0.99. The ECG signal quality obtained by the proposed noncontact electrodes across a T-shirt was exactly similar to that of the conventional ECG electrodes with conductive gels.

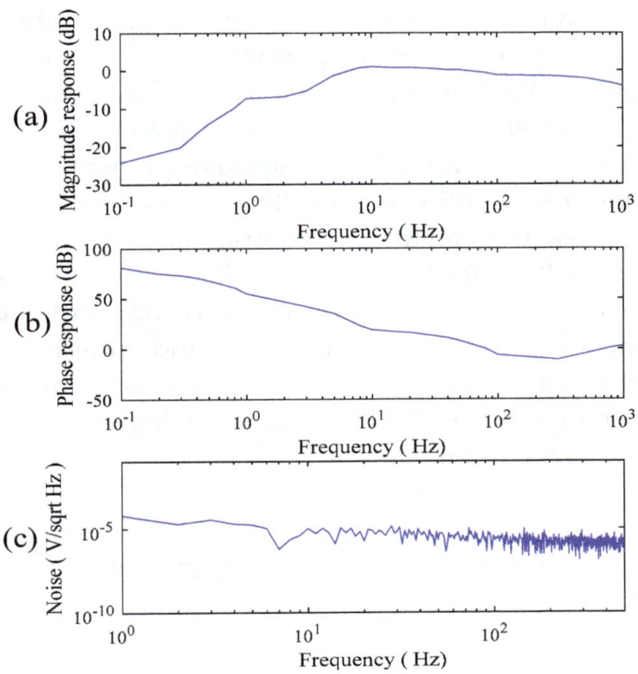

Figure 5. (**a**) The magnitude response, (**b**) phase response, and (**c**) referred noise spectrum of the proposed noncontact electrode.

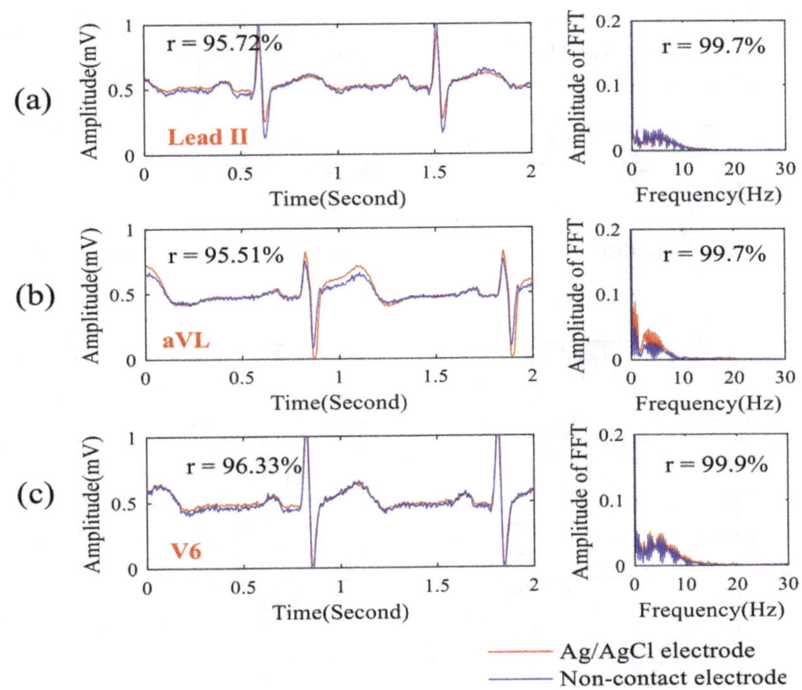

Figure 6. Comparisons between the ECG signals and their spectra obtained by different electrodes: (**a**) lead II, (**b**) aVL, and (**c**) V6.

4.2. *ECG Signal Quality of Wearable 12-Lead ECG Monitoring System under Different Conditions*

In this section, the influence of motion artifact on the ECG signal quality of the proposed system was first investigated. Figure 7a,b shows the ECG signals obtained by the proposed system while sitting and walking respectively. While walking, the motion artifact of walking causes the slight baseline swinging of the ECG signals, but its signal quality is still similar to that while sitting. Next, the ECG signals of patients in the emergency room were measured by the proposed system. Figure 8a–c shows the ECGs signal obtained from the patients with myocardial ischemia, installation pacemaker, and ventricular premature contraction, respectively. From the experimental results, the ECG features of Lead III T-wave inversion and the V6 ST-wave depression for myocardial ischemia [22] were measured by the proposed system. In Figure 8b, the pulse waves generated by installation pacemaker [23] in the front of each ECG cycle were also measured. For ventricular premature contraction, its ECG features can be reflected on the broadening QRS wave and the lack of P-wave [24], and the ECG signal in Figure 8c could also present these ECG features of ventricular premature contraction. Next, the effect of the cloth material, the effect of the thickness, and the influence of sweating on the ECG signal quality of the proposed system was also investigated. Figure 9a–d shows the ECG signal measured under different cloth conditions, including materials, thicknesses, and humidity. It shows that the amplitude of the ECG signal is slightly attenuated when the cloth thickness increased. In this experiment, the effect of selecting the cloth material on the ECG signal quality was unobvious. Moreover, the effect of sweating could improve the ECG signal quality.

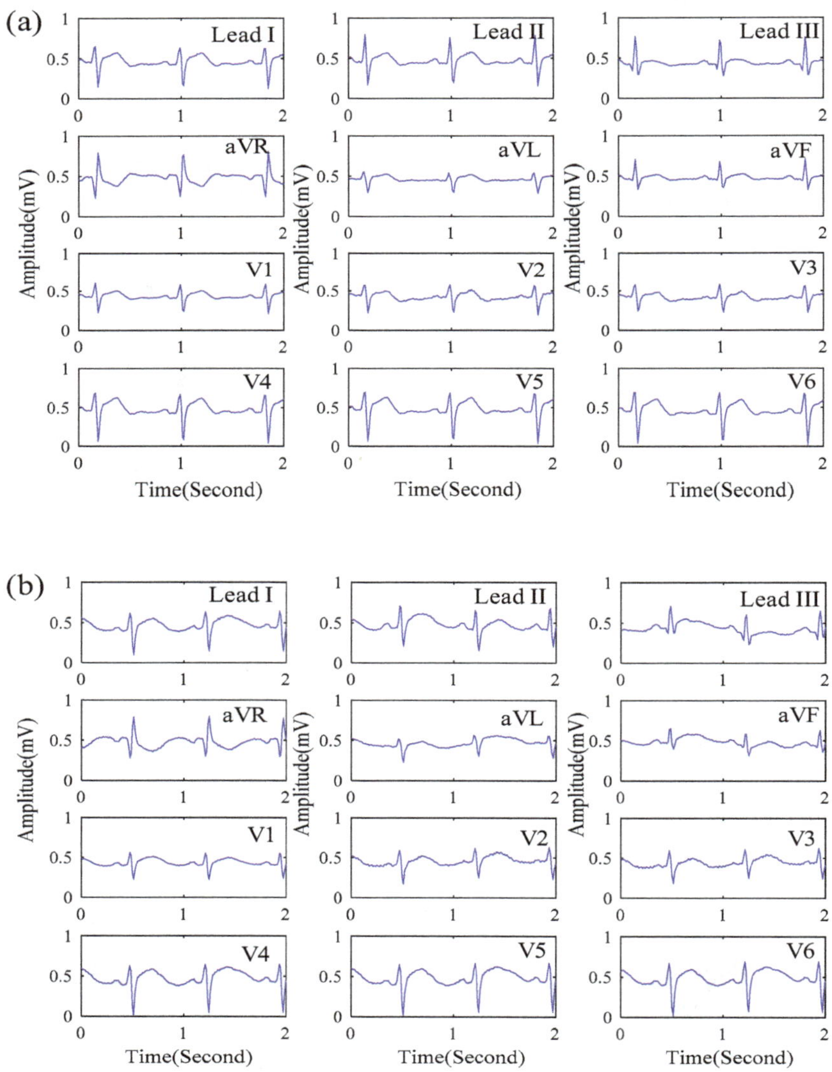

Figure 7. The 12-lead ECG signals obtained by the proposed system when (**a**) sitting and (**b**) walking.

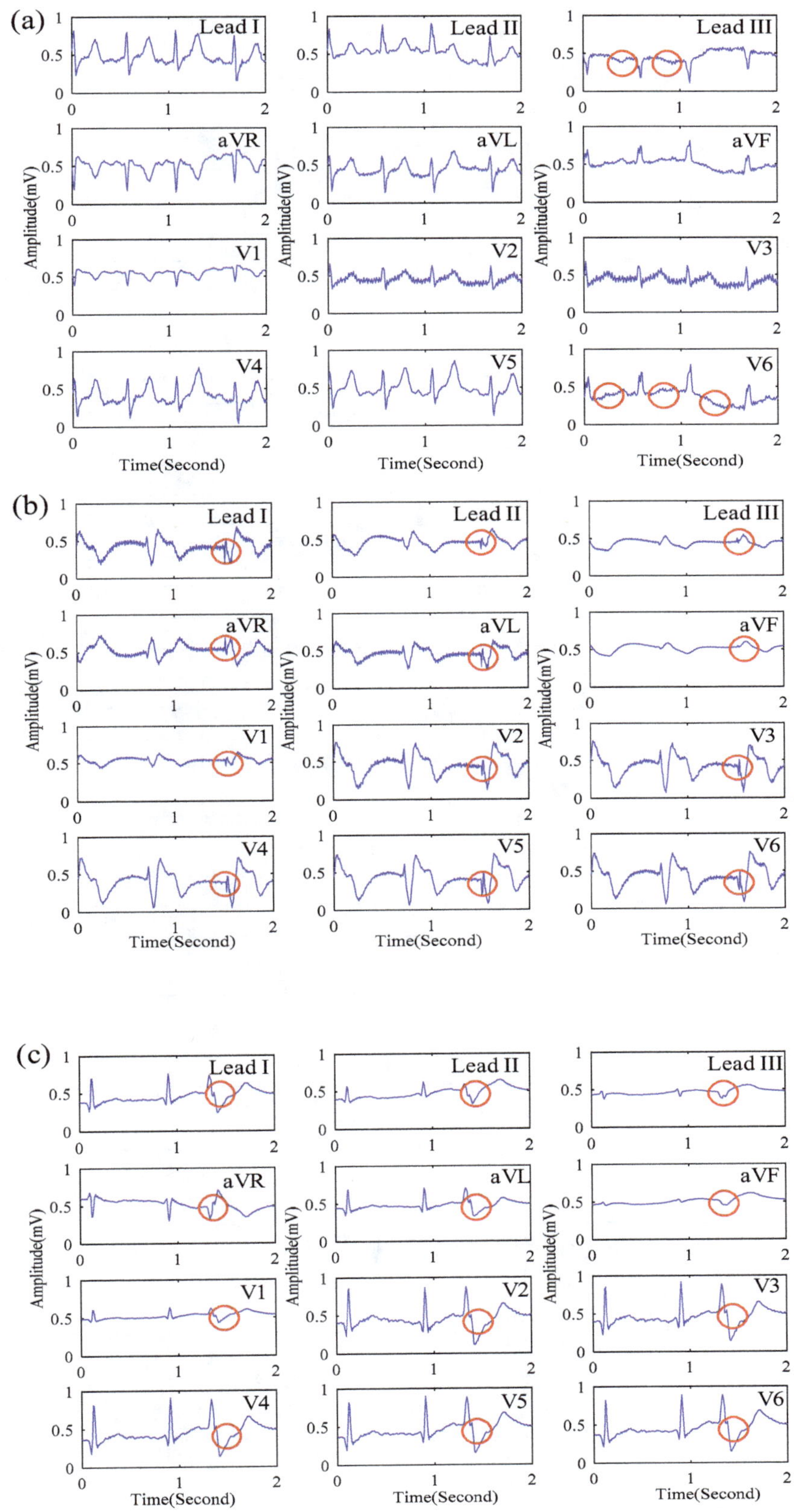

Figure 8. The ECG signal of patients with (**a**) myocardial infarction, (**b**) installation pacemaker, and (**c**) ventricular premature contraction obtained by the proposed system.

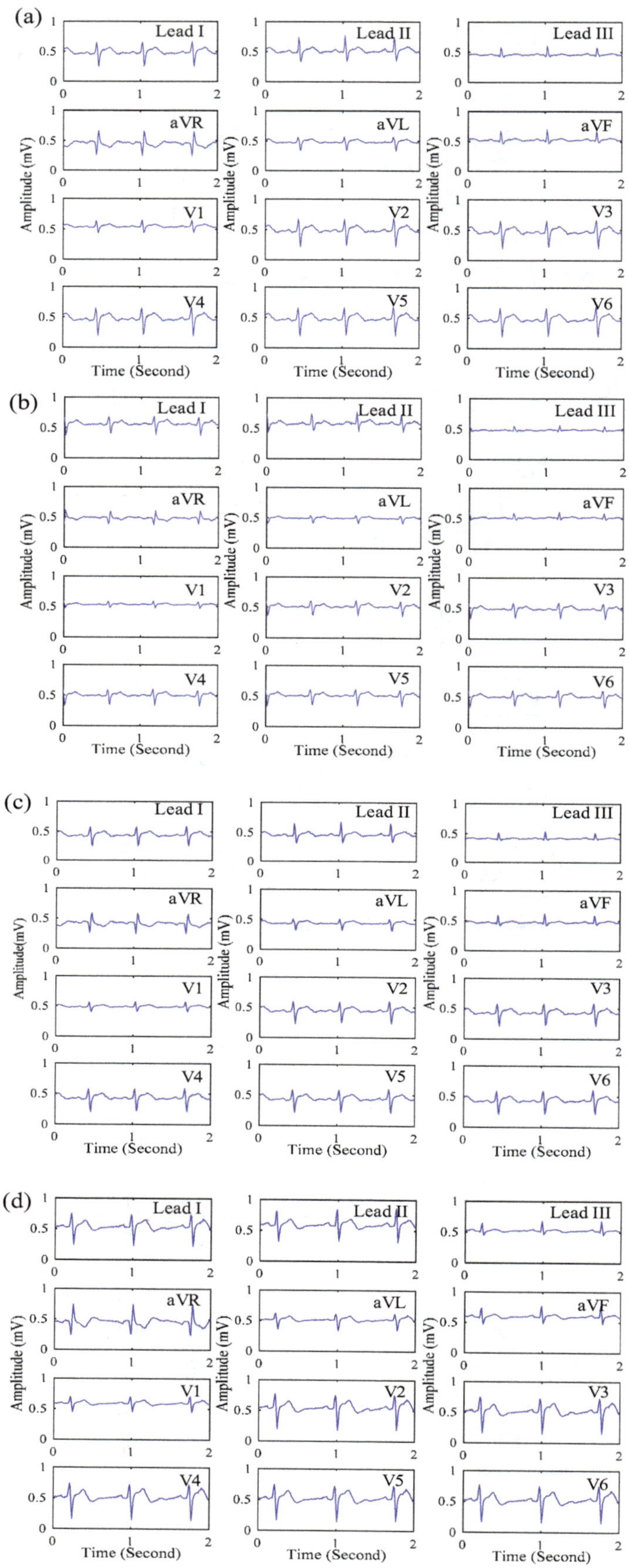

Figure 9. The 12-lead ECG signals obtained by the proposed system under different cloth conditions: (**a**) material: 100% cotton, thickness: 0.8 mm, dry; (**b**) material: 100% cotton, thickness: 1.4 mm, dry; (**c**) material: 80% cotton and 20% polyester, thickness: 0.8 mm, dry; (**d**) material: 100% cotton, thickness: 0.8 mm, sweating.

5. Discussion

In Figure 5a–c, in the frequency range between 0.1 Hz and 1000 Hz, the amplitude response of the proposed noncontact electrode is stable, and its phase response is linear. The whole referred noise of the proposed electrode is less than 10^{-5} V/Hz. From the above electrical specifications, the proposed noncontact electrode is suitable for measuring biopotentials, such as ECG, EEG, etc. In Figure 6a–c, the correlations between the EEG signals and spectra obtained by the proposed noncontact electrode and the conventional electrode with conductive gels are high. The influence of motion artifact on measuring the ECG signal was also investigated. The experimental results showed that the ECG signal quality was also good while walking, due to the fact that the flexibility of the wearable mechanical design might provide a suitable pressure to reduce the shifting of the noncontact electrodes. Moreover, the ECG features of myocardial ischemia, installation pacemaker, and ventricular premature contraction were also measured by the proposed system. Therefore, the reliability and practicability of the proposed system on measuring ECG were good. Moreover, the effect of the cloth condition on the ECG signal quality was also investigated. In Figure 9 a–d, it shows the amplitude of the ECG signal would be attenuated when the cloth thickness increased. Moreover, the effect of sweating could improve the ECG signal quality. This can be explained by the value of Cg in Equation (1) which would increase when the distance between the electrode and skin decreased or the humidity increased, due to the increase in dielectric.

Several dry and noncontact electrodes have been proposed in previous studies, and their specification comparison is summarized in Table 1. In 2013, Zhang et al. proposed a microneedle array (MNA) electrode [25]. The size of this MNA electrode was about 12×12 mm^2. Its substrate and microneedles were made of polydimethylsiloxane (PDMS) and silicon respectively, and finally, the MNA electrode was coated with poly-3,4-ethylenedioxythiophene/polystyrene sulfonate (PEDOT/PPS). This MNA electrode contained the properties of excellent flexibility, good conductivity, and semi-invasive measurement. The MNA electrode could directly penetrate the human stratum corneum to reduce the impedance of the skin-electrode interface and the electrode movement caused from the body friction. However, the manufacturing procedure of the MNA electrode is relatively complex, and its cost is also expensive. Under strenuous exercise, sweating might cause the falling off of the PEDOT/PSS coating, increase the skin-electrode interface impedance, and further affect the signal quality. In 2015, Weder et al. proposed an embroidered electrode [26]. The size of this embroidered electrode was about 70×20 mm^2. Here, polyethylene terephthalate (PET) yarn was used as the electrode substrate, and then, it was coated with silver/titanium (Ag/Ti) to provide a good biocompatibility and good conductivity. However, body hair might easily affect the measurement of this embroidered electrode. In 2011, Liao et al. proposed a spring probe dry electrode [27]. The size of this spring probe dry electrode was about 13×13 mm^2. A 13-mm-diameter copper piece was used as the substrate, and 17 gold-plated spring probes were soldered on the copper piece. The electrode was also coated with silicone. The comb telescopic structure of this electrode allowed it to pass through the hair layer and contact the skin directly. However, the skin-electrode interface impedance might be still higher and affect the signal quality [11]. In 2018, Castro et al. proposed a four-channel contactless capacitively coupled electrocardiography (ccECG) system for the extraction of sleep apnea features [28]. The ccECG system has the advantage of long-term physiological monitoring but the disadvantage of a high variation in the quality of the acquired signals due to its high sensitivity to motion artefacts. This system was only used in sleep apnea; it was not verified and did not guarantee a good performance of the ECG measurement under motion. Different from the above dry and noncontact electrodes, the proposed noncontact electrode could access biopotentials across the clothes without contacting the skin directly. Moreover, a flexible printed circuit board (PCB) was used as the substrate of the proposed electrode. The proposed electrode could easily be embedded into the clothes, and its flexibility could fit the body contour to provide a stable and good signal quality even under motion.

Table 1. The specification comparisons between different dry and noncontact electrodes and the proposed noncontact electrode.

	Zhang et al. [25]	Weder et al. [26]	Liao et al. [27]	Castro et al. [28]	Proposed Electrode
Area of electrode (cm^2)	1.44	14	1.69	-	6.16
Frequency band (Hz)	0.5–50	-	-	0.5–40	0.1–100
Input-referred noise (V/Hz)	-	-	-	-	6×10^{-5}
Electrode material	PEDOT/PSS	Ag/Ti	Gold, copper	Ag/AgCl	Copper
Noncontact electrode	No	No	No	Noncontact	Noncontact
Advantages	Excellent flexibility and conductivity, measurement under motion	Good biocompatibility and conductivity	Measurement in hairy site	Good measurement under slight motion (e.g., sleep)	Excellent flexibility, noncontact measurement under motion
Affecting factors	Influence of sweating	Influence of body hairs	Poor skin-electrode interface impedance	Not verified and guaranteed under motion	Thickness of clothing

In previous studies, several wearable 12-lead ECG systems have also been designed, and a comparison between the proposed system and other systems is listed in Table 2. In 2016, Boehm et al. proposed a 12-lead ECG T-Shirt [29], and its system size was about 70×65 mm^2. Ten active electrodes were embedded in a T-Shirt to greatly improve the convenience of use. However, it might be difficult to fit the body closely to affect the signal quality under motion. In 2015, Yasunori Tada et al. proposed a 12-lead ECG smart shirt [30], and its system size was about 90×28 mm^2. The system contained 10 dry foam electrodes, and conductive ink lines were also used as the ECG leads. The flexibility of the compressed shirt could help these foam electrodes contact the skin well to provide a good ECG signal quality, even under motion. However, these foam electrodes still have to contact the skin directly to acquire a biopotential, and body hairs might affect their measuring performance. In this study, the size of the proposed system was about 25×65 mm^2, and it contains 9 noncontact electrodes. Different from the above 12-lead ECG system, the flexible PCB was used as the substrate of the proposed noncontact electrodes and a wearable mechanical design was also designed to closely fit the body and provide a suitable pressure to reduce transversal motion and lateral motion. Thus, the proposed system could provide a good ECG signal quality under motion. Moreover, different from other wearable ECG monitoring systems, the proposed systems could access biopotentials across the clothes without contacting with the skin directly.

Table 2. The specification comparisons between the proposed 12-Lead ECG monitoring system and other systems.

	Anna Boehm et al. [29]	Yasunori Tada et al. [30]	Proposed System
Operation voltage	3.3 V	-	3.3 V
Amplifier gain	-	-	400 V/V
System of size	70×65 mm^2	90×28 mm^2	25×65 mm^2
Signal resolution	24 bits	-	12 bits
Frequency band (Hz)	2–20 Hz	-	0.1–100 Hz
Wireless transmission	-	XBee	Bluetooth
Power consumption	260 mW	-	150 mW
Advantages	Wearability, long-term monitoring	Wearability, measurement under motion	Wearability, noncontact measurement under motion
Affecting factors	Influence of motion	Influence of body hairs	Thickness of clothing

6. Conclusions

In this study, a wearable 12-lead noncontact electrocardiogram monitoring system was proposed and successfully applied in measuring the ECG signals of patients with myocardial ischemia and arrhythmia. From the experimental results, the magnitude and phase responses of the designed noncontact electrodes were suitable for measuring ECG signal, and its referred noise was less than 10^{-5} V/Hz. The proposed system could provide a good signal quality even while walking. Moreover, the ECG features of myocardial ischemia, installation pacemaker, and ventricular premature contraction could be measured by the proposed system. The properties of the noncontact electrode technique can effectively avoid contacting the wound of the subject. Moreover, the positions of the noncontact electrodes can be easily adjusted to reduce the influence of the individual body size difference. Therefore, the proposed system might be usefully applied in the applications of mobile ECG monitoring in the future.

Author Contributions: B.-S.L. (Bor-Shyh Lin) and B.-S.L. (Bor-Shing Lin) conceived the study idea, designed the framework and system architecture in this study, and modified the manuscript. K.-Y.H. implemented the system, collected data, analyzed the collected data, and wrote the draft. C.-C.H. provided conceptual advice, the design of the wearable device, and the domain knowledge of cardiology.

References

1. Searle, A.; Kirkup, L. A direct comparison of wet, dry and insulating bioelectric recording electrodes. *Physiol. Meas.* **2000**, *21*, 271–283. [CrossRef]
2. Griss, P.; Enoksson, P.; Tolvanen-Laakso, H.K.; Merilainen, P.; Ollmar, S.; Stemme, G. Micromachined electrodes for biopotential measurements. *J. Microelectromech. Syst.* **2001**, *10*, 10–16. [CrossRef]
3. Oh, T.I.; Yoon, S.; Kim, T.E.; Wi, H.; Kim, K.J.; Woo, E.J.; Sadleir, R.J. Nanofiber web textile dry electrodes for long-term biopotential recording. *IEEE Trans. Biomed. Circuits Syst.* **2013**, *7*, 204–211. [PubMed]
4. Taji, B.; Shirmohammadi, S.; Groza, V.; Batkin, I. Impact of skin–electrode interface on electrocardiogram measurements using conductive textile electrodes. *IEEE Trans. Instrum. Meas.* **2014**, *63*, 1412–1422. [CrossRef]
5. Yokus, M.A.; Jur, J.S. Fabric-based wearable dry electrodes for body surface biopotential recording. *IEEE Trans. Biomed. Eng.* **2016**, *63*, 423–430. [CrossRef]
6. Abu-Saude, M.J.; Morshed, B.I. Patterned Vertical Carbon Nanotube Dry Electrodes for Impedimetric Sensing and Stimulation. *IEEE Sensors J.* **2015**, *15*, 5851–5858. [CrossRef]
7. Wang, L.-F.; Liu, J.-Q.; Yang, B.; Yang, C.-S. PDMS-based low cost flexible dry electrode for long-term EEG measurement. *IEEE Sensors J.* **2012**, *12*, 2898–2904. [CrossRef]
8. Chen, Y.; Atnafu, A.D.; Schlattner, I.; Weldtsadik, W.T.; Roh, M.-C.; Kim, H.J.; Lee, S.-W.; Blankertz, B.; Fazli, S. A high-security EEG-based login system with RSVP stimuli and dry electrodes. *IEEE Trans. Inf. Forensics Secur.* **2016**, *11*, 2635–2647. [CrossRef]
9. Ueno, A.; Akabane, Y.; Kato, T.; Hoshino, H.; Kataoka, S.; Ishiyama, Y. Capacitive sensing of electrocardiographic potential through cloth from the dorsal surface of the body in a supine position: A preliminary study. *IEEE Trans. Biomed. Eng.* **2007**, *54*, 759–766. [CrossRef]
10. Pei, W.; Zhang, H.; Wang, Y.; Guo, X.; Xing, X.; Huang, Y.; Xie, Y.; Yang, X.; Chen, H. Skin-potential variation insensitive dry electrodes for ECG recording. *IEEE Trans. Biomed. Eng.* **2017**, *64*, 463–470. [CrossRef]
11. Huang, Y.-J.; Wu, C.-Y.; Wong, A.M.-K.; Lin, B.-S. Novel active comb-shaped dry electrode for EEG measurement in hairy site. *IEEE Trans. Biomed. Eng.* **2015**, *62*, 256–263. [CrossRef] [PubMed]
12. Laferriere, P.; Lemaire, E.D.; Chan, A.D. Surface electromyographic signals using dry electrodes. *IEEE Trans. Instrum. Meas.* **2011**, *60*, 3259–3268. [CrossRef]
13. Ribeiro, D.M.D.; Fu, L.S.; Carlos, L.A.D.; Cunha, J.P.S. A novel dry active biosignal electrode based on an hybrid organic-inorganic interface material. *IEEE Sensors J.* **2011**, *11*, 2241–2245. [CrossRef]
14. Chi, Y.M.; Jung, T.-P.; Cauwenberghs, G. Dry-contact and noncontact biopotential electrodes: Methodological review. *IEEE Rev. Biomed. Eng.* **2010**, *3*, 106–119. [CrossRef]
15. Yang, B.; Yu, C.; Dong, Y. Capacitively coupled electrocardiogram measuring system and noise reduction by singular spectrum analysis. *IEEE Sensors J.* **2016** *16*, 3802–3810. [CrossRef]

16. Zhou, W.; Song, R.; Pan, X.; Peng, Y.; Qi, X.; Peng, J.; Hui, K.; Hui, K. Fabrication and impedance measurement of novel metal dry bioelectrode. *Sens. Actuators A Phys.* **2013**, *201*, 127–133. [CrossRef]
17. Jung, H.-C.; Moon, J.-H.; Baek, D.-H.; Lee, J.-H.; Choi, Y.-Y.; Hong, J.-S.; Lee, S.-H. CNT/PDMS composite flexible dry electrodesfor long-term ECG monitoring. *IEEE Trans. Biomed. Eng.* **2012**, *59*, 1472–1479. [CrossRef]
18. Lin, C.-T.; Liao, L.-D.; Liu, Y.-H.; Wang, I.-J.; Lin, B.-S.; Chang, J.-Y. Novel dry polymer foam electrodes for long-term EEG measurement. *IEEE Trans. Biomed. Eng.* **2011**, *58*, 1200–1207.
19. Tseng, K.C.; Lin, B.-S.; Liao, L.-D.; Wang, Y.-T.; Wang, Y.-L. Development of a wearable mobile electrocardiogram monitoring system by using novel dry foam electrodes. *IEEE Syst. J.* **2014**, *8*, 900–906. [CrossRef]
20. Lin, B.-S.; Chou, W.; Wang, H.-Y.; Huang, Y.-J.; Pan, J.-S. Development of novel non-contact electrodes for mobile electrocardiogram monitoring system. *IEEE J. Transl. Eng. Health Med.* **2013**, *1*. [CrossRef]
21. Chen, Y.-C.; Lin, B.-S.; Pan, J.-S. Novel noncontact dry electrode with adaptive mechanical design for measuring EEG in a hairy site. *IEEE Trans. Instrum. Meas.* **2015**, *64*, 3361–3368. [CrossRef]
22. De Winter, R.J.; Tijssen, J.G. Non–ST-Segment Elevation Myocardial Infarction. *JACC Cardiovasc. Interv.* **2012**, *5*, 903–905. [CrossRef] [PubMed]
23. Murray, A.; Jordan, R.S.; Gold, R.G. Pacemaker assessment in the ambulant patient. *Heart* **1981**, *46*, 531–538. [CrossRef]
24. Talbi, M.L.; Charef, A. PVC discrimination using the QRS power spectrum and self-organizing maps. Comput. *Methods Programs. Biomed.* **2009**, *94*, 223–231. [CrossRef] [PubMed]
25. Zhang, H.; Pei, W.; Chen, Y.; Guo, X.; Wu, X.; Yang, X.; Chen, H. A motion interference-insensitive flexible dry electrode. *IEEE Trans. Biomed. Eng.* **2016**, *63*, 1136–1144. [CrossRef] [PubMed]
26. Weder, M.; Hegemann, D.; Amberg, M.; Hess, M.; Boesel, L.F.; Abächerli, R.; Meyer, V.R.; Rossi, R.M. Embroidered electrode with silver/titanium coating for long-term ECG monitoring. *Sensors* **2015**, *15*, 1750–1759. [CrossRef]
27. Liao, L.-D.; Wang, I.-J.; Chen, S.-F.; Chang, J.-Y.; Lin, C.-T. Design, fabrication and experimental validation of a novel dry-contact sensor for measuring electroencephalography signals without skin preparation. *Sensors* **2011**, *11*, 5819–5834. [CrossRef]
28. Castro, I.D.; Varon, C.; Torfs, T.; Huffel, S.V.; Puers, R.; Hoof, C.V. Evaluation of a multichannel non-contact ECG system and signal quality algorithms for sleep apnea detection and monitoring. *Sensors* **2018**, *18*, 577. [CrossRef]
29. Boehm, A.; Yu, X.; Neu, W.; Leonhardt, S.; Teichmann, D. A novel 12-lead ECG T-shirt with active electrodes. *Electronics* **2016**, *5*, 75. [CrossRef]
30. Tada, Y.; Amano, Y.; Sato, T.; Saito, S.; Inoue, M. A smart shirt made with conductive ink and conductive foam for the measurement of electrocardiogram signals with unipolar precordial leads. *Fibers* **2015**, *3*, 463–477. [CrossRef]

9

Quantile Coarsening Analysis of High-Volume Wearable Activity Data in a Longitudinal Observational Study

Ying Kuen Cheung [1,*], Pei-Yun Sabrina Hsueh [2], Ipek Ensari [3], Joshua Z. Willey [4] and Keith M. Diaz [3]

1. Department of Biostatistics, Mailman School of Public Health, Columbia University, New York, NY 10032, USA
2. IBM Watson Research Center, Yorktown Heights, NY 10598, USA; phsueh@us.ibm.com
3. Center for Behavioral Cardiovascular Health, Department of Medicine, Columbia University Medical Center, New York, NY 10032, USA; ie2145@cumc.columbia.edu (I.E.); kd2442@cumc.columbia.edu (K.M.D.)
4. Department of Neurology, Columbia University Medical Center, New York, NY 10032, USA; jzw2@cumc.columbia.edu

* Correspondence: yc632@cumc.columbia.edu

Abstract: Owing to advances in sensor technologies on wearable devices, it is feasible to measure physical activity of an individual continuously over a long period. These devices afford opportunities to understand individual behaviors, which may then provide a basis for tailored behavior interventions. The large volume of data however poses challenges in data management and analysis. We propose a novel quantile coarsening analysis (QCA) of daily physical activity data, with a goal to reduce the volume of data while preserving key information. We applied QCA to a longitudinal study of 79 healthy participants whose step counts were monitored for up to 1 year by a Fitbit device, performed cluster analysis of daily activity, and identified individual activity signature or pattern in terms of the clusters identified. Using 21,393 time series of daily physical activity, we identified eight clusters. Employment and partner status were each associated with 5 of the 8 clusters. Using less than 2% of the original data, QCA provides accurate approximation of the mean physical activity, forms meaningful activity patterns associated with individual characteristics, and is a versatile tool for dimension reduction of densely sampled data.

Keywords: citizen science; cluster analysis; physical activity; sedentary behavior; walking

---

1. Introduction

Physical activity has been shown to improve cardiovascular health, reduce risk of mortality [1–4] and is an important component of primary prevention for many chronic diseases and conditions such as Type 2 diabetes and obesity [5,6]. Walking, in particular, is recognized as an easily accessible, convenient, and familiar mode of physical activity, and thus is an appealing strategy for the promotion of health and well-being. As such there is impetus for examining walking behaviors as a predictor of multiple health outcomes in ambulatory, community-dwelling adults.

Advances in sensor technologies on wearable devices have enabled the continuous and accurate collection of step counts and other walking parameters over an extended period of time, thus providing a voluminous stream of data. The large amount of data provides an opportunity to better understand the daily physical activity patterns across populations. However, conventional analytical approaches focus on measuring physical activity patterns by predefined summary statistics such as total step counts and average minutes with activity on a given day. By summarizing physical activity at the daily level, however, these methods ignore between-day heterogeneity within a person, as they fail to capture the within-day patterns of activity. An understanding of within-day patterns of physical activity is of importance to facilitate individualized mobile experience, such as when push notifications and activity updates are being sent [7,8], and identifying changes in an individual's daily routines, thereby facilitating tailored behavior intervention [9,10]. Given the broad use of step-counting trackers to monitor and improve physical activity [11–25], analyzing sensor data beyond predefined daily features thus can have significant public health impact.

Multivariate finite mixture modeling (MFMM) is a clustering method, whose purpose is to identify homogeneous subgroups wherein the number of subgroups is not assumed to be known in the analysis. The MFMM analysis is model-based, data-driven, and aims to produce subgroups with features arising from the same statistical distribution; dividing the data into an optimal number of subgroups based on specific criteria such as the Bayesian information criterion [26]. Clustering algorithms utilizing MFMM methods have been applied to identify dietary patterns [27,28] and physical activity patterns based on questionnaire data [29]. These algorithms often entail prespecifying only a small-to-moderate number of features as input variables, as the computational complexity grows exponentially with the addition of more features [30]. In the present context where the goal is to examine the within-day activity patterns, hundreds of physical activity inputs can be recorded from sensors throughout a day (e.g., minute-by-minute step counts), existing clustering algorithms may prove to be computationally infeasible without properly reducing the dimension of the data in a pre-processing step.

Dimension reduction of sensor data continuously collected can be achieved by time series modeling of the data [31–34]. Typically, a time series is first transformed to a domain relevant to the scientific interest, and is then summarized by a few parameters (e.g., autocorrelation). These parameters in turn serve as input features in a clustering algorithm. In this article, we take a similar approach and propose a two-step method for analyzing sensor data as time series: the proposed method first transforms the daily physical activity data into a coarsened probability density function of quantiles of activity time, and then applies the MFMM analysis using the quantiles as input features. The method is thus called quantile coarsening analysis (QCA). This approach is motivated by the consideration that time of activity, as well as the amount of activity, is of primary interest in our application. As will be shown in *Statistical Analyses* below, the resolution or coarseness of dimension reduction can be set by users in accordance with the needs in their application; such flexibility distinguishes the proposed method from the traditional parametric modeling of time series data [35]. The purposes of this article are to demonstrate the feasibility of QCA in a data set of 21,393 time series of daily physical activity, and to examine its estimation properties under various degrees of coarseness.

2. Materials and Methods

2.1. Study Cohort

A single cohort, 12-month, intensive observational study was conducted in healthy adults with an objective to collect their personal daily stress and physical activity for associative analysis. The study was approved by Columbia University Medical Center's (CUMC) institutional review board. All participants provided informed consent. Access to the study dataset and information about the study's execution and materials is publicly available [36].

Potentially eligible participants were identified and screened at CUMC. The inclusion criteria were (i) aged 18 years or older; (ii) self-reported intermittent exerciser (i.e., exercise 6–11 times per month but did not have a regular workout schedule); (iii) having access to a personal computer and a smartphone. Exclusion criteria included individuals who (i) were unavailable for 12 continuous months; (ii) had serious medical comorbidity that would compromise their ability to engage in usual physical activity; (iii) had occupational work demands that required rigorous activity; or (iv) were unable to read and speak English. From January 2014 to July 2015, a total of 79 participants were enrolled and followed for 12 months. For the purpose of this article, we considered the physical activity data (described below). Details of enrollment, participant characteristics, and other association studies of stress level were previously reported [37]. Briefly, the data set for the present analysis consisted of 45 females and 34 males, with an overall mean age of 31.9 years (±9.5 years). In addition, we considered the following variables for association with physical activity: race/ethnicity (27 non-Hispanic whites vs. 52 others), education as an ordinal variable (13 having less than college vs. 34 completing college vs. 32 attaining graduate or professional degrees), employment status (64 full-time employed vs. 8 part-time), and partner status (32 having a partner or spouse vs. 45 being single).

2.2. Physical Activity

Physical activity was monitored continuously for up to 12 months using a wrist-worn Fitbit activity monitor (Fitbit Flex) [38]. The Fitbit device, containing an accelerometer and an altimeter, tracks the wearer's daily physical activity including steps, distance walked, and stairs climbed, and has been previously validated for measuring physical activity [39]. While the Fitbit devices (including the Fitbit Flex) have been demonstrated to have good validity for the objective measurement of physical activity, their accuracy has largely been reported for stepping-related physical activities (e.g., walking and running) [40]. Similar to other research-grade accelerometers, the Fitbit devices have poor accuracy for the measurement of cycling [41,42]. Furthermore, Fitbit instructs users to not swim with the Fitbit Flex because it is not waterproof [43], thus rendering it unable to assess swimming-based exercise.

Data from the devices were automatically uploaded to the Fitbit website whenever the device was within 15 feet of the base station, which was plugged into the participant's own personal computer. Participants were instructed to sync and charge their device every 5–7 days to ensure no loss of activity data. The Fitbit accelerometer recorded data in one-minute epochs, starting at 12:00 a.m. and ending at 23:59 p.m. every day, yielding a time series of 1440 minute-epochs per day per individual. The raw minute-by-minute step count data were extracted from the manufacturer's website using Fitabase (Small Steps Labs, San Diego, CA, USA) and were reduced using a novel QCA, described in *Statistical Analyses* below. Specifically, the raw data that was relevant to the present article included the step counts over one-minute intervals with a timestamp; data for each participant was converted to an "RDATA" file each associated with a unique participant ID. Based on the raw data, we calculated other predefined physical activity measurements, including total daily step counts, the duration in minutes of physical activity (PA, defined as having at least 50 steps in a minute), and activity midday (defined as the time when 50% of daily step counts were achieved).

2.3. Statistical Analyses

2.3.1. Quantile Coarsening Analysis (QCA)

Let $Y(t)$ denote the step counts at time t and $S(t) = \int_0^t Y(u)du$ be the cumulative activity up to time t $\in (0,\ t_{max})$. Then

$$T(p)\inf\{t : S(t) \geq p\ S(t_{max})\} \tag{1}$$

denotes the time where $100p$ percent of the total activity has been achieved and will be referred to as the $100pth$ quantile of the activity time [44]. Specifically, activity midday is defined by the 50th quantile, $T(0.5)$. The idea of QCA is to represent a time series $Y(t)$ using multiple quantiles $T(p_j)$ for a prespecified set of $p_1 < p_2 < \ldots < p_K$, together with the total daily counts $S(t_{max})$. The number K of quantiles determines the number of components used to represent $Y(t)$, and hence controls the resolution or coarseness of the approximation. Define the Kth order quantile-coarse function of $Y(t)$ as

$$C_K Y(t) = \frac{S(t_{max})}{(K+1)\{T(p_{j+1}) - T(p_j)\}} \text{ for } T(p_j) \leq t < T(p_{j+1}) \tag{2}$$

for $j = 0, \ldots, K$, with the convention that $T(0) = 0$ and $T(1) = t_{max}$. While p_j can be any values between 0 and 1, we consider an evenly spaced grid, i.e., setting $p_j = j/(K+1)$ for $j = 1, \ldots, K$. It can be easily shown that the quantile-coarse function is invariant under the quantile transformation. That is to say, applying the quantile transformation to $C_K Y(t)$ will result in the same quantile representation as applying the transformation to the original $Y(t)$, i.e., $C_K\{C_K Y(t)\} = C_K Y(t)$. As a result, there is no loss in information by converting between coarsened data and quantiles back and forth for any given K.

Our data set consisted of a total of 21,393 days of minute-by-minute step counts from 79 study participants. For each daily time series, we evaluated the quantile-coarse function. The mean time series $\overline{Y}(t)$ of each cluster was then approximated by the corresponding mean quantile-coarse function $\overline{C_K Y}(t)$. We calculated the integrated mean squared error:

$$\int_0^{t_{max}} \{\overline{C_K Y}(t) - \overline{Y}(t)\}^2 dt \tag{3}$$

to assess the accuracy of the quantile coarsening method under various coarseness values K.

2.3.2. Cluster Analysis

We performed cluster analysis using MFMM with the quantile-coarse function $C_K Y(t)$ as input. Specifically, we considered $K = 19$ so that each time series $Y(t)$ was represented by a total of 20 features, namely, $T(0.05)$, $T(0.10)$, $T(0.15)$, ... , $T(0.95)$, and $S(t_{max})$. Note that although we did not use common features such as PA minutes as direct inputs of the cluster analysis, these features were implicitly incorporated as they could be approximated from a quantile-coarse function. The number of clusters was determined based on the Bayesian information criterion [45]. After the MFMM analysis, physical activity features of each cluster were described using means and standard deviations, along with the mean time series $\overline{Y}(t)$ of each cluster.

2.3.3. Association Studies

In order to identify important factors affecting a participant's physical activity behaviors in terms of the identified clusters, association between the cluster membership and participant characteristics was assessed using generalized linear mixed model (GLMM) with a logit link in a univariate manner, with an adjustment for a weekend/weekday random effect nested within a subject random effect. For comparison purposes, we also examined the association of step-count based clusters with participant characteristics using the same GLMM approach.

3. Results

3.1. Physical Activity Clusters by Multivariate Finite Mixture Modeling

The MFMM analysis found an eight-cluster solution among the 21,393 series. Table 1 reports some summary physical activity measures in each cluster. The clusters were organized according to the average daily step counts, which were in concordance with PA duration. The least active cluster (Cluster 1) on average completed just below 1000 steps a day with 7.3 min in PA; this subgroup of activity either depicted a very sedentary pattern or effectively identified inactivity due to non-wear. The most active group (Cluster 8) had about 10,000 counts on average with 73 min in PA. The next two most active clusters (Clusters 6 and 7) had similar activity level to Cluster 8 and were within 1000 steps daily on average. However, activity midday in these clusters, ranging from noon to 3:00 p.m., occurred earlier than that of Cluster 8. While not as inactive as Cluster 1, Clusters 2 and 3 had low PA level when compared to the higher clusters, with different activity midday. Clusters 4 and 5 represented days of intermediate PA level.

Table 1. Physical activity clusters by multivariate finite mixture modeling.

Cluster ID	1	2	3	4	5	6	7	8
N	409	1302	2285	2751	7819	1678	2326	2823
Daily step counts	961	6227	6855	8037	8999	9379	9396	10,038
Activity midday [a]	11:30 a.m.	1:00 p.m.	2:00 p.m.	3:30 p.m.	2:00 p.m.	Noon	3:00 p.m.	5:00 p.m.
PA minutes [b]	7.3	42.3	45.6	52.8	59.9	65.9	65.1	72.7
Weekend [c]	37%	40%	39%	35%	16%	46%	30%	23%

[a] Time of day when 50% of daily counts were achieved; time was rounded to nearest half-hour. [b] Duration (in minutes) with ≥50 counts per minute. [c] Percent of time series in the cluster being on a weekend.

Figure 1 shows the mean activity curves of the clusters, and the superimposed cumulative activities of the clusters (lower right figure). These plots reveal additional cluster-defining features. Specifically, Cluster 2 was characterized by very early (i.e., late night) activity. Clusters 6 and 8 had peak activity averaged at around noon and 6:00 p.m. respectively, whereas Cluster 5 had multiple peaks throughout the day (at around 8:00 a.m., noon, and 5:00 p.m.).

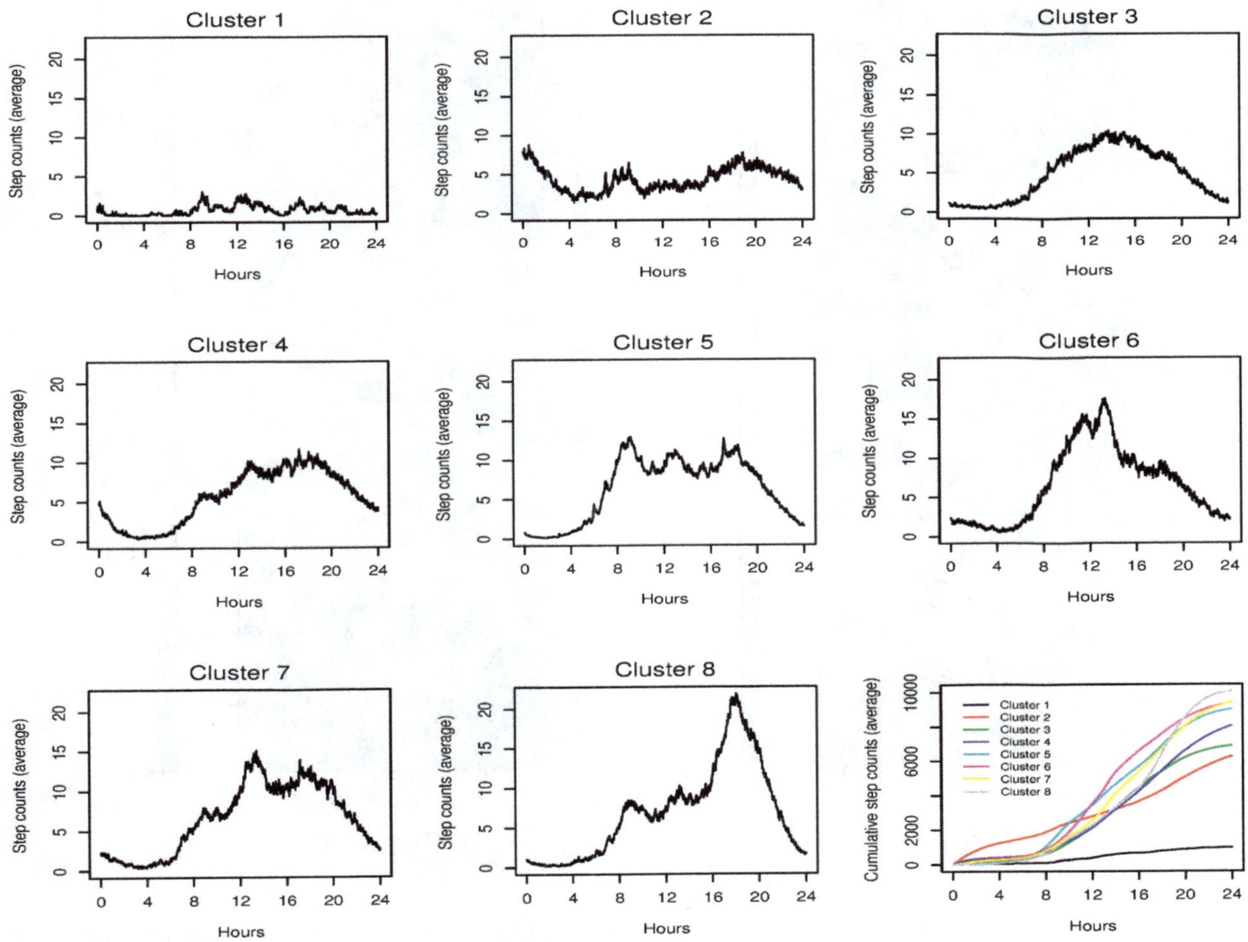

Figure 1. Mean activity of the 8 physical activity clusters by multivariate finite mixture modeling. Lower right: Superimposed cumulative step counts of the 8 clusters.

3.2. *Activity Patterns and the Weekends*

Table 1 also shows the proportion of daily activity falling on a weekend for each cluster, and demonstrates a range across the eight groups with ≥40% of time series in Clusters 2 and 6 occurring on a weekend, and 16% in Cluster 5 being on a weekend. Generally, it is also noted that the time series in the inactive clusters (Clusters 1–3) tended to fall on weekends.

Figure 2 further shows the PA patterns of the 79 participants were very different on weekdays and on weekends, with Cluster 5 being clearly a weekday phenomenon in most participants. It was consistent with the fact that Cluster 5 was characterized by spikes in activity around morning commute, lunch, and evening commute (Figure 1). At the same time, the heatmaps showed variations among the participants and that some did not follow this weekday/weekend differential (e.g., Participants 11 and 16). In addition, the PA patterns on the weekends were more dispersed than those on the weekdays, suggesting weekend activities were less structured and more heterogenous across participants.

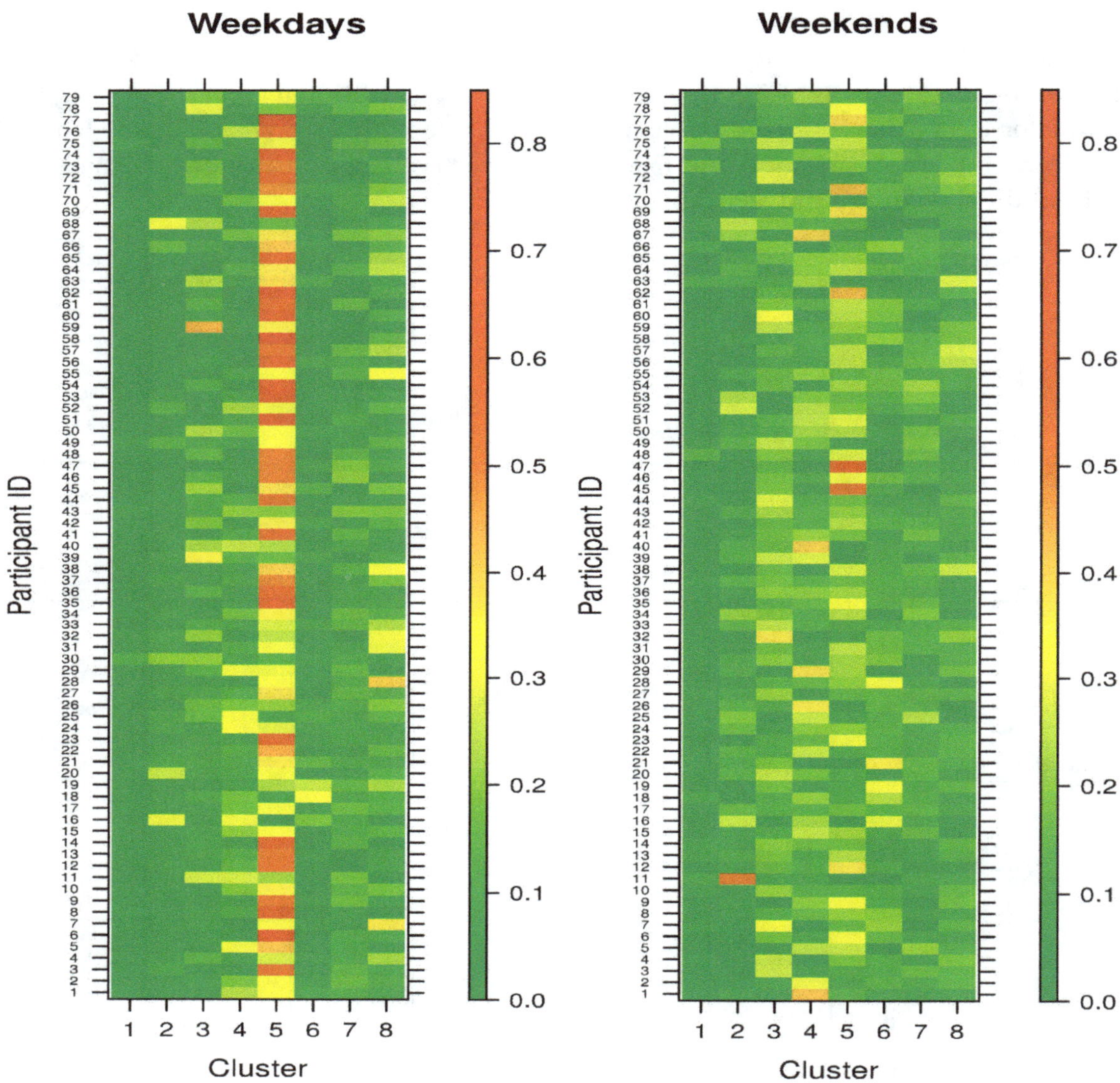

Figure 2. Heatmap of activity patterns of the 79 participants on weekdays and weekends. The color code indicates the proportion of days that a participant fell into each activity cluster.

3.3. Physical Activity Clusters and Participant Characteristics

Table 2 gives the association between each cluster and participant characteristics, in terms of odds ratio of falling into one activity cluster vs. the others using GLMM. In this cohort, employment and partner statuses were the most influential predictors of activity, each associated with 5 PA clusters. Specifically, Cluster 5 was highly significantly ($p < 0.01$) associated with being full-time employed and having a partner/spouse. Interestingly, the association between Cluster 5 and employment status was significant after adjusting for the weekend/weekday effect, suggesting that employment had a structural impact on an individual's behaviors and habits beyond the physical constraint it has during a workweek.

In contrast, Clusters 2 and 4, both having very early activity (Figure 1), were associated with singles with part-time jobs; having a younger age and receiving less education were also associated with these two clusters.

To a lesser extent, race/ethnicity was also predictive of an individual's activity behaviors. Specifically, non-Hispanic whites were more likely to engage in physical activities consistent with Clusters 5 and 8, and less with Cluster 2. Finally, it is interesting to note that the inactive cluster (Cluster 1) was not associated with any particular characteristics.

Table 2. Association (odds ratio) of physical activity clusters and participant characteristics.

Cluster ID	1	2	3	4	5	6	7	8
Age [a]	0.99	0.96 ***	0.99	0.98 *	1.02 *	1.01	1.00	1.01
Male (ref: Female)	0.77	0.94	0.80	1.37	0.86	1.04	1.02	0.95
NHW [b] (ref: others)	0.65	0.60 *	0.80	0.85	1.35 *	1.04	0.91	1.23 *
Education [c]	1.02	0.66 **	1.01	0.75 *	1.15	1.17	0.91	1.11
Full-time (FT) (ref: Part-time, PT)	1.17	0.44 *	0.93	0.42 ***	3.49 ***	0.57 **	1.01	1.41 *
Being single (ref: Partner/spouse)	0.74	2.37 ***	0.76*	1.72 ***	0.65 **	1.02	1.19 *	0.85

[a] Odds ratio per one-year increase in age. [b] NHW: Non-hispanic white. [c] Education as an ordinal variable: 0 = less than college; 1 = college graduate; 2 = above college. * ≤0.05, ** ≤0.01, *** ≤0.001.

3.4. *Accuracy of Approximation*

Table 3 gives the integrated mean squared errors of the quantile-coarse function using different values of K for estimating the mean activity of the 8 patterns. Accuracy improves as the original function $\overline{Y}(t)$ is represented with a larger number K of quantiles, with the initial improvement being most substantial. With K = 19, the mean squared error was about 3% on average of the error when daily activity was summarized using only the total daily counts (K = 0).

Table 3. Integrated mean squared errors in estimating the mean activity of the eight clusters.

K	1	2	3	4	5	6	7	8
0 [a]	563	3191	15,674	16,106	22,800	32,004	26,226	47,884
3	224	1690	5189	3926	13,473	8631	7356	15,360
9	59	609	880	908	2763	1519	2132	3084
19	29	255	253	342	676	506	626	826
39	19	131	98	135	181	188	211	237

[a] = 0 corresponds to approximation using daily step counts only; activity is assumed to be uniform throughout the day.

4. Discussion

We have proposed a novel QCA for reducing dimension of data collected from wearable devices, and for representing data in conjunction with downstream analyses such as MFMM and association studies. The proposed method contributes to the analysis and management of wearable data in two ways. First, quantile transformation lends itself to making inferences about the time of activity, which could be useful in distinguishing individuals and days from a single individual with differing patterns of PA accrual. Using data from an intensive, 12-month observational study, we were able to identify 8 unique clusters (or subgroups) that characterized the various types of PA accrual patterns observed at the day-level and were able to link these clusters with participant characteristics that provided important contextual information regarding the observed patterns. For example, we observed a "worker" cluster (Cluster 5) associated with employment status wherein spikes in activity were observed around times of day that typically coincide with morning commute, lunch, and evening commute. We also observed active clusters that accrued much of the activity earlier or later in the day (Clusters 6–8), possibly reflective of morning or evening exercise. On the other hand, it is interesting to note that the most active pattern (Cluster 8) accumulates steps late in the day and is associated with full-time employment, suggesting these are intentional leisure-time physical activities. This is consistent with the literature that individuals who meet physical activity guidelines are those who engage in leisure-time physical activity [46]. In contrast, when we performed cluster analysis using total step counts only (i.e., not including time of activity as inputs), all but one cluster had an activity midday at 2:30 p.m. (Table 1). And as a result, we identified fewer and weaker association between the step-count based clusters and participant characteristics (Table 2); this analysis did provide nuances about the nature of activity, which in turn could be useful for developing applications of individualized intervention.

Second, QCA facilitates large-scale data reduction, as quantile transformation requires only simple and scalable computations. We have demonstrated the method in a dataset of 21,393 time series (over 30 million minute-by-minute counts) from 79 participants for up to 1-year follow-up as a proof of concept. In real-life situations where deployment of mobile sensors such as Fitbit can occur at a much larger scale for a much longer duration, the large data volume will be a practical issue for storage and analyses and for the deployment of edge computing [47]. In a typical application, data are transmitted from the devices and stored externally on a server or in a cloud platform for specific analyses. Quantile coarsening in this context can be used as a data pre-processing step to minimize the volume of data transmission, storage, and persistence demand. As the size of the wearable devices tends to be small, their computational capacity is often limited. As such, continuous sensing may pose challenges to existing multi-modal analysis techniques using wearable devices. Since quantile transformation is easy to implement and can be computed independently of data from other individuals, simple scripts can be written to execute on the edge devices as well as on the server level. Depending on the purpose of the analysis, the end-user can specify the level of resolution in terms of the number K of quantiles needed. Our analyses show that the mean quantile-coarse function provides good approximation of the original mean function with only 20 data points per day per individual, representing less than 2% of the original amount of data (1440 data points). In addition, at the deployment time, QCA can also be applied on the incoming streams of data to compare to pre-stored cluster characteristics identified from the cluster analysis. This can lend support to the implementation of many other dynamic, just-in-time adaptive interventions that are key to persuasive reminder and sustainable behavioral changes [48].

The high volume of step count data offers the opportunities to tailor behavior intervention of each individual in a highly personalized manner. Specifically, we have created an activity behavior signature for each individual over time (Figure 2), which can serve as the basis of adaptive intervention. For instance, we could adapt the "dose" and time of push notifications if there are indications that an individual deviate from his/her own norm. The use of signature is broadly applicable to other behavioral intervention system such as centralized recommenders of health apps [49–51]. To allow for such tailored intervention, it is important to acknowledge individual behaviors are not monolithic, but heterogeneous. It is therefore important to note that our analysis goal was to identify clusters of daily activity as building blocks of each signature, as opposed to identify clusters of individuals. While within-day metrics (such as intensity and regularity [52]) have been examined to reflect enrich the heterogeneity in between-day activities of each individual, these approaches typically are semi-quantitative and are intended for visualization.

In the present article, we have shown the feasibility of QCA in a small cohort of relatively healthy individuals. The study design and analytical methods can be easily deployed to other populations. For example, the Northern Manhattan Study aims to assess risk factors for stroke and cardiovascular diseases, and has examined and analyzed the physical activity patterns of the cohort based on paper questionnaires [3,29]. It would be an interesting next step to follow up on these individuals to monitor and assess their mobility issues using wearables, and to provide additional information (signature) that contributes to cardiovascular risks.

We applied QCA to step count data. The method however is applicable to other data variety and supports monitoring of biometrics (e.g., heart rate, ambulatory blood pressure, etc.), location (e.g., indoor/outdoor), behaviors (e.g., medication adherence), exogenous factors such as weather, and user-input data via ecological momentary assessment. There is a growing trend towards self-monitoring on a daily basis with goals such as tracking health status, ameliorating exacerbations of chronic conditions, and avoiding episodic hospitalization; see [53–57] for example. As such, wearables devices are well-suited for this new approach to patient care, provided that they are capable of handling complex analysis efficiently (resulting in smaller and lighter devices with longer battery life). At the same time, we acknowledge that accelerometers are not capable of capturing some of the more common forms of aerobic exercise. Research- and commercial-grade accelerometers such as those made by Fitbit have poor accuracy for the measurement of cycling and cannot be worn while swimming due to not being waterproof [41,42]. However, given the versatility of the QCA, it shall provide useful unified analytical tools for the high data variety in multi-modal monitoring as sensing technologies advance.

Author Contributions: Conceptualization, Y.K.C. and K.M.D.; Methodology & Formal analysis, Y.K.C.; Resources, Y.K.C. and K.M.D.; Writing—Original Draft, Y.K.C.; Writing—Review & Editing, Y.K.C., P.-Y.S.H., I.E., J.Z.W. and K.M.D.

References

1. World Health Organization. *Global Health Risks: Mortality and Burden of Disease Attributable to Selected Major Risks*; WHO Press: Geneva, Switzerland, 2009.
2. Garcia, M.C.; Bastian, B.; Rossen, L.M.; Anderson, R.; Minino, A.; Yoon, P.W.; Faul, M.; Massetti, G.; Thomas, C.C.; Hong, Y.; et al. *Potentially Preventable Deaths among the Five Leading Causes of Death—United States, 2010 and 2014*; Morbidity and Mortality Weekly Report (MMWR): Atlanta, GA, USA, 18 November 2016; Volume 65, pp. 1245–1255.
3. Cheung, Y.K.; Moon, Y.P.; Kulick, E.R.; Sacco, R.L.; Elkind, M.S.V.; Willey, J.Z. Leisure-time physical activity and cardiovascular mortality in an elderly population in northern Manhattan: A prospective cohort study. *J. Gen. Int. Med.* **2017**, *32*, 168–174. [CrossRef] [PubMed]
4. Diaz, K.M.; Howard, V.J.; Hutto, B.; Colabianchi, N.; Vena, J.E.; Safford, M.M.; Blair, S.N.; Hooker, S.P. Patterns of sedentary behavior and mortality in U.S. middle-aged and older adults. *Ann. Int. Med.* **2017**, *167*, 465–475. [CrossRef] [PubMed]
5. Motl, R.W. Theoretical models for understanding physical activity behavior among children and adolescents—Social cognitive theory and self-determination theory. *J. Teach. Phys. Edu.* **2007**, *26*, 350–357. [CrossRef]
6. Bravata, D.M.; Smith-Spangler, C.; Sundaram, V.; Gienger, A.L.; Lin, N.; Lewis, R.; Stave, C.D.; Olkin, I.; Sirard, J.R. Using pedometers to increase physical activity and improve health. *JAMA* **2007**, *298*, 2296–2304. [CrossRef] [PubMed]
7. Consolvo, S.; McDonald, D.W.; Toscos, T.; Chen, M.Y.; Froehlich, J.; Harrison, B.; Klasnja, P.; LaMarca, A.; LeGrand, L.; Libby, R.; et al. Activity sensing in the wild: A field trial of UbiFit Garden. In Proceedings of the the SIGCHI Conference on Human Factors in Computing Systems, Florence, Italy, 5–10 April 2008; ACM Press: New York, NY, USA, 2008. [CrossRef]
8. Lin, J.J.; Mamykina, L.; Lindtner, S.; Delajoux, G.; Strub, H.B. Fish'n'Steps: Encouraging physical activity with an interactive computer game. In Proceedings of the 8th international conference on Ubiquitous Computing, Orange County, CA, USA, 17–19 September 2006; Dourish, P., Friday, A., Eds.; Springer: Berlin/Heidelberg, Germany, 2006; Volume 4206, pp. 261–278. [CrossRef]
9. Miller, A.D.; Mynatt, E.D. A School-based Pervasive Social Fitness System for Everyday Adolescent Health. In Proceedings of the SIGCHI Conference on Human Factors in Computing Systems, Toronto, ON, Canada, 26 April–1 May 2014; ACM Press: New York, NY, USA, 2014; pp. 823–2832. [CrossRef]

10. Munson, S.; Consolvo, S. Exploring goal-setting, rewards, self-monitoring, and sharing to motivate physical activity. In Proceedings of the 6th International. Conference on Pervasive Computing Technologies for Healthcare, San Diego, CA, USA, 21–24 May 2012; pp. 25–32. [CrossRef]
11. Pillay, J.D.; van der Ploeg, H.P.; Kolbe-Alexander, T.L.; Proper, K.I.; van Stralen, M.M.; Tomaz, S.A.; van Mechelen, W.; Lambert, E.V. The association between daily steps and health, and the mediating role of body composition: A pedometer-based, cross-sectional study in an employed South African population. *BMC Publ. Health* **2005**, *15*, 174. [CrossRef] [PubMed]
12. Evenson, K.R.; Wen, F.; Furberg, R.D. Assessing Validity of the Fitbit Indicators for U.S. Public Health Surveillance. *Am. J. Prev. Med.* **2017**, *53*, 931–932. [CrossRef] [PubMed]
13. Wang, J.B.; Cadmus-Bertram, L.A.; Natarajan, L.; White, M.M.; Madanat, H.; Nichols, J.F.; Ayala, G.X.; Pierce, J.P. Wearable Sensor/Device (Fitbit One) and SMS Text-Messaging Prompts to Increase Physical Activity in Overweight and Obese Adults: A Randomized Controlled Trial. *Telemed. E-Health* **2015**, *21*, 782–792. [CrossRef] [PubMed]
14. Bentley, F.; Tollmar, K.; Stephenson, P.; Levy, L.; Jones, B.; Robertson, S.; Price, E.; Catrambone, R.; Wilson, J. Health Mashups: Presenting Statistical Patterns between Wellbeing Data and Context in Natural Language to Promote Behavior Change. *ACM Trans. Comput. Hum. Interact.* **2013**, *20*, 1–27. [CrossRef]
15. Yoon, S.; Schwartz, J.E.; Burg, M.M.; Kronish, I.M.; Alcantara, C.; Julian, J.; Parsons, F.; Davidson, K.W.; Diaz, K.M. Using Behavioral Analytics to Increase Exercise: A Randomized N-of-1 Study. *Am. J. Prev. Med.* **2018**, *54*, 559–567. [CrossRef] [PubMed]
16. Cadmus-Bertram, L.A.; Marcus, B.H.; Patterson, R.E.; Parker, B.A.; Morey, B.L. Randomized Trial of a Fitbit-Based Physical Activity Intervention for Women. *Am. J. Prev. Med.* **2015**, *49*, 414–418. [CrossRef] [PubMed]
17. Auffray, C.; Balling, R.; Barroso, I.; Bencze, L.; Benson, M.; Bergeron, J.; Bernal-Delgado, E.; Blomberg, N.; Bock, C.; Conesa, A. Making sense of big data in health research: Towards an EU action plan. *Genome Med.* **2016**, *8*, 71. [CrossRef] [PubMed]
18. Cheung, Y.; Hsueh, P.; Qian, M.; Yoon, S.; Meli, L.; Diaz, K.M.; Schwartz, J.E.; Kronish, I.M.; Davidson, K.W. Are nomothetic or ideographic approaches superior in predicting daily exercise behaviors? Analyzing N-of-1 mHealth data. *Methods Inf. Med.* **2017**, *56*, 452–460. [CrossRef] [PubMed]
19. Hsiao, M.; Hsueh, P.; Ramakrishnan, S. Personalized adherence activity recognition via model-driven sensor data assessment. *Stud. Health Technol. Inf.* **2012**, *180*, 1050–1054.
20. Kim, Y.; Welk, G.J.; Braun, S.I.; Kang, M. Extracting Objective Estimates of Sedentary Behavior from Accelerometer Data: Measurement Considerations for Surveillance and Research Applications. *PLoS ONE* **2015**, *10*, e0118078. [CrossRef] [PubMed]
21. Swan, M. The Quantified Self: Fundamental Disruption in Big Data Science and Biological Discovery. *Big Data* **2013**, *1*, 85–99. [CrossRef] [PubMed]
22. Dijkhuis, T.B.; Blaauw, F.J.; van Ittersum, M.W.; Velthuijsen, H.; Aiello, M. Personalized Physical Activity Coaching: A Machine Learning Approach. *Sensors* **2018**, *18*, 623. [CrossRef] [PubMed]
23. Du, H.; Venkatakrishnan, A.; Youngblood, G.M.; Ram, A.; Pirolli, P. A Group-Based Mobile Application to Increase Adherence in Exercise and Nutrition Programs: A Factorial Design Feasibility Study. *JMIR MHealth UHealth* **2016**, *4*, e4. [CrossRef] [PubMed]
24. Burg, M.M.; Schwartz, J.E.; Kronish, I.M.; Diaz, K.M.; Alcantara, C.; Duer-Hefele, J.; Davidson, K.W. Does Stress Result in You Exercising Less? Or Does Exercising Result in You Being Less Stressed? Or Is It Both? Testing the Bi-directional Stress-Exercise Association at the Group and Person (N of 1) Level. *Ann. Behav. Med.* **2017**, *51*, 799–809. [CrossRef] [PubMed]
25. Hartman, S.J.; Nelson, S.H.; Weiner, L.S. Patterns of Fitbit Use and Activity Levels Throughout a Physical Activity Intervention: Exploratory Analysis from a Randomized Controlled Trial. *JMIR MHealth UHealth* **2018**, *6*, e29. [CrossRef] [PubMed]
26. McLachlan, G.; Peel, D. *Finite Mixture Models*; John Wiley & Sons, Inc.: Hoboken, NJ, USA, 2005.
27. Hu, F.B.; Rimm, E.; Smith-Warner, S.A.; Feskanich, D.; Stampfer, M.J.; Ascherio, A.; Sampson, L.; Willett, W.C. Reproducibility and validity of dietary patterns assessed with a food-frequency questionnaire. *Am. J. Clin. Nutr.* **1999**, *69*, 243–249. [CrossRef] [PubMed]
28. Hu, F.B. Dietary pattern analysis: A new direction in nutritional epidemiology. *Curr. Opin. Lipidol.* **2002**, *13*, 3–9. [CrossRef] [PubMed]

29. Cheung, Y.K.; Yu, G.; Wall, M.M.; Sacco, R.L.; Elkind, M.S.V.; Willey, J.Z. Patterns of leisure-time physical activity using multivariate finite mixture modeling and cardiovascular risk factors in the Northern Manhattan Study. *Ann. Epidemiol.* **2015**, *25*, 469–474. [CrossRef] [PubMed]
30. Inaba, M.; Katoh, N.; Imai, H. Applications of weighted Voronoi diagrams and randomization to variance-based k-clustering. In Proceedings of the 10th ACM Symposium on Computational Geometry, Stony Brook, NY, USA, 6–9 June 1994; pp. 332–339. [CrossRef]
31. Fan, J.; Yao, Q. *Nonlinear Time Series: Nonparametric and Parametric Methods*; Springer: Berlin, Germany, 2003.
32. Fryzlewicz, P.; Oh, H.S. Thick pen transformation for time series. *J. R. Stat. Soc. Ser. B* **2011**, *73*, 499–529. [CrossRef]
33. Tsay, R.S. Some methods for analyzing big dependent data. *J. Bus. Econ. Stat.* **2016**, *34*, 673–688. [CrossRef]
34. Lim, Y.; Oh, H.S.; Cheung, Y.K. Functional clustering of accelerometer data via transformed input variables. Unpublished manuscript.
35. Box, G.E.P.; Jenkins, G.M.; Reinsel, G.C. *Time Series Analysis*; John Wiley & Sons, Inc.: Hoboken, NJ, USA, 2008.
36. Diaz, K. Ecological Link of Psychosocial Stress to Exercise: Personalized Pathways. Available online: https://osf.io/kmszn/ (accessed on 11 September 2018).
37. Burg, M.M.; Schwartz, J.E.; Kronish, I.M.; Diaz, K.M.; Alcantara, C.; Duer-Hefele, J.; Davidson, K.W. Does stress result in you exercising less? Or does exercising result in you being less stressed? Or it is both? Testing the bi-directional stress-exercise association at the group and person (n of 1) level. *Ann. Behav. Med.* **2017**, *51*, 799–809. [CrossRef] [PubMed]
38. Fitbit Flex. Available online: http://www.fitbit.com (accessed on 11 September 2018).
39. Diaz, K.; Krupka, D.J.; Chang, M.J.; Peacock, J.; Ma, Y.; Goldsmith, J.; Schwartz, J.E.; Davidson, K.W. Fitbit: An accurate and reliable device for wireless physical activity tracking. *Int. J. Cardiol.* **2015**, *185*, 138–140. [CrossRef] [PubMed]
40. Evenson, K.R.; Goto, M.M.; Furberg, R.D. Systematic review of the validity and reliability of consumer-wearable activity trackers. *Int. J. Behav. Nutr. Phys. Act.* **2015**, *12*, 159. [CrossRef] [PubMed]
41. Sasaki, J.E.; Hickey, A.; Mavilia, M.; Tedesco, J.; John, D.; Kozey Keadle, S.; Freedson, P.S. Validation of the Fitbit wireless activity tracker for prediction of energy expenditure. *J. Phys. Act. Health* **2015**, *12*, 149–154. [CrossRef] [PubMed]
42. Wallen, M.P.; Gomersall, S.R.; Keating, S.E.; Wisloff, U.; Coombers, J.S. Accuracy of heart rate watches: Implications for weight management. *PLoS ONE* **2016**, *11*, e0154420. [CrossRef] [PubMed]
43. Fitbit Flex. Available online: https://staticcs.fitbit.com/content/assets/help/manuals/manual_flex_en_US.pdf (accessed on 11 September 2018).
44. Koenker, R. *Quantile Regression (Econometric Society Monographs)*; Cambridge University Press: Cambridge, UK, 2005.
45. Fraley, C.; Raftery, A.E. How many clusters? Which clustering method? Answers via model based cluster analysis. *Comput. J.* **1998**, *41*, 578–589. [CrossRef]
46. Nang, E.E.K.; Khoo, E.Y.; Salim, A.; Tai, E.S.; Lee, J.; Van Dam, R.M. Patterns of physical activity in different domains and implications for intervention in a multi-ethnic Asian population: A cross-sectional study. *BMC Public Health* **2010**, *10*, 644.
47. Garcia Lopez, P.; Montresor, A.; Epema, D.; Datta, A.; Higashino, T.; Iamnitchi, A.; Barcellos, M.; Felber, P.; Riviere, E. Edge-centric computing: Vision and challenges. *ACM SIGCOMM Comput. Commun. Rev.* **2015**, *45*, 37–42. [CrossRef]
48. Klasnja, P.; Hekler, E.B.; Shiffman, S.; Boruvka, A.; Almirall, D.; Tewari, A.; Murphy, S.A. Microrandomized trials: An experimental design for developing just-in-time adaptive interventions. *Health Psychol.* **2015**, *34*, 1220–1228. [CrossRef] [PubMed]
49. Mohr, D.C.; Cheung, K.; Schueller, S.M.; Brown, C.H.; Duan, N. Continuous evaluation of evolving behavioral intervention technologies. *Am. J. Prev. Med.* **2013**, *45*, 517–523. [CrossRef] [PubMed]
50. Cheung, K.; Ling, W.; Karr, C.J.; Weingardt, K.; Schueller, S.M.; Mohr, D.C. Evaluation of a recommender app for apps for the treatment of depression and anxiety: An analysis of longitudinal user engagement. *J. Am. Med. Inf. Assoc.* **2018**, *25*, 955–962. [CrossRef] [PubMed]
51. Hu, X.; Hsueh, P.S.; Qian, M.; Chen, C.-H.; Diaz, K.M.; Cheung, Y.K. A First Step Towards Behavioral Coaching for Managing Stress: A Case Study on Optimal Policy Estimation with Multi-stage Threshold Q-learning. *AMIA Annu. Symp. Proc.* **2017**, *2017*, 930–939.

52. Marschollek, M. A semi-quantitative method to denote generic physical activity phenotypes from long-term accelerometer data—The ATLAS index. *PLoS ONE* **2013**, *8*, e63522. [CrossRef] [PubMed]
53. Rodriguez-Paras, C.; Tippey, K.; Brown, E.; Sasangohar, F.; Creech, S.; Kum, H.-C.; Lawley, M.; Benzer, J.K. Posttraumatic Stress Disorder and Mobile Health: App Investigation and Scoping Literature Review. *JMIR MHealth UHealth* **2017**, *5*, e156. [CrossRef] [PubMed]
54. Kiral-Kornek, I.; Roy, S.; Nurse, E.; Mashford, B.; Karoly, P.; Carroll, T.; Payne, D.; Saha, S.; Baldassano, S.; O'Brien, T.; et al. Epileptic Seizure Prediction Using Big Data and Deep Learning: Toward a Mobile System. *EBioMedicine* **2018**, *27*, 103–111. [CrossRef] [PubMed]
55. Garcia-Alamino, J.M.; Ward, A.M.; Alonso-Coello, P.; Perera, R.; Bankhead, C.; Fitzmaurice, D.; Heneghan, C.J. Self-monitoring and self-management of oral anticoagulation. *Cochrane Database Syst. Rev.* **2010**, *7*, CD003839. [CrossRef]
56. Roditi, D.; Robinson, M.E. The role of psychological interventions in the management of patients with chronic pain. *Psy. Res. Behav. Manag.* **2011**, *4*, 41–49. [CrossRef] [PubMed]
57. Wells, N.; Pasero, C.; McCaffery, M. Improving the Quality of Care Through Pain Assessment and Management. In *Patient Safety and Quality: An Evidence-Based Handbook for Nurses. Agency for Healthcare Research and Quality (US)*; NCBI: Bethesda, MD, USA, 2008. Available online: http://www.ncbi.nlm.nih.gov/pubmed/21328759 (accessed on 6 September 2018).

10

Allumo: Preprocessing and Calibration Software for Wearable Accelerometers Used in Posture Tracking

Alexis Fortin-Côté [1,2], Jean-Sébastien Roy [1,3], Laurent Bouyer [1,3], Philip Jackson [1,2] and Alexandre Campeau-Lecours [1,4,*]

1 Center for Interdisciplinary Research in Rehabilitation and Social Integration, Quebec City, QC G1M 2S8, Canada; alexis.fortin-cote.1@ulaval.ca (A.F.-C.); Jean-Sebastien.Roy@fmed.ulaval.ca (J.-S.R.); Laurent.Bouyer@rea.ulaval.ca (L.B.); Philip.Jackson@psy.ulaval.ca (P.J.)
2 School of Psychology, Université Laval, Quebec City, QC G1V 0A6, Canada
3 Department of Rehabilitation, Université Laval, Quebec City, QC G1V 0A6, Canada
4 Department of Mechanical Engineering, Université Laval, Quebec City, QC G1V 0A6, Canada
* Correspondence: Alexandre.Campeau-Lecours@gmc.ulaval.ca

Abstract: Inertial measurement units have recently shown great potential for the accurate measurement of joint angle movements in replacement of motion capture systems. In the race towards long duration tracking, inertial measurement units increasingly aim to ensure portability and long battery life, allowing improved ecological studies. Their main advantage over laboratory grade equipment is their usability in a wider range of environment for greater ecological value. For accurate and useful measurements, these types of sensors require a robust orientation estimation that remains accurate over long periods of time. To this end, we developed the Allumo software for the preprocessing and calibration of the orientation estimate of triaxial accelerometers. This software has an automatic orientation calibration procedure, an automatic erroneous orientation-estimate detection and useful visualization to help process long and short measurement periods. These automatic procedures are detailed in this paper, and two case studies are presented to showcase the usefulness of the software. The Allumo software is open-source and available online.

Keywords: accelerometer; calibration; inertial measurement units; human movement

---

1. Introduction

Wearable sensors are increasingly being used in research and clinical practice to assess the pose and posture of individuals. For instance, physical rehabilitation may require objective movement measurements over extended periods of time to perform a comprehensive assessment of the patient. Being able to obtain quantitative measurements outside of controlled environments, such as a laboratory, through the use of wearable sensors could help in the diagnosis and treatment of patients. For instance, stride parameters are measured through GPS and inertial measurement unit (IMU) data [1], as well as gait and posture analyzed from pressure-sensitive insoles and IMU data [2]. Navigation estimates using IMUs with [3] and without GPS [4] have also been studied. IMU sensors have proven to be effective in orientation estimation, such as trunk orientation and lower limb kinematics [5] and in measuring the shoulder joint angles [6]. Accelerometers can also be used for impact detection and gait timing [7–9]. They have also been used in harsher conditions such as swimming [10]. As the number of contexts using these types of sensors increases, so does the need to improve orientation estimation accuracy. A static accuracy assessment of the Xsens IMU sensors [11] for 3D orientation positioning has been published [12]. Validation of the Xsens movement measurement [13] reported good correlation (0.96) between Xsens movement and vision-based measurements. Further assessment of accuracy for joint rotation for field-based occupational studies [14] reported measurement errors varying from 4° to 12°. A recent systematic review reported that IMU should be considered as a valid tool to assess the whole body range of motion, and underlined the importance of the calibration step [15] to obtain such levels of accuracy.

Indeed, calibration is an important step to capture accurate pose estimates, especially for joint angle measurement [16]. The published procedure for pose calibration to align an IMU to another motion-capture system, which is presented in [17], and a pose calibration procedure for 3D knee joint angle [18]. Furthermore, Lotter et al. [19] published a procedure for in-use calibration of triaxial accelerometers that shares similarities with our proposed automatic orientation estimation algorithm, such as relying on the fact that the magnitude of the gravity acceleration vector measured with the accelerometer is constant and equals to 1g under quasi-static conditions. They use those assumptions to calibrate the tension readings of the triaxial acceleration (an offset and scaling for each axis). In our proposed automatic orientation algorithm, the same assumptions are leveraged to determine the orientation of the accelerometer reference frame with respect to the fixed, world reference frame. A review of several calibration methods of the former style for motion analysis is available in [20].

In the context of a project to collect mobility data, an important challenge occurs during the assessment of IMU data obtained in the field. Indeed, while the typical use case is a relatively short acquisition duration (minutes to hours long), larger scale mobility projects aim to record data over long periods of time. Corresponding time series data sets are thus quite large and require a tedious and time-consuming manual preprocessing task, during which the accuracy of the pose estimate can decrease. This concern was also raised in [21]. In mobility data, file duration can span over several weeks of continuous recording at 60 Hz (three data channels per accelerometer). While this data file size may not be considered large in a big data context, the amount of manual preprocessing required using the existing commercial tools precludes them from being used at the scale required for many projects. As participants remove and install the equipment, a manual recalibration of the orientation estimate of the devices is required and can be difficult in the field. Whereas some analyses such as automatic activity recognition does not require a known orientation [22], posture monitoring does, and therefore requires this recalibration step. Manual adjustments of the orientation estimate using only the data stream and without direct monitoring from an external observer in the field are impracticable. Furthermore, uncontrolled events such as unwanted shifts of the sensor on the participant may result in erroneous readings stemming from an inaccurate calibration. These also require identification and a subsequent sensor recalibration, which is also manually impracticable using the raw data stream. Identifying such erroneous readings is difficult with the available commercial tools, as they tend to only present time series plots of the data, a counter-intuitive method for detecting erroneous orientation estimate by most observers.

To help in the calibration of the orientation estimate of IMUs used for joint angle measurement, we present a tool for visualization and preprocessing to be used in human posture monitoring and assessment. The development goal of the software presented here was to expedite the identification and recalibration of the orientation estimate of triaxial accelerometer readings by showing an intuitive graphical interface to the observer. An animated humanoid avatar illustrates the estimated posture of the participant along the data stream. It makes it easier to identify erroneous orientation estimates since abnormal postures of the body will be displayed (e.g., wrong limb orientation, walking at a skewed angle).

This paper is structured as follows: first is the presentation and description of the automatic calibration of the orientation estimate, erroneous orientation-estimate detection and activity detection algorithms; second is an overview of the software followed by two case studies to show typical usage of the software.

2. Software Overview

The main software, of which the interface in presented in Figure 1, boasts several features useful for the preprocessing and assessment of IMU data. It features a real-time playback visualization of a humanoid model for easy diagnostics of improbable orientation estimate or wrongly positioned sensors. It helps to identify potential problems by displaying captured motion on an avatar model. For instance, a mis estimated orientation measurement could show a skewed trunk angle or unrealistic leg movement. It can also display a matching video to help with the visual comparison of the movement. Options in the settings are available to synchronize the video playback with the animated human shape motion. There is also a live display of the variables of interest, such as torso and leg joint angles, with respect to the vertical axis. For long duration data acquisitions, the software provides convenient time selection features that allow the definition of a specific working window.

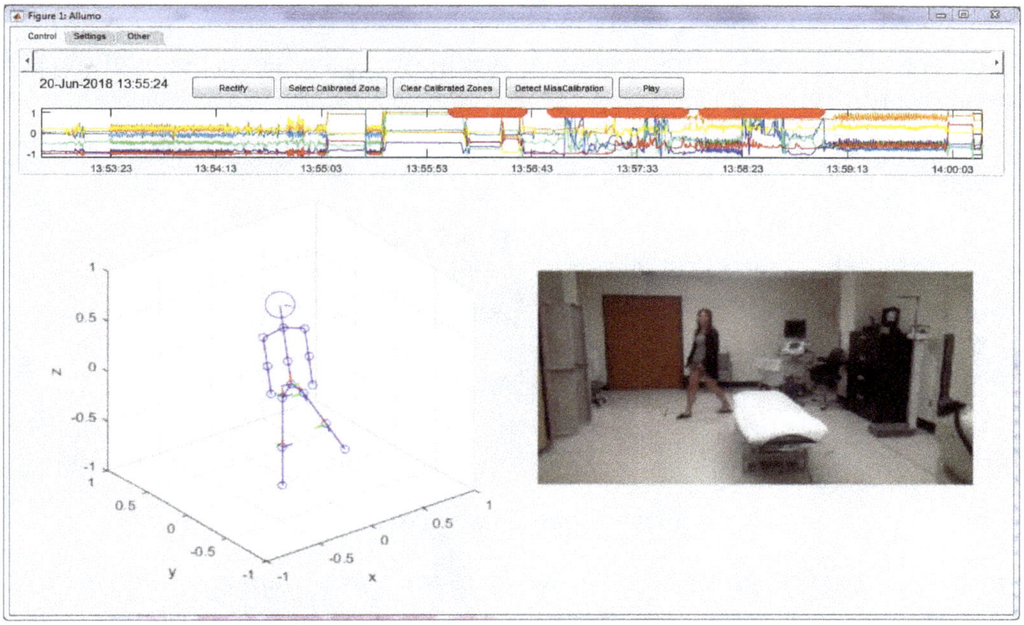

Figure 1. Main interface of the software.

The software also features an interface for manual selection of reference positions that is useful for the initialization of the orientation estimate of short recordings when reference points (neutral position) are known, e.g., a recording that begins with still sensors positioned in a known orientation. To improve the accuracy of the reference point measure, a section (window) of the signal can be marked as the reference orientation so that an averaging can be performed to reduce measurement noise during the reference position in the recording. To further help with this task, an algorithm, used for the automatic detection of erroneous orientation estimates, was implemented and is described in Section 4. Since manual adjustment of the initial orientation estimate can be complex and time-consuming, one of the software's main features is the automatic calibration of the sensor initial orientation through automatic detection of motionless neutral positions (quasi-static), based on filtering and singular value decomposition, all of which are further described in Section 3. A basic automatic activity detection feature, used to distinguish between idling, walking and running, is also available.

Lastly, the software allows the importation of raw accelerometer values from multiple file formats such as Actigraph GT3x, comma-separated values (csv) files, and Excel spreadsheets. It allows the exportation of the calibrated accelerometer values to a convenient csv or Excel file format for uploading to most analytics programs.

3. Automatic Calibration Algorithm

We define the calibration of the orientation estimate of the triaxial accelerometer as "identifying the rotation matrix that aligns the mobile reference frame originating at the accelerometer with the fixed (world) reference frame". In other words, the orientation of the mobile reference frame $\mathscr{R}$, with respect to the fixed reference frame $\mathscr{F}$, is defined by the rotation matrix $\mathbf{R}$ as seen in Figure 2. This therefore defines the three rotational degrees of freedom (DOF) of the accelerometer. This allows for the full orientation of an arbitrarily placed sensor to be estimated. To this end, the automatic calibration algorithm leverages the gravitational force $\mathbf{g}$, which is constant in the fixed reference frame, to constrain two of the three DOF, and a variance analysis to constrain the third DOF, fully defining the matrix $\mathbf{R}$. The measured acceleration matrix is defined as

$$\mathbf{A} = \begin{bmatrix} a_{x1} & a_{y1} & a_{z1} \\ \vdots & \vdots & \vdots \\ a_{xm} & a_{ym} & a_{zm} \end{bmatrix} \in \mathbb{R}^{m\times 3}, \tag{1}$$

where a_{xi}, a_{yi}, a_{zi}, are the ith measurements along the $x_{\mathcal{R}}, y_{\mathcal{R}}, z_{\mathcal{R}}$ axes respectively, and m is the index of the last measurement.

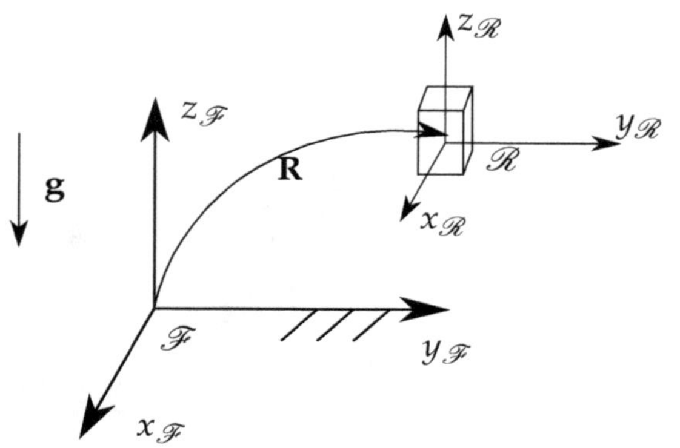

Figure 2. Geometric representation of the accelerometer.

The automatic calibration algorithm works by using three main assumptions. First, when the participant is at rest, he/she is in the neutral position most of the time (e.g., standing upright). Second, the gravity vector can be measured without bias most of the time, meaning that no steady state acceleration should be present outside of gravity, i.e., the system is not in free fall or under centrifugal acceleration. Third, most of the variance in the movement occurs in the plane that is parallel to the gravitational force and in the forward-facing direction $x_{\mathcal{F}}$ (e.g., walking). If these conditions are not met, a manual assisted option is available (see Section 4).

When those assumptions are observed, the algorithm works as follows. The first step is to find the direction of the gravitational force acting on the sensor. To this end, raw accelerometer data are filtered with a bidirectional low-pass filter with a cutoff frequency (COF) of 1/10 Hz to remove impacts, high-frequency noise and human limb movements to keep only low-frequency signals indicative of a steady state acceleration, which should correspond to a large extent to the neutral position. To accurately identify the direction of the gravity vector, the only data points kept for averaging are those where no movement is perceived (quasi-static). Those data points are found using a high-pass filter with the same COF of 1/10 Hz, filtering over the acceleration vector magnitude (l2 norm) instead of over each component, to identify where the signal lies closer to zero. A 2-s Hann window filter is used to further smooth the acceleration magnitude signal and keep only substantially long periods of quasi-static movements. The gravitational acceleration direction is then averaged across these sections with low movements. Knowing the unit vector $\hat{\mathbf{g}}$, which represents the direction of the measured gravitational acceleration, a matrix $\mathbf{R}'$ such as

$$\mathbf{g} = \mathbf{R}'\hat{\mathbf{g}}, \tag{2}$$

that aligns the $z_{\mathcal{R}}$ axis to the $z_{\mathcal{F}}$ axis can be derived, therefore establishing two DOFs. To establish the last DOF, raw acceleration measurements are transformed with matrix $\mathbf{R}'$ so that the measured gravitational acceleration aligns with the negative $z_{\mathcal{F}}$ direction, leaving acceleration on the $x_{\mathcal{R}}, y_{\mathcal{R}}$ planes as the only result of the accelerometer motion. The principal axis of motion is then computed using singular-value decomposition of the acceleration matrix $\mathbf{A}$ to find the largest singular value, σ_1, and its corresponding singular vector, $\mathbf{v}_1$, such as

$$\mathbf{A} = \mathbf{U}\boldsymbol{\Sigma}\mathbf{V}, \tag{3}$$

with $\mathbf{U} \in \mathbb{R}^{m\times m}$, containing the left-singular vectors, $\boldsymbol{\Sigma} \in \mathbb{R}^{m\times 3}$ containing the singular values $\sigma_1 \ldots \sigma_3$ and $\mathbf{V} \in \mathbb{R}^{3\times 3}$ containing the right-singular vectors including the vector of interest $\mathbf{v}_1$. The singular vector $\mathbf{v}_1$, which corresponds to the largest singular value, σ_1, is considered to be the forward-facing direction and therefore allows to establish the last DOF which, in turn, allows the full computation of $\mathbf{R}$. Note that since the direction of the singular vector can be positive or negative, this leaves the distinction between forward and backward undefined, and is thus a known shortcoming of the method that needs to be corrected manually.

4. Automatic Erroneous-Orientation Detection

When the automatic orientation estimation calibration cannot be used (assumption not met), the automatic erroneous orientation-estimate detection provides an alternative assisted orientation estimation calibration option. It is based on the same assumption as the automatic calibration algorithm, but is only used as a tool for the detection of periods when manual orientation adjustment is necessary. The user can then manually discriminate between erroneous orientation estimates and other movements that may trigger the erroneous orientation-estimate detection, such as lying down for a long period of time. The algorithm operates by checking whether the gravitational acceleration aligns correctly with the negative $z_{\mathscr{F}}$ direction. Using a bidirectional low-pass filter, it isolates the gravitational measurement, as described in Section 3, and flags sections of the accelerometer measurements in which the angle between the measured direction of gravity and the $z_{\mathscr{F}}$ direction is larger than a user-defined threshold value. This way, the algorithm can help detect whether or not a sensor has moved since the last adjustment. A visual cue is presented to the user so that he/she can act on the flagged section by manually adding reference orientation point as presented in Section 2, or removing the section altogether.

5. Activity Detection

A basic activity detection algorithm is implemented in the software. It differentiates between three different states: idling, walking or running. Again, using a low-pass filter followed by a Hann window filter over the acceleration vector magnitude (l2 norm) generates an activity intensity signal. By using simple threshold values, the discrimination between idling, walking and running can be achieved.

6. Case Studies

6.1. Demonstration in the Laboratory

A participant wearing two Actigraph GT3X accelerometers, one placed on the left thigh and the other on his back, was asked to perform a 15-min routine with a mix of standing, walking, running and lying down. The activity was captured on video to qualitatively assess the pose estimates of reported by the software. During the routine, the orientation of the sensors on the body was deliberately altered at three different times to test the algorithm's erroneous orientation-estimate detection. This resulted in 5 sections of signal being flagged using the erroneous orientation-estimate detection tool. The three deliberate orientation change and both time the participant lay down for an extended period of time had been correctly flagged. Using the playback of the humanoid visualization, the user can easily identify whether the detection is caused by an erroneous orientation estimate or a real change in steady-state operation such as going from a standing vertical to a horizontal orientation. This demonstration showed good performance in correctly identifying miscalibrated orientation estimates and was able to process the signal by applying the correct orientation adjustment parameters during each segment. With the correct adjustment applied, the user can look at the avatar and easily distinguish certain movements performed by the participant such as sitting, crouching and lying down. The activity detection algorithm was also able to correctly identify the two running events, the six walking events and the corresponding idling sequences between those.

6.2. Demonstration in the Field

In this data collection, the software has been used in the analysis of data from two expeditions lasting 39 and 32 days, respectively. During those expeditions, two participants wore two Actigraph GT3X accelerometers; one of the accelerometers was placed on the pelvis and the other on the left thigh. Both were affixed on shorts so that they moved along with the body. Data acquisition was performed over the 71 days for a total of around 1700 h of recording. Participants wore the sensors for the major part of the days and removed them during most sleep hours. Manual initialization of the orientation estimate for those types of extended periods is impractical. The automatic calibration algorithm was therefore used for each day of acquisition. After automatic calibration is performed, relevant data can be extracted, such as the amount of time walking or running and the trunk angle. The calibrated accelerometer's data can then be exported for further processing. Table 1 shows an example of which data can be obtained for 1 hour segments of a day of recording and the corresponding logbook entries. By comparing the ratio of walking and running detection to corresponding entries, an overall assessment of the activity detection can be made. It can be seen that high trunk angle correlates with nap time and that running detection correlates with high-intensity activities. Walking proportion also varies sensibly with reported activities.

Table 1. Data summary samples for a 1-h expedition segment.

	Walking	Running	Trunk Angle	Logbook Entry
segment 1	7.40%	0.19%	6.28°	Jumping jacks as a warm-up following by work at the computer
segment 2	7.20%	0.00%	71.21°	Lying down for 50 min
segment 3	4.42%	0.00%	3.53°	Work at the computer (mostly siting)
segment 4	12.78%	35.84%	10.61°	30 min jogging followed by work at the laboratory
segment 5	6.89%	0.00%	83.14°	50 min nap (lying down)
segment 6	17.08%	0.83%	6.17°	Helicopter outing and walk ashore
segment 7	9.87%	0.02%	5.47°	Diner and relaxation on board

7. Conclusions

This paper presented a graphical software for preprocessing raw accelerometer data in the context of posture tracking. The software allows the visualization of measured posture on a humanoid form to easily identify errors in measurements or in the orientation estimate of the device in long duration, in the field, experiment. The paper also presented a novel algorithm for automatic calibration of the orientation estimate that can be used when manual initialization of the orientation estimate is impractical. A simple erroneous orientation-estimate detection and basic activity detection algorithms are implemented in the software. Two case studies were used to show typical usage of the software. The software is open-source and available at https://github.com/alexisfcote/allumo.

Author Contributions: Conceptualization, A.F.-C.; Data curation, A.F.-C.; Software, A.F.-C.; Supervision, L.B., P.J. and A.C.-L.;Writing—original draft, A.F.-C.;Writing—review & editing, A.F.-C., J.-S.R., L.B., P.J. and A.C.-L. All authors have read and agreed to the published version of the manuscript.

References

1. Tan, H.; Wilson, A.M.; Lowe, J. Measurement of stride parameters using a wearable GPS and inertial measurement unit. *J. Biomech.* **2008**, *41*, 1398–1406. [CrossRef] [PubMed]
2. Benocci, M.; Rocchi, L.; Farella, E.; Chiari, L.; Benini, L. A wireless system for gait and posture analysis based on pressure insoles and Inertial Measurement Units. In Proceedings of the 2009 3rd International Conference on Pervasive Computing Technologies for Healthcare, London, UK, 1–3 April 2009; pp. 1–6. [CrossRef]
3. Brodie, M.; Walmsley, A.; Page, W. Fusion motion capture: A prototype system using inertial measurement units and GPS for the biomechanical analysis of ski racing. *Sports Technol.* **2008**, *1*, 17–28. . [CrossRef]
4. Bebek, O.; Suster, M.A.; Rajgopal, S.; Fu, M.J.; Huang, X.; Cavusoglu, M.C.; Young, D.J.; Mehregany, M.; van den Bogert, A.J.; Mastrangelo, C.H. Personal Navigation via High-Resolution Gait-Corrected Inertial Measurement Units. *IEEE Trans. Instrum. Meas.* **2010**, *59*, 3018–3027. [CrossRef]
5. Bonnet, V.; Mazzà, C.; Fraisse, P.; Cappozzo, A. Real-time Estimate of Body Kinematics During a Planar Squat Task Using a Single Inertial Measurement Unit. *IEEE Trans. Biomed. Eng.* **2013**, *60*, 1920–1926. [CrossRef] [PubMed]
6. Poitras, I.; Bielmann, M.; Campeau-Lecours, A.; Mercier, C.; Bouyer, L.J.; Roy, J.S. Validity of Wearable Sensors at the Shoulder Joint: Combining Wireless Electromyography Sensors and Inertial Measurement Units to Perform Physical Workplace Assessments. *Sensors* **2019**, *19*, 1885. [CrossRef] [PubMed]
7. Peruzzi, A.; Croce, U.D.; Cereatti, A. Estimation of stride length in level walking using an inertial measurement unit attached to the foot: A validation of the zero velocity assumption during stance. *J. Biomech.* **2011**, *44*, 1991–1994. [CrossRef] [PubMed]
8. Bergamini, E.; Picerno, P.; Pillet, H.; Natta, F.; Thoreux, P.; Camomilla, V. Estimation of temporal parameters during sprint running using a trunk-mounted inertial measurement unit. *J. Biomech.* **2012**, *45*, 1123–1126. [CrossRef] [PubMed]
9. Bergamini, E.; Guillon, P.; Camomilla, V.; Pillet, H.; Skalli, W.; Cappozzo, A. Trunk Inclination Estimate During the Sprint Start Using an Inertial Measurement Unit: A Validation Study. *J. Appl. Biomech.* **2013**, *29*, 622–627. [CrossRef] [PubMed]
10. Dadashi, F.; Millet, G.; Aminian, K. Inertial measurement unit and biomechanical analysis of swimming: An update. *Swiss Soc. Sports Med.* **2013**, *61*, 21–26,
11. Roetenberg, D.; Luinge, H.; Slycke, P. *Xsens MVN: Full 6DOF Human Motion Tracking Using Miniature Inertial Sensors*; Xsens Technologies: Enschede, The Netherlands, 2009; pp. 1–7.
12. Brodie, M.; Walmsley, A.; Page, W. The static accuracy and calibration of inertial measurement units for 3D orientation. *Comput. Methods Biomech. Biomed. Eng.* **2008**, *11*, 641–648. [CrossRef] [PubMed]
13. Zhang, J.T.; Novak, A.C.; Brouwer, B.; Li, Q. Concurrent validation of Xsens MVN measurement of lower limb joint angular kinematics. *Physiol. Meas.* **2013**, *34*, N63–N69. [CrossRef] [PubMed]
14. Schal, M.C., Jr.; Fethke, N.B.; Chen, H.; Oyama, S.; Douphrate, D.I. Accuracy and repeatability of an inertial measurement unit system for field-based occupational studies. *Ergonomics* **2016**, *59*, 591–602. [CrossRef] [PubMed]
15. Poitras, I.; Dupuis, F.; Bielmann, M.; Campeau-Lecours, A.; Mercier, C.; Bouyer, L.J.; Roy, J.S. Validity and Reliability of Wearable Sensors for Joint Angle Estimation: A Systematic Review. *Sensors* **2019**, *19*, 1555. [CrossRef] [PubMed]
16. Luinge, H.; Veltink, P.; Baten, C. Ambulatory measurement of arm orientation. *J. Biomech.* **2007**, *40*, 78–85. [CrossRef] [PubMed]
17. Chardonnens, J.; Favre, J.; Aminian, K. An effortless procedure to align the local frame of an inertial measurement unit to the local frame of another motion capture system. *J. Biomech.* **2012**, *45*, 2297–2300. [CrossRef] [PubMed]
18. Favre, J.; Aissaoui, R.; Jolles, B.; de Guise, J.; Aminian, K. Functional calibration procedure for 3D knee joint angle description using inertial sensors. *J. Biomech.* **2009**, *42*, 2330–2335. [CrossRef] [PubMed]
19. Lötters, J.; Schipper, J.; Veltink, P.; Olthuis, W.; Bergveld, P. Procedure for in-use calibration of triaxial accelerometers in medical applications. *Sens. Actuators A Phys.* **1998**, *68*, 221–228. [CrossRef]
20. Nez, A.; Fradet, L.; Laguillaumie, P.; Monnet, T.; Lacouture, P. Comparison of calibration methods for accelerometers used in human motion analysis. *Med. Eng. Phys.* **2016**, *38*, 1289–1299. [CrossRef] [PubMed]

21. Cheung, Y.; Hsueh, P.Y.; Ensari, I.; Willey, J.; Diaz, K. Quantile Coarsening Analysis of High-Volume Wearable Activity Data in a Longitudinal Observational Study. *Sensors* **2018**, *18*, 3056. [CrossRef] [PubMed]
22. Yurtman, A.; Barshan, B.; Fidan, B. Activity Recognition Invariant to Wearable Sensor Unit Orientation Using Differential Rotational Transformations Represented by Quaternions. *Sensors* **2018**, *18*, 2725. [CrossRef] [PubMed]

11

Methods for the Real-World Evaluation of Fall Detection Technology

Robert W. Broadley, Jochen Klenk, Sibylle B. Thies, Laurence P. J. Kenney and Malcolm H. Granat

1 School of Health Sciences, University of Salford, Salford, M6 6PU, UK; s.thies@salford.ac.uk (S.B.T.); l.p.j.kenney@salford.ac.uk (L.P.J.K.); m.h.granat@salford.ac.uk (M.H.G.)

2 Department of Clinical Gerontology, Robert-Bosch-Hospital, 70376 Stuttgart, Germany; jochen.klenk@rbk.de

3 Institute of Epidemiology and Medical Biometry, Ulm University, 89081 Ulm, Germany

* Correspondence: r.broadley@edu.salford.ac.uk

Abstract: Falls in older adults present a major growing healthcare challenge and reliable detection of falls is crucial to minimise their consequences. The majority of development and testing has used laboratory simulations. As simulations do not cover the wide range of real-world scenarios performance is poor when retested using real-world data. There has been a move from the use of simulated falls towards the use of real-world data. This review aims to assess the current methods for real-world evaluation of fall detection systems, identify their limitations and propose improved robust methods of evaluation. Twenty-two articles met the inclusion criteria and were assessed with regard to the composition of the datasets, data processing methods and the measures of performance. Real-world tests of fall detection technology are inherently challenging and it is clear the field is in its infancy. Most studies used small datasets and studies differed on how to quantify the ability to avoid false alarms and how to identify non-falls, a concept which is virtually impossible to define and standardise. To increase robustness and make results comparable, larger standardised datasets are needed containing data from a range of participant groups. Measures that depend on the definition and identification of non-falls should be avoided. Sensitivity, precision and F-measure emerged as the most suitable robust measures for evaluating the real-world performance of fall detection systems.

Keywords: accidental falls; fall detection; real-world; signal analysis; performance measures; wearable sensors; non-wearable sensors; accelerometers; cameras

---

1. Introduction

Falls in older adults and their related consequences pose a major healthcare challenge that is set to grow over the coming decades [1]. Approximately 30 percent of those over the age of 65 experience one or more falls each year, which rises to around 45 percent in those over 80 [2]. Roughly six percent of older adult falls result in fractured bones [3,4]. Falls are estimated to cost the UK over one billion pounds each year, with fractures being the most costly fall related injury [5].

Even when the injuries are not so serious, fallers often struggle to get up unaided [6,7], sometimes leading to a 'long-lie' where the faller remains trapped on the floor for an extended period of time. Long-lies can lead to dehydration, pressure sores, pneumonia, hypothermia and death [8–11]. Further to the physical consequences, the fear of falling can impact on older adults' quality of life. A fear of falling is associated with a decline in physical and mental health, and an increased risk of falling [12]. Estimates suggest that between 25 and 50 percent of older adults are fearful of falling and half of these will limit their activities as a result [13,14].

One method used to address the severe consequences associated with falling is the use of a push button alarm system, which can ensure help is received quickly, and reduce the risk of a long-lie. However, studies have shown that 80 percent of fallers do not or cannot activate their alarm following a fall, meaning an alternative approach is needed [6,15]. As a result, there has been extensive research into automatic detection of falls and a broad range of approaches have been developed.

In order to understand the efficacy of the automated fall detection systems, it is important to have a robust method of testing performance. Key to the assessment of these systems is the evaluation of reproducibility and experimental validity [16]. There are two types of experimental validity: internal and external. Internal validity is the extent to which the results truly reflect the capability of the tested system, and were not influenced by other confounding factors or systematic errors. External validity is the extent to which the results can be generalised across people and environments.

External validity has been a central issue in tests of fall detection systems. The poor external validity has been caused by the use of laboratory simulated falls conducted by young healthy adults. The accidental, unexpected and uncontrolled nature of a fall makes it challenging to simulate. When a person simulates a fall the movement is expected, deliberate and carried out in a safe space where injury is highly unlikely. Therefore, reflexes to prevent or lessen the severity of the fall are likely to be suppressed leading to a different pattern of movement. When 13 previously published approaches were tested using real-world fall data, the performance was found to be considerably worse (mean sensitivity and specificity of 0.57 and 0.83, respectively) than had originally been reported from testing using simulations (mean sensitivity and specificity of 0.91 and 0.99, respectively) [17].

Despite the challenge associated with simulating falls, the vast majority of studies have used simulated fall data (for recent reviews see [18,19]). The use of laboratory simulated falls has been an accepted approach due to the challenge associated with recording real-world falls. The rarity of falls means that recording them is both costly and time consuming. Bagala et al. [17] estimated that to collect 100 falls, 100,000 days of activity would need to be recorded, assuming a fall incidence of one fall per person every three years. Despite this challenge, the focus is now moving to real-world fall data due to the external validity issues inherent in simulated fall based testing. Real-world data, by its very nature provides high ecological validity and therefore contributes to higher external validity.

The use of real-world data, while a significant step forward, does not make the test robust. Other factors such as cohort selection and size are important for external validity. In addition, the use of real-world data does not increase the internal validity, in fact, the level of variation and abundance of confounding factors creates a greater risk of systematic errors. Therefore, careful consideration and planning of both the data collection and test procedure is vital to ensure the validity of results.

All methods of testing fall detection systems share the same basic framework which shapes the whole method from data collection through to data processing. Therefore, a basic understanding of this framework is needed to understand the best method to evaluate fall detector performance. Fall detection is a case of binary classification; each movement is classified as either a fall (positive case) or non-fall (negative case). For each movement there are four possible outcomes:

- True Positive (TP)—Correctly detected fall
- True Negative (TN)—Non-fall movement not detected as a fall
- False Positive (FP)—Classified as a fall when none occurred
- False Negative (FN)—A fall which was not detected

These four values can be represented as a table comparing the actual data with the system's predictions, this is known as a confusion matrix (Figure 1). All further measures can be calculated from either a complete confusion matrix or a subset of one. Therefore, studies should aim to collect data and process it in such a way that as many of these four values as possible can be calculated.

		Predicted		
		Fall	Non-Fall	
Actual	Fall	True Positives (TP)	False Negatives (FN)	No. Actual Falls (P)
	Non-Fall	False Positives (FP)	True Negatives (TN)	No. Actual Non-Falls (N)

Figure 1. Example confusion matrix.

The aim of this review is to identify the methods which have previously been used to evaluate fall detector performance using real-world data and investigate how the differences in these methods of evaluation effect the results. The review covers the methods of data collection and processing as well as the performance measures which have been used for evaluation. In this review, we aim to identify the strengths and limitations of current approaches and propose a more robust approach of evaluation based on the findings.

2. Methods

A systematic search was conducted in August 2017 and repeated in March 2018, using the following on-line literature databases: Medline, Cinahl, Pubmed, Web of Science and IEEE Xplore. The search aimed to find all records where a fall detection technology (hardware or software) had been tested using real-world falls. The search strategy used is shown in Table 1. Papers were excluded where no fall detection technology was tested, where tests used fall simulations, or the technology was not aimed at older adults. Only articles available in English were included.

Table 1. Example Search Strategy for PubMed.

	fall*-detect*[Title/Abstract] OR fall*-sensor*[Title/Abstract] OR fall*-alarm*[Title/abstract]
AND	real-world[Title/Abstract] OR real-life[Title/Abstract] OR free-living[Title/Abstract] OR community-dwelling[Title/Abstract] OR home-dwelling[Title/Abstract] OR domestic-environment[Title/Abstract] OR long-term-care[Title/Abstract] OR care-home[Title/Abstract] OR nursing-home[Title/Abstract] OR hospital[Title/Abstract]

The studies which met the inclusion criteria were assessed with regard to the method used to test the fall detection system. The focus was to assess the robustness of these tests and we therefore did not assess the systems' design or performance. For a comparison of wearable systems see [17] and for a comparison of non-wearable systems see [20]. All included studies tested fall detection technology using real-world fall data. Where studies reported on both tests using simulated data and tests using real-world data, only the methods used for the real-world portion of the data were considered.

First we reviewed the information studies provided about their participants, how they collected data and the volume of data collected. Next, we examined the methods used to identify fall events and to process the data. Finally, we evaluated the use of each applicable performance measure.

3. Results

The systematic search returned 259 unique records. Following application of the selection criteria, 22 papers were identified for analysis. The full breakdown of the literature identification process, including the reasons for exclusion, is shown in Figure 2. Table 2 provides a breakdown of the 22 included papers with regard to participant groups, devices used, participant numbers, numbers of recorded falls, the quantity and processing of non-fall data and finally, the performance measures reported. The following sections provide further detail to complement Table 2.

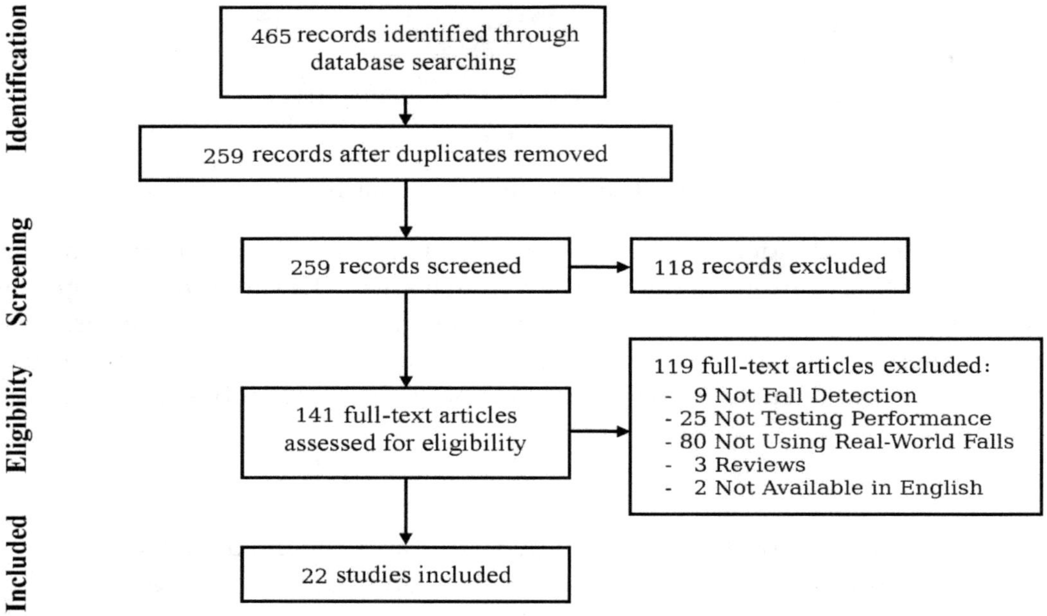

Figure 2. Flow diagram of the systematic search.

Table 2. Summary of papers evaluating fall detection systems using real-world falls.

Author	Participant Group	Additional Information	Device Type	Number of Participants	Number of Falls	Quantity of Non-Fall Data and Method of Preparation		Performance Measures
Aziz [21]	Residents of a long-term care facility who had experienced at least one fall in the previous year	Age, mobility assessment	Accelerometer	9	1	214 h	Data were divided into 2.5 s time windows with a 1.5 s overlap. The 30 s of data following a fall event were ignored.	**Sensitivity**, Specificity, **FPRT**, TP, FP, FN
	Patients at a hospital geriatrics department with Progressive Supranuclear Palsy	Age	Accelerometer	10	9	178 h		
Bagala [17]	Patients with Progressive Supranuclear Palsy	Age, gender, height, weight	Accelerometer	9	29 the number from each group was not provided	A total of 168 h from seven of the participants. Recordings were divided into 60 s windows and only the 1170 windows where max(RSS) – min(RSS) > 1.01 g were included		**Sensitivity**, **Specificity**, **FPRT**, Precision NPV, Accuracy
	Community dwelling older adult	None	Accelerometer	1				

Table 2. *Cont.*

Author	Participant Group	Additional Information	Device Type	Number of Participants	Number of Falls	Quantity of Non-Fall Data and Method of Preparation	Performance Measures
Bloch [22]	Patients at a geriatric rehabilitation ward with an identified risk of falling	Age	Working alarm composed of an accelerometer and infrared sensor	10	8	A total of 196 days. Data was processed on-line and the analysis compared the alarm times to reported fall times. Assumed 30 fall like events per day to estimate of the number of non-fall events.	**Sensitivity**, **Specificity**, Precision, NPV, TP
Bourke [23]	Patients at a geriatric rehabilitation unit	None	Accelerometer and gyroscope	42	89	A total of 3466 events extracted using a dynamic detection algorithm and further reduced to 367 events where: max(RSS) > 1.05 g Total length of recorded data was not given.	**Sensitivity**, **Specificity**, Accuracy, ROC AUC

Table 2. *Cont.*

Author	Participant Group	Additional Information	Device Type	Number of Participants	Number of Falls	Quantity of Non-Fall Data and Method of Preparation	Performance Measures
Chaudhuri [24]	Community dwelling older adults	None	Working alarm consisting of an accelerometer, magnetometer, and gyroscope	18	14	A total of 1452.6 days. Details of data preparation not given.	Sensitivity, Specificity, Precision, NPV, Confusion Matrix
Chen [25]	Community dwelling older adults living in geriatric rehabilitation centres	Age, gender, height, weight	Accelerometer	22	22	A total of 22 events. Only data from a 1200 s window around the falls was used, data up to 1 s before each fall were used as non-fall events.	Sensitivity, FPR, Accuracy, Confusion matrix

Table 2. *Cont.*

Author	Participant Group	Additional Information	Device Type	Number of Participants	Number of Falls	Quantity of Non-Fall Data and Method of Preparation	Performance Measures
Debard [26]	Older adults	Age	Camera	4	25	A total of 14,000 h. Only data for the 20 min up to and including the falls were used, this was divided into 2 min windows.	**Sensitivity**, Specificity, **Precision**, Confusion matrix
Debard [27]	Older persons (two community dwelling, one in a nursing home and four in assisted living), two of which did not fall and were excluded	Age, mobility assessment, walking aid use	Camera	7	29	Over 21,000 h recorded. Only data from the 24 h prior to each fall were used which was divided into 1 s windows.	Sensitivity, Precision, PR Curve, PR AUC, TP, FP, FN

Table 2. *Cont.*

Author	Participant Group	Additional Information	Device Type	Number of Participants	Number of Falls	Quantity of Non-Fall Data and Method of Preparation	Performance Measures
Debard [28]	Older persons (two community dwelling, one in a nursing home and four in assisted living), two of which did not fall and were excluded	Age, mobility assessment, walking aid use	Camera	7	29	Over 21,000 h recorded. Only data from the 24 h prior to each fall were used which was divided into 1 s windows.	**Sensitivity**, Precision, PR Curve, **PR AUC**, TP, FP, FN, **FPRT**
Feldwieser [29]	Community dwelling older adults	Age, height, weight, mobility assessments, cognitive assessments	Accelerometer	28	12	A total of 1225.7 days (average daily user wear time 8.1 ± 4.8 h). Details of data preparation not given.	**TP**, FP, FPRT
Gietzelt [30]	Older adults with recurrent falls	Age, gender, mobility assessments, cognitive assessments	Accelerometer and camera	3	4	A total of 10 days. Details of data preparation not given.	TP, FPRT

Table 2. *Cont.*

Author	Participant Group	Additional Information	Device Type	Number of Participants	Number of Falls	Quantity of Non-Fall Data and Method of Preparation	Performance Measures
Godfrey [31]	Older adult with Parkinson's disease	Age, BMI, balance assessment	Accelerometer	1	1	A total of 7 days. No preparatory steps.	TP, FPRT
Hu [32]	Community dwelling older adults with a history of falls	Age, gender, height, weight	Accelerometer and Gyroscope	5	20	A total of 70 days, divided into sliding windows. Window size was varied from 5 to 30 min.	Sensitivity, Specificity
Kangas [33]	Residents of elderly care units	Age, gender, mobility assessments, cognitive assessments	Accelerometer	16	15	A total of 1105 days (average daily user wear time 14.2 ± 6.3 h). Data processed on line, 14 s raw acceleration data where recorded when acceleration of all three axes fell below 0.75 g.	**Sensitivity, FPRT**, TP, FP

Table 2. *Cont.*

Author	Participant Group	Additional Information	Device Type	Number of Participants	Number of Falls	Quantity of Non-Fall Data and Method of Preparation	Performance Measures
Lipsitz [34]	Residents of a long-term care facility who had at least once in the previous 12 months	Age, gender, height, weight, BMI, prevalence of 21 comorbidities	Working alarm system using an accelerometer	62	89	A total of 9300 days. Working alarm, raw sensor data not stored, analysis compared the alarm times to reported fall times.	Sensitivity, Precision, TP, FP, FN
Liu [35]	Older adult	None	Doppler radar	1	6	A total of 7 days. No preparatory steps.	TP, FPRT

Table 2. *Cont.*

Author	Participant Group	Additional Information	Device Type	Number of Participants	Number of Falls	Quantity of Non-Fall Data and Method of Preparation	Performance Measures
Palmerini [36]	Patients with Progressive Supranuclear Palsy staying in a geriatric rehabilitation unit	Age, gender	Accelerometer	1	12	A total of 168 h from four of the participants. Recordings were divided into 60 s windows and only the 1170 windows where max(RSS) − min(RSS) > 1.01 g were included	Sensitivity, Specificity, FPR, FPRT, Informedness, ROC Curve, **ROC AUC**, FP
	Community dwelling patients with Progressive Supranuclear Palsy	Age, gender	Accelerometer	6	16		
	Community dwelling older adult	Age, gender	Accelerometer	1	1		
Rezaee [37]	Nursing home residents	None	Camera	Not given	48	A total of 163 normal movements extracted from video sequences totalling 57,425 frames. Details of identification not given.	**Sensitivity**, **Accuracy**, **FPR**, Confusion matrix

Table 2. *Cont.*

Author	Participant Group	Additional Information	Device Type	Number of Participants	Number of Falls	Quantity of Non-Fall Data and Method of Preparation		Performance Measures
Skubic [20]	Residents of an older adult independent living facility	Age, gender	Doppler radar	1	13	10 days	Details of data preparation not given for any of the datasets.	Sensitivity, FPRT, TP, FP
	Residents of an older adult independent living facility	Age, gender	Kinect	16	9	3,339 days		
	Resident of an older adult independent living facility	Age, gender, mobility device use	Kinect	1	142	601 days		
	Residents of assisted living apartments	Gender	Kinect	67	67	10,707 days		
Soaz [38]	Older adult	Age, gender	Accelerometer	1	1	3.5 h	No preparatory steps.	Sensitivity, **FPRT**, FP
	Older adults	Age, gender	Accelerometer	14	0	996 h		

Table 2. *Cont.*

Author	Participant Group	Additional Information	Device Type	Number of Participants	Number of Falls	Quantity of Non-Fall Data and Method of Preparation	Performance Measures
Stone [39]	Residents of an older adult independent living facility	Age, gender	Kinect	16	9	A total of 3339 days. Device only stored data for periods where motion was detected.	Sensitivity, FPRT
Yu [40]	FARSEEING data used previously in [17,23] no further details provided	None	Accelerometer	22	22	A total of 2618 normal activities extracted as 1 s windows from the 2 min surrounding the fall signals.	**Sensitivity**, **Precision**, Specificity

Notes: Performance measures reported in the articles abstract are shown in bold. Where a working alarm system was tested this is stated in the Device Type column, otherwise the test was carried out off-line, using the collected dataset. Soaz [38] focused on estimating the false alarm rate, however one real fall was recorded by chance and was included. RSS = Root Sum of Squares; FPRT = False Positive Rate Over Time; NPV = Negative Predictive Value; ROC Curve = Receiver Operating Characteristic Curve; ROC AUC = Area Under ROC Curve; PR Curve = Precision Recall Curve; PR AUC = Area Under Precision Recall Curve; TP = True Positives; FP = False Positives; FN = False Negatives; TN = True Negatives.

3.1. *Participant Descriptions*

The level of detail provided about participants varied considerably. All but three [31,38,40] of the articles stated whether participants were community dwelling, in long-term care or hospital patients. Five articles did not provide any additional descriptive information on the participants [23,24,35,37,40]. The other eighteen articles describe participant's age, twelve also provide gender information and six provide details of height and weight or BMI [17,25,29,31,32,34]. Four articles provided information on specific medical conditions, three recruited participants with Progressive Supranuclear Palsy [17,21,36] and one included a single older adult with Parkinson's disease [31]. Lipsitz et al. [34] provided the most in-depth description with a breakdown of the proportion of participants with a range of 21 comorbidities. Eight articles reported results of mobility assessments [21,27–31,33,38], three articles provided information on walking aid use [20,27,28] and three articles additionally reported results of cognitive assessments [29,30,33]. None of the other 15 articles reported standardised measures of cognitive or mobility status.

3.2. *Method of Data Collection*

All studies used the same general approach of monitoring participants with one or more sensor devices. Studies can be classified into two main categories, those using wearable technology (e.g. accelerometers or gyroscopes) and those using non-wearable technology (e.g. fixed cameras or Kinect sensors). Both approaches have advantages and disadvantages with regard to fall detection. For example, wearable devices are always with the user, however they may forget to wear the device. In contrast, non-wearable devices have a limited capture area but the user can safely forget about them. For a full discussion on the advantages and disadvantages of different sensor types refer to recent reviews [19,41].

Fifteen studies used wearable technology and ten used non-wearable, Table 2 shows full details of the devices used in each study. Accelerometers are the most common choice of sensor and have been used in 15 of the studies [17,21–25,29–34,36,38,40]. Eight studies tested some form of optical sensor [20,22,26–28,30,37,39], making them the most common choice of non-wearable devices. One additional study deployed an optical sensor as part of their system, but this did not record any falls so they could not test it [29].

Studies can be further classified based on whether the device used was capable of processing data on-line and raising an alarm when it detected a fall. Three studies deployed functioning wearable alarm systems [24,33,34], one study deployed a system combining wearable and non-wearable devices [22], no studies deployed an alarm system solely using non-wearable devices. Two of the studies which tested working alarm systems did not store the raw sensor data, only recording when the alarm went off [22,34], one article did not state if the raw sensor data was stored [24]. The raw sensor data can be used for future development and testing, and therefore the favoured approach is to store this data.

The availability of the collected data is important for future work and the direct comparison of approaches. None of the studies used publicly available datasets nor made their real-world fall data publicly available. Two studies [25,40] made use of a subset of the FARSEEING repository, which is available on request. The FARSEEING project is a real-world fall repository project funded by the European Union. Four studies [17,21,23,36] were conducted by members of the FARSEEING project or in collaboration with members, and also used data from the FARSEEING repository. No other studies provide any information on the availability of their datasets.

3.3. *Number of Participants and Falls, and the Volume of Non-Fall Data*

There is a large range in the number of participants included, with most studies using small cohorts. One article did not provide any information on the number of participants [37]. Three studies had just a single participant [31,35,38] and one study [20] used data from only one participant in parts of their analysis. The maximum number of participants was 62 [34] and the median was nine (IQR 4–18).

There was an equally large range in the number of fall events recorded. Two studies included just a single real fall [31,38] and in one of the two datasets used by Aziz et al. [21] only one fall was recorded. The maximum number of falls was 89, which was achieved in two separate studies [23,34]. The median number of falls contained in the datasets used was 17.5 (IQR 8.25–29).

Where reported, the length of the monitoring period varied considerably and comparison is made difficult by the inconsistent choice of reported metrics. Thirteen articles provided the total length of the recorded data, but did not provide details of the proportion where the system was recording participant's movement (participant in the capture area or wearing the device) [20–22,24,26–28,30,32,34,35,38,39]. The median length of total recorded data, from studies which provided it, was 592 days (IQR 21–1474). Only three articles provided information on device wear time, in these studies the mean wear times were 8.1 [29], 14.2 [33] and 24 [31] h per day. None of the articles on non-wearable devices provided information on the proportion of time during which participants were in the capture area.

Six articles did not clearly state the time period over which participants were monitored or the amount of data captured, instead they provided the number of extracted non-fall events [17,23,25,36,37,40]. The number of non-fall events used in these studies ranged from 22 [25] to 3466 [23].

3.4. Method of Fall Identification and Validation

One of the main challenges in recording real-world falls is ensuring every fall that occurs is identified accurately. How fall events are identified is influenced by both the choice of device and whether the system is capable of raising alarms in real-time. The device used determines the type and detail of information available for retrospective verification of fall times and types. A camera, for example, provides a greater level of information compared to an accelerometer; assuming the video footage is not highly pre-processed, for privacy reasons, before being stored. Where working alarm systems are deployed, all detected falls can be quickly verified, providing additional robustness over a single reporting method such as staff incident reports.

Four studies [22,24,33,34] deployed a functioning wearable alarm system. As the alarm systems were being validated, a second reporting system was still needed to identify falls which did not trigger an alarm. Three of the studies used staff incident reports in addition to the alarm system [22,33,34]. It was unclear what secondary method of fall identification was used in one of the studies [24]. Of the 18 studies which analysed the data retrospectively, three identified falls using staff reports [17,21,39], five used participant self-report [29–32,38] and ten did not state how falls were identified [20,23,25–28,35–37,40].

Where self-report of falls is used it is important to consider the cognitive ability of participants, especially their memory. Only two of the five studies which used self-report provide results of assessments of cognitive ability [29,30]. Both of these studies used a Mini Mental State Exam [42]. Feldwieser et al. [29] found no signs of cognitive impairment and Gietzelt et al. [30] found that one of their three participants had cognitive impairment, but does not report how they accounted for this.

It is important to consider that reported fall times might not be accurate and that some falls may not be reported, or may be reported by more than one member of staff with different timestamps. This could, for example, be due to delays in completing the report, delays in the faller being discovered, participant recall problems or staff naturally prioritising helping the faller over checking and reporting the time. Only three articles describe methods to check reported fall times [17,21,32]. Two of these [17,21] used datasets from the FARSEEING repository where expert analysis of the sensor signals in combination with fall reports was used to pinpoint the fall signal. Hu et al. [32] reported correlating self-reported fall times with the signals, but provided no details on how this was carried out.

3.5. Methods of Data Processing

There are two approaches for testing real-world fall detection systems, the key difference is how the data is prepared. The first approach is based on simply identifying when falls occur in continuous user movement or a stream of sensor data, we call this the continuous data approach. The second approach is based on a fall detector classifying events as either a fall or not a fall, we call this the event based approach. The following sections explain each of these approaches and review their use. In five studies it was unclear which approach was used [20,24,29,30,39].

3.5.1. Continuous Data Approach

The continuous data approach mirrors real-world usage of fall alarm systems where user movement is the input and fall times or alarms are the output. This approach is therefore the primary way of testing deployed fall alarm systems but can also be used for retrospective testing using existing data. The fall detection systems sensors convert movement into a stream of raw data which is then processed by the software component of the system. In this approach all aspects of data processing are part of the fall detection software and are tested as a single unit. To test performance the systems predictions are compared to the actual verified fall times. This comparison allows quantification of the number of true positives (actual and predicted timestamps match), false positives (predicted fall with no actual fall) and false negatives (fall occurred but none was predicted).

True negatives can be quantified if the times when non-falls occurred were recorded, however, non-falls are not defined. In the strictest sense non-falls are everything which is not a fall, but that does not enable their occurrence to be quantified. It is not possible to count when a fall doesn't occur without arbitrarily dividing the time-series data into events, and counting the events where no fall occurred. Such a method of dividing the data would fall under the event based testing approach. In the continuous data approach any segmenting of the data for processing purposes is part of the fall detection system, not the test procedure.

Six studies used the continuous data approach [22,31,33–35,38]. Bloch et al. [22] processed the data using the continuous data approach, and then used an assumption of thirty 'fall-like' events per day to calculate a number of true negatives (30 × number of days the sensor was in use). The other five studies did not attempt to quantify TN.

3.5.2. Event Based Approach

The event based approach has its roots in tests using laboratory based simulation datasets. When data is collected in the laboratory a predefined set of movements or events is simulated, the times of these events is known and therefore they can be easily extracted. To test performance all the events must first be labelled as either a fall or not a fall using the record of event times. For each event the label is compared to the software's predictions allowing a complete confusion matrix to be generated.

In real-world data, events are less clearly defined than in simulated data since there is no complete record of the movements which occurred. The creation of events from real-world data has been based on arbitrary rules rather than identification of the underlying movements of the users. The events are labelled using reported fall times, where no fall occurred the event is considered a non-fall. As this method always yields non-fall events, true negatives can be quantified, unlike in the continuous approach.

Eleven studies used the event based approach [17,21,23,25–28,32,36,37,40]. The predominant method to create events was based on time windows, where the data is sliced using constant time intervals, for example each 60 seconds of data is one event. However, there is no consensus on what constitutes an event and in practice, a method of reducing the volume of data is often used, for example, to exclude data where no movement was recorded. The time windows can overlap allowing the same data to be processed multiple times, although the rationale for this is not clear.

To create events, one study used 2.5 s windows with a 1.5 s overlap and kept all the events [21]. Two studies divided the data into 60 s windows and used a movement detection algorithm to select events [17,36]. Bourke et al. [23] also used a movement detection algorithm to select events but does not describe the windowing technique. Two studies used the same dataset where the 24 hours prior to each fall was divided into one second windows [27,28]. One study used self-reported wear time to reduce the dataset prior to dividing into windows, but does not provide any details about the windowing technique [32].

Three studies used only a limited section of data from around each fall. Debard et al. [26] divided up the 20 minutes of data prior to a fall into two minute windows. Chen et al. [25] only used data from 20 minutes surrounding each fall and used the section of data up to one second prior to impact as non-fall events. Yu et al. [40] divided the two minutes around each fall into one second windows, removed the one second window where the fall occurred and used the remaining windows as non-fall events.

3.6. Definition of Performance Measures and Review of Their Use

3.6.1. Sensitivity

Sensitivity (also known as recall and true positive rate) is the proportion of falls which are correctly detected (Equation (1)). The inverse of sensitivity is miss rate (false negative rate) which quantifies the proportion of falls not detected (Equation (2)). Sensitivity is by far the most commonly reported statistic; it was reported in 18 of the articles [17,20–28,32–34,36–40] and could be calculated from the information given in the other four [29–31,35].

$$\text{Sensitivity} = \frac{TP}{TP + FN} = \frac{TP}{P} \tag{1}$$

$$\text{Miss Rate} = \frac{FN}{FN + TP} = \frac{FN}{P} = 1 - \text{Sensitivity} \tag{2}$$

3.6.2. Specificity

Specificity (also known as true negative rate) is the proportion of non-fall events which are correctly detected (Equation (3)). It quantifies the ability to avoid false positives (false alarms). The inverse of specificity is false positive rate, which is the proportion of non-fall events mistakenly detected as falls (Equation (4)). Nine articles reported specificity [17,21–24,26,32,36,40] and two reported false positive rate [36,37]. It is unclear whether Chen et al. [25] reported specificity or false positive rate, as the reported number of TN and FP suggest that what they report as specificity is in fact false positive rate. Specificity could be calculated from the information provided in a further two of the studies [27,28].

$$\text{Specificity} = \frac{TN}{TN + FP} = \frac{TN}{N} \tag{3}$$

$$\text{False Positive Rate} = \frac{FP}{FP + TN} = \frac{FP}{N} = 1 - \text{Specificity} \tag{4}$$

3.6.3. False Positive Rate over Time

False Positive Rate over Time (FPRT) has become a popular measure in real-world tests of fall detection. This measure provides information on the frequency of false alarms. Twelve articles report the number of false positives either per hour or per day [17,20,21,28–31,33,35,36,38,39] and it could be calculated from the information provided in seven others [24–27,32,34,37].

3.6.4. Precision

Precision (also known as positive predictive value) is the proportion of alarms which are true falls (Equation (5)). It therefore provides the probability that an alarm will be an actual fall and not a false alarm. For example, a precision of 0.5 means that half of alarms will be actual falls, and half will be false alarms (1 false positive for every detected fall). Eight articles reported precision [17,22,24,26–28,34,40] and it could be calculated from the information provided in all of the other articles.

$$\text{Precision} = \frac{TP}{TP + FP} \tag{5}$$

3.6.5. Negative Predictive Value

Negative Predictive Value (NPV) is the proportion of events classified as non-falls which are true non-fall events (Equation (6)). NPV therefore provides information about the ability to correctly classify non-fall events. NPV will be high if a system correctly ignores many times more non-fall events than the number of falls it fails to detect. Therefore, for false negatives to have any notable effect, the number of falls and non-falls must be approximately equal. However, in real-world fall data falls are usually much less frequent than non-fall events, which limits the insights yielded from NPV as systems typically score over 0.99 out of 1 [17,22,24]. Three articles reported NPV in their results [17,22,24]. NPV could also be calculated from the information provided in eleven of the other articles [21,23,25–28,32,34,36,37,40].

$$\text{Negative Predictive Value} = \frac{TN}{TN + FN} \tag{6}$$

3.6.6. Accuracy

Accuracy is the proportion of predictions which were correct (Equation (7)). Accuracy is a measure which summarises the whole confusion matrix in a single value. Accuracy's major limitation is the inability to handle imbalanced datasets, for example, in real-world fall data where there are many more non-fall events than falls. Similar to NPV, accuracy is dominated by the larger group and the effect is proportional to the size of the imbalance. Therefore, in real-world fall detection studies, accuracy is skewed towards the correct detection of non-fall events over the correct detection of falls. For example, in eight of the algorithms tested by Bagala et al. [17] the accuracies were greater than 0.9 with sensitivities below 0.6, in one case an accuracy of 0.96 with a sensitivity of 0.14. Four articles reported accuracy [17,23,25,37] and it could be calculated from the results provided in seven of the other articles [21,24,26–28,36,40].

$$\text{Accuracy} = \frac{TP + TN}{P + N} \tag{7}$$

3.6.7. F-Measure

F-measure (also known as F-score) is the harmonic mean of sensitivity and precision (Equation (8)). F-measure, therefore, considers all outcomes except true negatives (non-falls). In fall detection, the priorities are detected falls (TP), missed falls (FN) and false alarms (FP). F-measure considers all of these outcomes and therefore provides a good overview of performance. No articles report a value for F-measure, however it could be easily calculated from their results as eight articles [17,22,24,26–28,34,40] reported both sensitivity and precision and all but two [32,39] reported enough information to calculate both sensitivity and precision.

$$\text{F-measure} = 2 \times \frac{\text{Precision} \times \text{Sensitivity}}{\text{Precision} + \text{Sensitivity}} \tag{8}$$

3.6.8. Informedness

Informedness (also known as Youden's J Statistics or Youden's Index) is a statistic which combines sensitivity and specificity (Equation (9)). It is the probability that predictions are informed versus a pure guess. Informedness is linked to the proportion of cases classified correctly. However, unlike accuracy, it is robust to an imbalance in the number of fall and non-fall events. This is achieved through equal weighting of sensitivity and specificity which are in turn the proportions of falls detected and non-falls correctly ignored. The value ranges from negative one to positive one. Zero indicates predictions are no better than guessing, positive one indicates perfect predictions and negative one indicates all predictions are the opposite of the true value. In cases where the value is negative, the output classes can simply be swapped over. One study reported informedness [36], however, 12 other articles reported both sensitivity and specificity or false positive rate, or the information necessary to calculate them [17,21–28,37,40], so informedness could be calculated from their results.

$$\text{Informedness} = \text{Sensitivity} + \text{Specificity} - 1 \tag{9}$$

3.6.9. Markedness

Markedness is a statistic which combines precision and NPV (Equation (10)). Markedness is linked with the proportion of predictions which are correct. It combines the proportion of correct positive and negative predictions with equal weighting and is therefore unaffected by imbalance in the number of positive and negative predictions. As with informedness, the result is a value between negative and positive one. No articles reported markedness, but twelve did report enough information for markedness to be calculated [17,21–28,36,37,40].

$$\text{Markedness} = \text{Precision} + \text{NPV} - 1 \tag{10}$$

3.6.10. Matthews Correlation Coefficient

Matthews Correlation Coefficient (MCC) is the geometric mean of informedness and markedness (Equations (11) and (12)). It should be noted that Equation (11) only works if informedness and markedness are both positive, Equation (12) works in all cases. MCC considers both the proportion of events classified correctly and the proportion of correct predictions and is therefore robust to imbalanced datasets. The result is a value between negative and positive one as with both informedness and markedness. None of the articles reported MCC, enough information to calculate MCC was given in 14 articles [17,21–28,32,34,36,37,40].

$$\text{MCC} = \sqrt{\text{Informedness} \times \text{Markedness}} \tag{11}$$

$$\text{MCC} = \frac{TP \times TN - FP \times FN}{\sqrt{(TP + FP)(TP + FN)(TN + FP)(TN + FN)}} \tag{12}$$

3.6.11. Receiver Operating Characteristic Curve

A Receiver Operating Characteristic (ROC) Curve is a plot of sensitivity versus false positive rate as the primary threshold of the classifier is adjusted. ROC curves can therefore be used to understand the trade-off between sensitivity and false positive rate and optimise a primary threshold. There could be debate as to which balance of sensitivity and false positives is optimal, therefore a ROC curve provides useful insight. However, it is difficult to compare systems robustly based on a curve. Consequently, it is in the optimisation where ROC curves are best used, rather than final results, as only the optimised version will be deployed.

ROC curves can be reduced to a single number by calculating the area under the curve (AUC). AUC has been found to be a poor measure for comparing classifiers, particularly where the sample size is small [43–45]. Two studies have used ROC analysis and reported AUC [23,36].

3.6.12. Precision-Recall Curve

A precision-recall (PR) curve is similar to a ROC curve, the difference is that precision is used instead of false positive rate and the term recall is used in place of sensitivity. PR curves are preferred over ROC curves when there is a large imbalance in the data [46]. Calculating AUC for PR curves is more challenging than for ROC curves as precision does not increase linearly, meaning linear interpolation yields incorrect results [46]. Two studies reported PR AUC [27,28], although it is unclear how PR AUC was calculated in these studies.

4. Discussion

This is the first review to be conducted on the methods used to evaluate real-world performance of fall detection systems. Ensuring a sound method is critical for meaningful results, therefore reflecting on the way studies are conducted and seeking improvements to the method is vital in emerging areas of research where no consensus has yet been reached. The real-world testing of fall detection systems is currently in its infancy and this is reflected in our findings. The method is highly variable across studies, which makes comparing the results difficult if not impossible. The following three sections discuss the key issues and make recommendations for future studies.

4.1. Data Collection and Preparation

One major aspect which leads to variation between studies is the participant groups and the differences in the movements and behaviours captured by the sensor systems. If insufficient detail is gathered about participants it is challenging to reproduce the findings as differing results could be due to differing participant characteristics. In addition, one may want to collect new data comparable to that used in a previous study for the purpose of comparing the performance of a new system using different sensors with previously tested systems. Information gathered about participants was both inconsistent and insufficient to allow the data collection to be reproduced.

A comprehensive consensus process has previously been carried out by the FARSEEING consortium [47]. As part of the consensus process the group identified a minimum set of clinical measures which they deemed essential for the interpretation of real-world fall data. The measures included age, height, weight, gender, fall history, assistive device use as well as assessments of mobility, cognitive impairments and visual impairments. None of the reported studies have implemented these recommendations.

Cognitive and mobility tests provide useful information about fall risk and the likelihood of false positives caused by events such as 'falling into a chair' or improper use of the device. Compared to standard metrics such as age, height and weight, assessments of mobility and cognition provide a much deeper insight into participant's fall risk and movement characteristics. Therefore, standardised cognitive and mobility assessments should be prioritised. Deeper insights into participant's movements could be achieved though continuous profiling using activity monitoring software to process the recorded dataset. However, development and validation of activity monitoring software may be a barrier unless an existing activity monitoring system is used for the data collection. Where such profiling is possible details should be reported to enhance the interpretation of results.

Another critical aspect of the test is the size of the dataset. Currently, the datasets used are generally small, have been collected with a low number of participants and contain only a few falls. Small datasets reduce the validity of the test and hinder reproducibility. Where the dataset is small either due to few participants, a low incidence of falls or both, it is possible that only a limited subset of movements and fall types were captured. In such cases comparisons of results to tests of other systems is difficult as the dataset may be the main cause of differences in reported performance. Further, the generalisability of results is questionable where the sample size is small. The small datasets are one factor which makes it difficult to understand which systems perform the best and therefore where future development should focus. The other main factors are the different populations recruited for studies and the limited insights into how this effects the fundamental aspect of the data—the movements captured.

Due to the known challenges in recording fall signals, the only feasible way for most researchers to gain access to a large number of fall signals is through collaboration. In addition, if systems are tested using the same data, the results are directly comparable. Therefore, large shared test datasets are needed to allow the performance of fall detection software to be compared. To facilitate the sharing of datasets, the FARSEEING consortium have established a data repository which currently contains over 300 fall signals [48]. However, more studies are needed to generate datasets that can be added to the repository and used for robust testing of devices and development of improved software.

Even with shared data, there is still an issue of how to ensure all fall signals are accurately identified. We have identified that the method used to identify the fall signals is poorly described in published studies, leaving a large gap in our understanding of how the dataset was prepared. The current prevailing method to identify fall signals is expert signal analysis to verify participant or staff reported fall times. There is a risk that not all falls are reported, leading to real falls being included as non-fall data. Expert signal analysis cannot overcome the issue of under reporting, but does at least give greater confidence that inaccurate reported times were corrected and all included fall signals were real falls.

Expert signal analysis, while clearly better than no verification, could lead to bias. Currently there is an insufficient understanding of fall signals due to a limited number of recorded falls and a lack of research into the profile of the signals. Our limited understanding could lead to atypical falls not being verified and thus excluded. There is a risk that systems are designed to detect certain signal profiles as falls and only these profiles are being verified as falls. Therefore the results could be artificially improved through restricting the test data.

Unless a gold standard fall reporting system is used, such as video analysis, studies will be limited in their ability to verify fall signals, under reporting of falls will remain a concern and there is a risk of bias in the verification process needed to compensate for the inaccuracies of the 'silver standard' reporting system. The current lack of standardised method or gold standard, and the lack of reporting how fall signals were identified and verified, inhibits understanding of results. A consensus is needed on the process for fall signal identification and studies should clearly report their methods.

4.2. Data Processing

Two approaches were identified for preparing sensor signals for fall detection system testing and we named these the continuous data approach and the event based approach. Both approaches have issues surrounding what constitutes a non-fall. In the continuous data approach the issue is centred around the definition and identification of non-falls. In the event based approach non-fall events can be defined as any event which is not a fall. However, events could be defined as anything which is either a fall event or non-fall event, and since falls are defined, the issue returns to what constitutes a non-fall.

The strictest definition of non-falls as everything which is not a fall is not particularly useful. This definition does not allow non-falls to be quantified in the continuous data approach and provides no indication of how the data should be divided into events for the event based approach. A more helpful concept is that of fall-like movements, a subset of non-falls which share characteristics with falls. The FARSEEING consortium defined a fall as "an unexpected event in which the person comes to rest on the ground, floor or lower level" [49]. A fall-like movement could therefore, by removing the unexpected clause, be defined as "any event in which the person comes to rest on the ground, floor or lower level".

With a definition for fall-like events these could be recorded, at least theoretically, in the same manner as falls and therefore, allow true negatives to be quantified robustly. In reality it is not feasible for a researcher to record the times of all fall-like movements in the same way that falls are recorded, due to the vast quantity which would occur. An automated system would be more practical, although it is unlikely to be easier to develop automated fall-like detection than automated fall detection systems. Consequently, researchers must consider if the development of fall-like movement detection systems is worth the investment, simply to extend the testing of fall-detection systems. Given that a robust evaluation of fall detection systems can be achieved without the need for true negatives, and hence non-fall or fall-like movements, we suggest that automated fall-like movement detection is unlikely to bring benefits which outweigh the required investment.

4.3. Performance Measures

It is challenging to compare results across studies or determine the current state-of-the-art due to disparity in the choice of measures reported and challenges calculating unreported measures. The measures used to report and interpret performance vary widely across studies and not all studies report the basic results from which all measures can be calculated (TP, FP, FN and TN). Where TP, FP, FN and TN are not reported these can only be estimated, due to rounding of the reported results. Using one of the tests reported by Bourke et al. [23] as an example, the number of FP could be any value between 18 and 51 based on the reported specificity of 0.99 with 3466 total non-falls. To facilitate the calculation of additional measures, future studies should report TP, FP, FN and TN if these can be calculated robustly and are used in the calculation of the reported performance measures.

In addition to reporting enough information to allow further measures to be calculated, it is important that the headline measures give a true reflection of performance and allow robust comparisons to be made with other systems. Sensitivity has been a mainstay in previous studies, it is an important aspect of system performance. Sensitivity only quantifies the ability to detect falls, it does not consider false positives. The question is therefore which measure to pair sensitivity with to provide understanding of the ability to avoid false positives. In addition, a single combined measure which considers both aspects is important in order to understand the overall level of performance.

Specificity has been the most common choice of measure to quantify the ability to avoid false alarms in laboratory based testing [19] and it has remained a common choice in real-world tests. Specificity considers how well non-fall events are classified, it could therefore be considered sensitivity's natural counterpart. The weakness of specificity in the context of real-world fall detection is the reliance on non-falls, which are poorly defined and troublesome to identify.

The need for researchers to design or select methods for non-fall identification opens up a considerable possibility of bias. A method could be used which suits the specific system and dataset causing distortion of the results and hindering comparisons with other systems. In the case of specificity, the difficulty of the test is very much determined by the definition of a non-fall; the more inclusive the definition, the more non-fall events and therefore the higher the score for the same number of false positives. This effect can be seen in the study of Bourke et al. [23], where tests were conducted twice using different definitions of non-falls. With the most restrictive definition of non-falls, specificity ranged from 0.83 to 0.91. With the more open definition, specificity was consistently 0.98 or greater. Expanding the definition includes more movements which are less fall-like, thus it creates an easier test.

It is hard to prevent bias in selecting a definition of non-falls as it is likely unintentional. One solution is to remove the need to select a method on a study by study basis, however, standardising the method is challenging. Since there is currently no clear way to standardise non-fall identification, the best option may simply be to avoid them altogether. A solution might be standard publicly available datasets, with an agreed method to identify non-fall events. In such a case, the results are comparable to each other, but not to other studies using other datasets or methods.

Using standard data is challenging due to the vast array of sensors which could be used and the huge number of combinations. It is simply not possible to have a single dataset used to test all systems. Furthermore, it seems impossible to identify all types of relevant non-fall movements needed for a universal standard dataset. Any measures which rely on non-falls (specificity, NPV, accuracy, informedness, markedness, MCC and ROC AUC) are subject to the above problems and therefore should not be used as a primary measure. Where measures reliant on non-falls are used the methods should be described in detail and their limitations should be made clear to avoid confusion and misinterpretation.

The issues surrounding non-falls substantially reduces the options for quantifying the ability to avoid false positives and gauge overall performance. There are four possible measures which do not rely on non-falls, these are FPRT, precision, F-measure and PR AUC.

FPRT is a useful measure to understand the frequency of false alarms, however differences in the datasets affect the calculation. Wear time or time in the capture area must be considered, as false positives will, most likely, be far lower when the device is not in use. Another consideration is which hours of the day the device is in use; false positive rate during night time hours would be very different to day time hours. Reporting of times when the device was monitoring participants was found to be inadequate. Of the 11 articles which reported FPRT only two clearly reported wear time or time in the capture area [29,33] and none reported any details on the distribution of this time throughout the day.

Our findings suggest that there is a lack of an agreed and clearly defined method to calculate FPRT. Only one study clearly states that FPRT was calculated using solely the time a participant was being monitored by the device [33]. None of the other studies appear to have taken usage time into account when calculating FPRT. If usage time is not considered or reported it is unclear what extent device usage, or lack thereof affected the result. An unused system is unlikely to produce false positives. The issues in identifying wear time or time in the capture area could make FPRT an unreliable measure to compare across studies. Although users and clinicians may find the rate of false positives over time useful, it might be better to use a rate of something other than time.

Precision is an alternative to specificity and FPRT, it quantifies the false positives (FP) in relation to detected falls (TP). TP and FP should, for any reasonable level of performance, be in the same order of magnitude, therefore precision is resilient to the imbalance in the data. Further, the ratio between TP and FP is unlikely to be notably affected by usage time, if a device is used half of the time, TP and FP would be expected to be half compared to full device usage. Therefore, compared to FPRT, precision is far less affected by device usage, or lack thereof. The proportion of fall predictions which were true falls could be more useful than FPRT since frequent false positives may be acceptable to a frequent faller, assuming the falls are detected. Precision should be the primary measure of the ability to avoid false positives.

Sensitivity and precision together quantify the ability to detect falls and avoid false alarms, therefore providing a complete portrayal of performance. In addition to sensitivity and precision it is important to have a single measure which can quantify the trade-off between them. PR AUC is one possible option, however it considers the performance of multiple sub-optimum versions of the system as the system's parameters are adjusted. Since only the optimised system can be deployed, it is the optimised version which should be the focal point of the evaluation. F-measure, the harmonic mean of sensitivity and precision, appears to be the most suitable single measure for objective comparison. This trio of measures has two major advantages in robustness: (1) it does not rely on non-falls and (2) it is resistant to issues surrounding wear time and time in the capture area. Future studies should report sensitivity, precision and F-measure, and F-measure should be used as the standard for comparing systems.

5. Summary and Conclusions

As focus in fall detection performance evaluation shifts from simulated to real-world fall data, one must consider if the approach used for evaluating on simulations is optimum for real-world data.

Through examining the published articles on evaluation of real-world fall detection, two issues have become apparent:

1. The approaches to quantifying performance are inconsistent and many studies use measures which provide limited representation of performance.
2. The number of falls is generally small and study populations are diverse, making comparison between the datasets and results difficult.

It is critical that a consensus is reached on the most appropriate method to evaluate real-world performance of fall detection systems.

To address the issues with the datasets there needs to be greater collaboration and sharing of data. The FARSEEING consortium have made substantial steps to facilitate data sharing and have recorded over 300 falls through collaboration between six institutions [48]. Six of the 22 studies published to date have used parts of this data to develop or test approaches to fall detection [17,21,23,25,36,40], highlighting the importance of this data. However, further work is still needed to grow the volume of available data, record more falls, improve standardisation and further develop fall detection technology. Only through collaboration will the collection of a dataset large enough for robust development and testing become possible.

To address the issues surrounding how performance is quantified studies should avoid the need for non-falls. The concept is poorly defined and standardisation seems to be extremely problematic. The concept of non-falls is only needed to allow the calculation of measures such as specificity and accuracy, both of which are common in simulation based studies [19]. However, quantification of the difference in false alarm rate between simulated and real-world tests is not possible due to the disparity of the data. Therefore, traditional measures such as specificity and accuracy are of little value. Continued use of these traditional measures may lead to confusion and improper interpretation of performance. Measures which do not depend on non-falls should be used instead of these traditional measures. Sensitivity and precision should be the cornerstones of the evaluation with F-measure used for the objective comparison of systems.

Author Contributions: Conceptualization, R.W.B.; Methodology, R.W.B.; Formal Analysis, R.W.B.; Investigation, R.W.B.; Data Curation, R.W.B.; Writing-Original Draft Preparation, R.W.B.; Writing-Review & Editing, J.K., M.H.G., L.P.J.K., S.B.T.; Supervision, M.H.G., L.P.J.K., S.B.T.; Funding Acquisition, M.H.G., L.P.J.K., S.B.T.

Abbreviations

The following abbreviations are used in this manuscript:

P	Positive cases
N	Negative cases
TP	True Positives
FP	False Positives
FN	False Negatives
TP	True Positives
NPV	Negative Predictive Value
FPRT	False Positive Rate over Time
MCC	Mathews Correlation Coefficient
ROC	Receiver Operating Characteristic
PR	Precision-Recall
AUC	Area Under Curve
RSS	Root Sum of Squares
IQR	InterQuartile Range

References

1. World Health Organisation. *WHO Global Report on Falls Prevention in Older Age*; World Health Organization: Geneva, Switzerland, 2007.
2. Department of Health (UK). *Falls and Fractures: Effective Interventions in Health and Social Care*; Technical Report; Department of Health (UK): London, UK, 2009.
3. Luukinen, H.; Koski, K.; Honkanen, R.; Kivelä, S.L. Incidence of Injury-Causing Falls among Older Adults by Place of Residence: A Population-Based Study. *J. Am. Geriatr. Soc.* **1995**, *43*, 871–876, doi:10.1111/j.1532-5415.1995.tb05529.x.
4. Tinetti, M.E.; Speechley, M.; Ginter, S.F. Risk Factors for Falls among Elderly Persons Living in the Community. *N. Engl. J. Med.* **1988**, *319*, 1701–1707, doi:10.1056/NEJM198812293192604.
5. Heinrich, S.; Rapp, K.; Rissmann, U.; Becker, C.; König, H.H. Cost of Falls in Old Age: A Systematic Review. *Osteoporos. Int.* **2010**, *21*, 891–902, doi:10.1007/s00198-009-1100-1.
6. Fleming, J.; Brayne, C. Inability to Get up after Falling, Subsequent Time on Floor, and Summoning Help: Prospective Cohort Study in People over 90. *BMJ* **2008**, *337*, a2227, doi:10.1136/bmj.a2227.
7. Treml, J.; Husk, J.; Lowe, D.; Vasilakis, N. *Falling Standards, Broken Promises: Report of the National Audit of Falls and Bone Health in Older People 2010*; Technical Report; Royal College of Physicians: London, UK, 2010.
8. King, M.B.; Tinetti, M.E. Falls in Community-Dwelling Older Persons. *J. Am. Geriatr. Soc.* **1995**, *43*, 1146–1154, doi:10.1111/j.1532-5415.1995.tb07017.x.
9. Lord, S.R.; Sherrington, C.; Menz, H.B. *Falls in Older People : Risk Factors and Strategies for Prevention*; Cambridge University Press: Cambridge, UK, 2001.
10. Nevitt, M.C.; Cummings, S.R.; Kidd, S.; Black, D. Risk Factors for Recurrent Nonsyncopal Falls: A Prospective Study. *JAMA* **1989**, *261*, 2663–2668.
11. Wild, D.; Nayak, U.S.; Isaacs, B. How Dangerous Are Falls in Old People at Home? *Br. Med. J. (Clin. Res. Ed.)* **1981**, *282*, 266–268, doi:10.1136/bmj.282.6260.266.
12. Scheffer, A.C.; Schuurmans, M.J.; Van Dijk, N.; Van Der Hooft, T.; De Rooij, S.E. Fear of Falling: Measurement Strategy, Prevalence, Risk Factors and Consequences among Older Persons. *Age Ageing* **2008**, *37*, 19–24, doi:10.1093/ageing/afm169.
13. Howland, J.; Lachman, M.E.; Peterson, E.W.; Cote, J.; Kasten, L.; Jette, A. Covariates of Fear of Falling and Associated Activity Curtailment. *Gerontologist* **1998**, *38*, 549–555, doi:10.1093/geront/38.5.549.
14. Murphy, S.L.; Williams, C.S.; Gill, T.M. Characteristics Associated with Fear of Falling and Activity Restriction in Community-Living Older Persons. *J. Am. Geriatr. Soc.* **2002**, *50*, 516–520, doi:10.1046/j.1532-5415.2002.50119.x.
15. Heinbüchner, B.; Hautzinger, M.; Becker, C.; Pfeiffer, K. Satisfaction and Use of Personal Emergency Response Systems. *Z. Gerontol. Geriatr.* **2010**, *43*, 219–223, doi:10.1007/s00391-010-0127-4.
16. Baker, M. 1,500 Scientists Lift the Lid on Reproducibility. *Nature* **2016**, *533*, 452–454, doi:10.1038/533452a.
17. Bagala, F.; Becker, C.; Cappello, A.; Chiari, L.; Aminian, K.; Hausdorff, J.M.; Zijlstra, W.; Klenk, J. Evaluation of Accelerometer-Based Fall Detection Algorithms on Real-World Falls. *PLoS ONE* **2012**, *7*, e37062, doi:10.1371/journal.pone.0037062.
18. Schwickert, L.; Becker, C.; Lindemann, U.; Marechal, C.; Bourke, A.; Chiari, L.; Helbostad, J.L.; Zijlstra, W.; Aminian, K.; Todd, C.; et al. Fall Detection with Body-Worn Sensors : A Systematic Review. *Z. Gerontol. Geriatr.* **2013**, *46*, 706–719, doi:10.1007/s00391-013-0559-8.
19. Chaudhuri, S.; Thompson, H.; Demiris, G. Fall Detection Devices and Their Use with Older Adults: A Systematic Review. *J. Geriatr. Phys. Ther.* **2014**, *37*, 178–196, doi:10.1519/JPT.0b013e3182abe779.
20. Skubic, M.; Harris, B.H.; Stone, E.; Ho, K.C.; Su, B.Y.; Rantz, M. Testing Non-Wearable Fall Detection Methods in the Homes of Older Adults. In Proceedings of the 2016 38th Annual International Conference of the IEEE Engineering in Medicine and Biology Society (EMBC), Orlando, FL, USA, 16–20 August 2016; pp. 557–560, doi:10.1109/EMBC.2016.7590763.
21. Aziz, O.; Klenk, J.; Schwickert, L.; Chiari, L.; Becker, C.; Park, E.J.; Mori, G.; Robinovitch, S.N. Validation of Accuracy of SVM-Based Fall Detection System Using Real-World Fall and Non-Fall Datasets. *PLoS ONE* **2017**, *12*, e0180318, doi:10.1371/journal.pone.0180318.

22. Bloch, F.; Gautier, V.; Noury, N.; Lundy, J.E.; Poujaud, J.; Claessens, Y.E.; Rigaud, A.S. Evaluation under Real-Life Conditions of a Stand-Alone Fall Detector for the Elderly Subjects. *Ann. Phys. Rehabil. Med.* **2011**, *54*, 391–398, doi:10.1016/j.rehab.2011.07.962.

23. Bourke, A.K.; Klenk, J.; Schwickert, L.; Aminian, K.; Ihlen, E.A.F.; Mellone, S.; Helbostad, J.L.; Chiari, L.; Becker, C. Fall Detection Algorithms for Real-World Falls Harvested from Lumbar Sensors in the Elderly Population: A Machine Learning Approach. In Proceedings of the 2016 38th Annual International Conference of the IEEE Engineering in Medicine and Biology Society (EMBC), Orlando, FL, USA, 16–20 August 2016; pp. 3712–3715, doi:10.1109/EMBC.2016.7591534.

24. Chaudhuri, S.; Oudejans, D.; Thompson, H.J.; Demiris, G. Real World Accuracy and Use of a Wearable Fall Detection Device by Older Adults. *J. Am. Geriatr. Soc.* **2015**, *63*, 2415–2416, doi:10.1111/jgs.13804.

25. Chen, K.H.; Hsu, Y.W.; Yang, J.J.; Jaw, F.S. Enhanced Characterization of an Accelerometer-Based Fall Detection Algorithm Using a Repository. *Instrum. Sci. Technol.* **2017**, *45*, 382–391, doi:10.1080/10739149.2016.1268155.

26. Debard, G.; Karsmakers, P.; Deschodt, M.; Vlaeyen, E.; Van Den Bergh, J.; Dejaeger, E.; Milisen, K.; Goedeme, T.; Tuytelaars, T.; Vanrumste, B. Camera Based Fall Detection Using Multiple Features Validated with Real Life Video. In Workshop Proceedings of the 7th International Conference on Intelligent Environments, The Netherlands, 2011; Volume 10, pp. 441–450, doi:10.3233/978-1-60750-795-6-441.

27. Debard, G.; Mertens, M.; Deschodt, M.; Vlaeyen, E.; Devriendt, E.; Dejaeger, E.; Milisen, K.; Tournoy, J.; Croonenborghs, T.; Goedeme, T.; et al. Camera-Based Fall Detection Using Real-World versus Simulated Data: How Far Are We from the Solution? *J. Ambient Intell. Smart Environ.* **2016**, *8*, 149–168, doi:10.3233/AIS-160369.

28. Debard, G.; Mertens, M.; Goedeme, T.; Tuytelaars, T.; Vanrumste, B. Three Ways to Improve the Performance of Real-Life Camera-Based Fall Detection Systems. *J. Sens.* **2017**, doi:10.1155/2017/8241910.

29. Feldwieser, F.; Gietzelt, M.; Goevercin, M.; Marschollek, M.; Meis, M.; Winkelbach, S.; Wolf, K.H.; Spehr, J.; Steinhagen-Thiessen, E. Multimodal Sensor-Based Fall Detection within the Domestic Environment of Elderly People. *Z. Gerontol. Geriatr.* **2014**, *47*, 661–665, doi:10.1007/s00391-014-0805-8.

30. Gietzelt, M.; Spehr, J.; Ehmen, Y.; Wegel, S.; Feldwieser, F.; Meis, M.; Marschollek, M.; Wolf, K.H.; Steinhagen-Thiessen, E.; Govercin, M. GAL@Home: A Feasibility Study of Sensor-Based in-Home Fall Detection. *Z. Gerontol. Geriatr.* **2012**, *45*, 716–721, doi:10.1007/s00391-012-0400-9.

31. Godfrey, A.; Bourke, A.; Del Din, S.; Morris, R.; Hickey, A.; Helbostad, J.L.; Rochester, L.; Godfrey, A.; Bourke, A.; Del Din, S.; et al. Towards Holistic Free-Living Assessment in Parkinson's Disease: Unification of Gait and Fall Algorithms with a Single Accelerometer. In Proceedings of the Annual International Conference of the IEEE Engineering in Medicine And Biology Society, Orlando, FL, USA , 16–20 August 2016; pp. 651–654, doi:10.1109/EMBC.2016.7590786.

32. Hu, X.; Dor, R.; Bosch, S.; Khoong, A.; Li, J.; Stark, S.; Lu, C. Challenges in Studying Falls of Community-Dwelling Older Adults in the Real World. In Proceedings of the 2017 IEEE International Conference on Smart Computing (SMARTCOMP), Hong Kong, China, 29–31 May 2017; pp. 1–7, doi:10.1109/SMARTCOMP.2017.7946993.

33. Kangas, M.; Korpelainen, R.; Vikman, I.; Nyberg, L.; Jamsa, T. Sensitivity and False Alarm Rate of a Fall Sensor in Long-Term Fall Detection in the Elderly. *Gerontology* **2015**, *61*, 61–68, doi:10.1159/000362720.

34. Lipsitz, L.A.; Tchalla, A.E.; Iloputaife, I.; Gagnon, M.; Dole, K.; Su, Z.Z.; Klickstein, L. Evaluation of an Automated Falls Detection Device in Nursing Home Residents. *J. Am. Geriatr. Soc.* **2016**, *64*, 365–368, doi:10.1111/jgs.13708.

35. Liu, L.; Popescu, M.; Skubic, M.; Rantz, M. An Automatic Fall Detection Framework Using Data Fusion of Doppler Radar and Motion Sensor Network. In Proceedings of the Annual International Conference of the IEEE Engineering in Medicine and Biology Society, Chicago, IL, USA, 26–30 August 2014; pp. 5940–5943, doi:10.1109/EMBC.2014.6944981.

36. Palmerini, L.; Bagala, F.; Zanetti, A.; Klenk, J.; Becker, C.; Cappello, A. A Wavelet-Based Approach to Fall Detection. *Sensors* **2015**, *15*, 11575–11586, doi:10.3390/s150511575.

37. Rezaee, K.; Haddadnia, J.; Delbari, A. Intelligent Detection of the Falls in the Elderly Using Fuzzy Inference System and Video-Based Motion Estimation Method. In Proceedings of the 2013 8th Iranian Conference on Machine Vision and Image Processing (MVIP), Zanjan, Iran, 10–12 September 2013; pp. 284–288, doi:10.1109/IranianMVIP.2013.6779996.

38. Soaz, C.; Lederer, C.; Daumer, M. A New Method to Estimate the Real Upper Limit of the False Alarm Rate in a 3 Accelerometry-Based Fall Detector for the Elderly. In Proceedings of the 2012 Annual International Conference of the IEEE Engineering in Medicine and Biology Society, San Diego, CA, USA, 28 August–1 September 2012; pp. 244–247, doi:10.1109/EMBC.2012.6345915.
39. Stone, E.E.; Skubic, M. Fall Detection in Homes of Older Adults Using the Microsoft Kinect. *IEEE J. Biomed. Health Inform.* **2015**, *19*, 290–301, doi:10.1109/JBHI.2014.2312180.
40. Yu, S.; Chen, H.; Brown, R.A. Hidden Markov Model-Based Fall Detection with Motion Sensor Orientation Calibration: A Case for Real-Life Home Monitoring. *IEEE J. Biomed. Health Inform.* **2017**, doi:10.1109/JBHI.2017.2782079.
41. Delahoz, Y.S.; Labrador, M.A. Survey on Fall Detection and Fall Prevention Using Wearable and External Sensors. *Sensors* **2014**, *14*, 19806–19842, doi:10.3390/s141019806.
42. Folstein, M.F.; Folstein, S.E.; McHugh, P.R. "Mini-Mental State": A Practical Method for Grading the Cognitive State of Patients for the Clinician. *J. Psychiatr. Res.* **1975**, *12*, 189–198, doi:10.1016/0022-3956(75)90026-6.
43. Hand, D.J. Measuring Classifier Performance: A Coherent Alternative to the Area under the ROC Curve. *Mach. Learn.* **2009**, *77*, 103–123, doi:10.1007/s10994-009-5119-5.
44. Hanczar, B.; Hua, J.; Sima, C.; Weinstein, J.; Bittner, M.; Dougherty, E.R. Small-Sample Precision of ROC-Related Estimates. *Bioinformatics* **2010**, *26*, 822–830, doi:10.1093/bioinformatics/btq037.
45. Lobo, J.M.; Jiménez-Valverde, A.; Real, R. AUC: A Misleading Measure of the Performance of Predictive Distribution Models. *Glob. Ecol. Biogeogr.* **2008**, *17*, 145–151, doi:10.1111/j.1466-8238.2007.00358.x.
46. Davis, J.; Goadrich, M. The Relationship between Precision-Recall and ROC Curves. In Proceedings of the 23rd International Conference on Machine Learning, Pittsburgh, PA, USA, 25–29 June 2006; pp. 233–240.
47. Klenk, J.; Chiari, L.; Helbostad, J.; Zijlstra, W.; Aminian, K.; Todd, C.; Bandinelli, S.; Kerse, N.; Schwickert, L.; Mellone, S. Development of a Standard Fall Data Format for Signals from Body-Worn Sensors. *Z. Gerontol. Geriatr.* **2013**, *46*, 720–726.
48. Klenk, J.; Schwickert, L.; Palmerini, L.; Mellone, S.; Bourke, A.; Ihlen, E.A.F.; Kerse, N.; Hauer, K.; Pijnappels, M.; Synofzik, M.; et al. The FARSEEING Real-World Fall Repository: A Large-Scale Collaborative Database to Collect and Share Sensor Signals from Real-World Falls. *Eur. Rev. Aging Phys. Act.* **2016**, *13*, 8, doi:10.1186/s11556-016-0168-9.
49. Becker, C.; Schwickert, L.; Mellone, S.; Bagala, F.; Chiari, L.; Helbostad, J.L.; Zijlstra, W.; Aminian, K.; Bourke, A.; Todd, C.; et al. Proposal for a Multiphase Fall Model Based on Real-World Fall Recordings with Body-Fixed Sensors. *Z. Gerontol. Geriatr.* **2012**, *45*, 707–715, doi:10.1007/s00391-012-0403-6.

12

In-Ear Pulse Rate Measurement: A Valid Alternative to Heart Rate Derived from Electrocardiography?

Stefanie Passler *, Niklas Müller and Veit Senner

Technical University of Munich, Department of Mechanical Engineering, Professorship of Sport Equipment and Materials, Boltzmannstraße 15, D-85747 Garching, Germany

* Correspondence: stefanie.passler@tum.de

Abstract: Heart rate measurement has become one of the most widely used methods of monitoring the intensity of physical activity. The purpose of this study was to assess whether in-ear photoplethysmographic (PPG) pulse rate (PR) measurement devices represent a valid alternative to heart rate derived from electrocardiography (ECG), which is considered a gold standard. Twenty subjects (6 women, 14 men) completed one trial of graded cycling under laboratory conditions. In the trial, PR was recorded by two commercially available in-ear devices, the Dash Pro and the Cosinuss°One. They were compared to HR measured by a Bodyguard2 ECG. Validity of the in-ear PR measurement devices was tested by ANOVA, mean absolute percentage errors (MAPE), intra-class correlation coefficient (ICC), and Bland–Altman plots. Both devices achieved a MAPE $\leq$5%. Despite excellent to good levels of agreement, Bland–Altman plots showed that both in-ear devices tend to slightly underestimate the ECG's HR values. It may be concluded that in-ear PPG PR measurement is a promising technique that shows accurate but imprecise results under controlled conditions. However, PPG PR measurement in the ear is sensitive to motion artefacts. Thus, accuracy and precision of the measured PR depend highly on measurement site, stress situation, and exercise.

Keywords: photoplethysmography; heart rate; consumer-wearable devices; in-ear; validation; optical pulse rate monitoring; pulse rate

---

1. Introduction

As a result of the development of mobile heart rate monitors, heart rate has become one of the most widely used methods for controlling the general state of health and, particularly, the intensity of physical activity [1]. In 1938, Hertzman [2] first introduced photoplethysmography (PPG) as an alternative to electrocardiographic (ECG) heart rate monitoring. Since then, PPG has gained increasing popularity [3] and, with increasing technological improvements, it is used as an alternative pulse rate measurement method in wearable devices. In his review article, Toshiyo Tamura [4] provides an overview of the parameters that influence PPG signals. Besides the wavelength of light, contact force, motion artefacts, ambient temperature, and light intensity, the anatomical measurement location also influences PPG signals. Currently, PPG signals can be measured at the wrist [5–7], upper and lower arm [8–10], finger [11], esophageal region [12], forehead [13,14], and the ear, respectively. Ear-worn devices are defined as devices worn in or on the ear. Specifically, pulse rate measurement at the earlobe [15], the external ear cartilage [16,17], the superior and inferior auricular region [18–21], and the external auditory canal [22–24] has already been discussed in several studies as an alternative to ECG heart rate monitoring. Besides wrist-worn devices, ear-worn devices are probably the most common application of PPG.

The measuring principle of a PPG sensor is based on optical variations in pulsatile blood-flow volume. A PPG sensor includes a light-emitting diode (LED) and a photodetector (PD). The arrangement of these two components determines the mode of PPG. There are two modes, transmission and reflectance. In transmission mode, the PD, located opposite to the LED, captures the light transmitted through the tissue. Especially in medicine, this mode is frequently used. In it, the finger is the most common measurement location. A clip enables the opposite positioning of LED and PD. However, blood flow in the extremities, e.g., in the fingers, can be severely impaired due to circulatory disorders, for example. This may lead to unreliable and invalid measurement of the pulse rate. In reflectance mode, the PD captures the light reflected from bony structures, tissue, and blood vessels. Moreover, LED and PD are located next to each other. Thus, the reflectance mode is hardly limited to certain anatomical measurement locations [25,26]. Obviously, this is a reason for the suitability of PPG's reflectance mode in wearable devices. However, the intensity of the reflected or backscattered light is strongly dependent on the anatomical conditions of the measuring location [13]. On the forehead, where skin is very thin, but many blood vessels are present, a reliable signal can usually be recorded. On anatomical locations with a lower density of blood vessels and bony structures, the detected light intensity is usually lower.

Common wavelengths of PPG are between 500 nm and 1100 nm. This corresponds to the range from green-yellow to infrared light. The absorption rate of the light is mainly influenced by the pigment melanin and the water content in the tissue. The correlation between melanin and the absorption rate can be described as inversely proportional; the longer the wavelength, the more light is absorbed by melanin [27]. Water absorbs light in the ultraviolet and upper infrared range, whereas red and near infrared (NI) light is slightly absorbed by water [28]. This shows that the spectrum from NI to infrared light should be used for measuring deeper tissue structures. Hence, the transmission mode of PPG often uses wavelengths of 500–600 nm. Because of the stronger plethysmography signal, the green spectrum of light is more suited for optical pulse rate measurement [9]. The use of green LEDs allows a more accurate detection of the pulse rate [9,29–31].

The main difference between heart rate and pulse rate is the duration the pulse wave takes to complete the distance from the heart to the measurement site. This time is named the pulse transit time (PTT). It is determined as the time lag between the peak of the R-wave on the ECG and the peak value of the corresponding pulse at the measurement site, measured by PPG.

Altogether, several studies show that PPG is a promising method with regard to its use in wearable devices, especially when applied on the ear. However, most of the above-mentioned studies evaluated non-commercial devices, applied on the ear. So far, to our knowledge, no comprehensive studies have been published on the validity of commercial in-ear pulse rate monitoring devices using PPG. Thus, detailed validation of in-ear pulse rate monitoring devices using PPG is still pending.

The purpose of this study is to evaluate the validity of two consumer-wearable in-ear devices with respect to an ECG. Within the scope of this study, heart rate and PPG signals were first recorded simultaneously and then the rate variability of the two methods was compared.

2. Materials and Methods

2.1. Participants

Twenty healthy subjects (men = 14, women = 6) participated in the study and provided their written informed consent. Study protocol was proceeded under medical supervision of the Department of Prevention, Rehabilitation, and Sports Medicine of the Technical University of Munich. Additionally, the study was conducted in accordance with the Declaration of Helsinki. Participants who were eligible received detailed information on the purpose and methods of the study, as well as on data treatment and confidentiality according to the General Data Protection Regulation (2016/679) of the European Parliament and the Council of 27 April 2016 [32] and its Corrigendum of 23 May 2018 [33]. The characteristics of the sample population are shown in Table 1.

Table 1. Participant characteristics. Values are means ± standard deviation.

	Male (N = 14)	Female (N = 6)	All Participants (N = 20)
Age (years)	22.1 ± 1.8	22.5 ± 2.1	22.3 ± 2.0
Body mass (kg)	74.6 ± 8.4	57.8 ± 4.2	69.6 ± 11.0

2.2. *Instruments*

Within the scope of this study, the validity of the Cosinuss°One and the Dash Pro in-ear pulse rate measurement devices was investigated.

2.2.1. The Dash Pro

The Dash Pro (Bragi, Munich, Germany) is a wireless headset, equipped with sensor technology that is able to provide real-time feedback of recorded movements and pulse rate. The device consists of left and right headphones that communicate wirelessly with each other. The Dash Pro measures pulse rate in the external auditory canal using infrared light by reflection measurement. The device itself is available in one size, but can be fitted to the user's ear with interchangeable silicone caps in sizes XS to L. Figure 1a shows the Dash Pro with a silicone cap in size M. The blue arrows mark the diodes that allow heart rate detection by reflection measurement. Figure 1b shows the right device, worn in the right ear of a participant.

Figure 1. (**a**) The Dash Pro with silicone cap in size M; blue arrows show the LEDs for pulse rate detection. (**b**) Right Dash Pro, worn in the right ear.

For the comparison of the two in-ear pulse rate measurement devices, they had to be worn simultaneously. Therefore, the right Dash Pro has a self-sufficient and independent single-use mode.

2.2.2. Cosinuss°One

The second in-ear pulse rate measurement device evaluated in this study was the Cosinuss°One (Cosinuss, Munich, Germany). For comparison with the Dash Pro, the Cosinuss°One was used in the participant's left ear. Cosinuss°One measures the pulse rate in the external auditory canal by means of reflection measurement. Green light is used for this purpose. Measurement accuracy is ±1 bpm, as specified by the manufacturer. To optimize the fit and minimize movement artefacts, the device is available in sizes S to L. Individual size could be determined by means of the Cosinuss° app, using a value representing the received signal strength of the PO sensor. At a signal quality above 60%, size can be considered suitable. Figure 2a shows the Cosinuss°One. The two LEDs used for the reflection measurement in the external auditory canal are marked with blue arrows. Figure 2b shows the Cosinuss°One worn in the left ear of a participant.

(a) (b)

Figure 2. (**a**) Cosinuss°One; blue arrows show the LEDs for pulse rate detection. (**b**) Left Cosinuss°One, worn in the left ear.

2.2.3. Criterion Measure ECG—Bodyguard 2

Bodyguard 2 (Firstbeat Technologies Oy, Jyväskylä, Finland) was used as criterion measure. This ECG is not a medical device, but a sports-oriented electrocardiogram suitable for long-term and exercise ECG. Heart rate is recorded with two electrodes and processed with an integrated algorithm to correct artefacts. Compared to a clinical standard ECG, the Bodyguard 2 indicates 99.98% agreement [34].

2.3. Experimental Protocol

In order to evaluate the two in-ear pulse rate measurement devices as comprehensively as possible, their validity was evaluated during rest and under stress on a bicycle ergometer (Excalibur sport, Lode, Groningen, The Netherlands). Protocol started with a 10-min rest measurement in lying position, followed by a standardized, self-designed exercise protocol in a controlled laboratory setting. Prior to measurement under stress, each participant was instructed to cycle at a stress of 50 W for a 3-min warm-up period. Measurement under stress then started. The stress pattern of the protocol depended on the subject and was calculated from his/her weight in order to achieve an appropriate, comparable increase in intensity and thus heart rate for each subject. The number of watts per kilogram of body weight per minute increased uniformly by 0.4 W and 0.3 W in male and female subjects, respectively, starting from 50 W. The aim of this test protocol was to record a stress phase of at least 10 min and to measure a heart rate range of approximately 100–170 bpm. In order to ensure that participants did not stop prematurely because of maximum exhaustion, the duration of the protocol was set to 20 min. Formulas (1) and (2) show the calculation of the individual target stress of male and female participants.

$$\text{Target stress for males} = 50\ \text{W} + (\text{weight} \times 0.4 \times 20\ \text{min}), \tag{1}$$

$$\text{Target stress for females} = 50\ \text{W} + (\text{weight} \times 0.3 \times 20\ \text{min}). \tag{2}$$

The participants were instructed to cycle at a self-chosen number of rounds per minute (rpm) up to the individual maximum stress and to stop by hand signal in case of exhaustion. Upon completion, participants cooled down by cycling at a stress of 50 W for 3 min. During the entire data recording, participants were instructed to speak as little as possible, since jaw movements can lead to movement artefacts [21].

Regarding the use of all devices, care was taken to follow user guidelines as suggested by the manufacturers.

2.4. Data Analysis

ECG data were sampled at 1000 Hz and the heart rate was calculated from the time between R-R intervals, then exported as a text file at 1 s intervals. Data from optical pulse rate measurement of the in-ear devices was sampled at 100 Hz. The Cosinuss°One and the Dash Pro report the currently measured pulse rate to the respective mobile device app. For further analyses, data files of both in-ear devices were downloaded at 5 s intervals. Afterwards, data files of the in-ear and ECG devices were synched using the respective timestamps of each data acquisition.

To ensure the synchronization of the in-ear and the ECG devices, their timestamps have to be reliable and identical. Therefore, all data files were recorded in the Unix timestamp format (UTC). This format counts time in milliseconds since 1 January 1970. In contrast, the Dash Pro counts time in milliseconds since 1 January 2015. This represents an overall time discrepancy of 45 years or a shift by up to 40 s within 24 h. This correction was carried out immediately before each examination.

Time-synched data from each device were concurrently and continuously acquired for each participant throughout the entire test protocol. In accordance to the validation study of Spierer et al. [31], a 5 s time interval was defined as sufficiently accurate for detecting significant variations in heart rate measurement. Hence, every fifth value of the heart rate was used for further analysis.

Figure 3 presents heart and pulse rate during the entire test protocol, including the change from lying position to cycling.

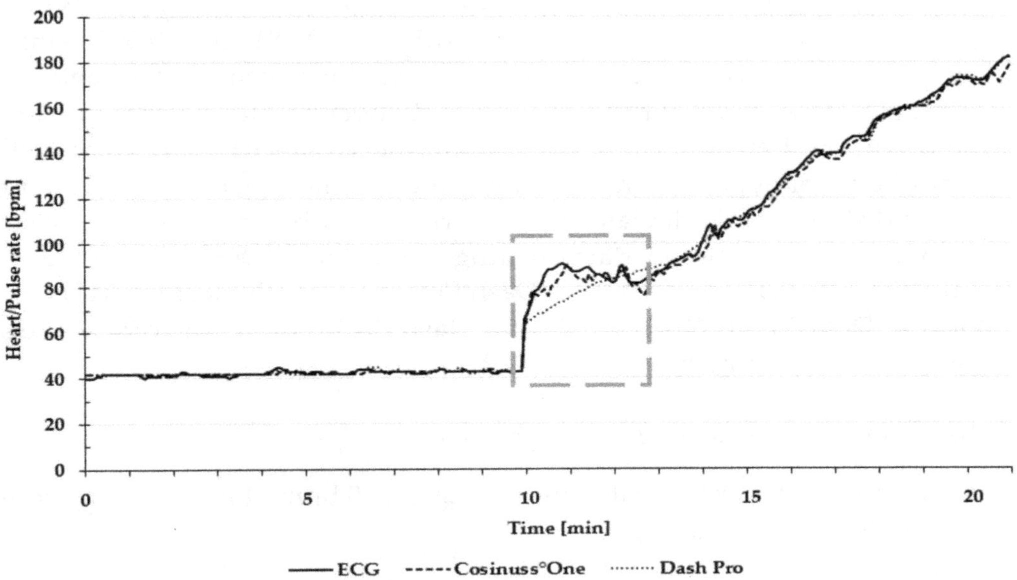

Figure 3. Exemplary presentation of pulse and heart rate during the entire test protocol. The dashed frame indicates the change from lying position to cycling. Heart rate of the ECG is depicted as a solid line; the pulse rate of Cosinuss°One is depicted as the dashed line; and the pulse rate of Dash Pro is depicted as the dotted line.

Motion artefacts, due to the change of body position and the re-adjustment of the sensors, resulted in strong signal noise, which can be seen in the dashed frame of Figure 3. Consequently, this data was not taken into account in the statistical evaluation.

Statistical analyses were conducted using IBM's SPSS Statistics software version 24 (IBM, Armonk, NY, USA). Descriptive statistics were used to characterize the sample population. The validity of the in-ear pulse rate measurement devices was determined by means of several statistical tests. Looking more closely at the term of validity, a distinction should be made between accuracy and precision. In the present study, accuracy was tested by MAPE and ICC values, whereas precision was identified by the limits of agreement of the Bland–Altman analysis.

Mean absolute percentage errors (MAPE) compared to the criterion measure were calculated as indicators of measurement error. MAPE, representing the error as a percentage of the overall mean relative to the ECG, does not have a standardized threshold for determining the accuracy of measurements. In the present study, a MAPE of ≤5% [35] was used as the criterion value for accuracy. To further investigate the level of agreement, Bland–Altman plots [36] were prepared. These plots serve as a visual illustration of variance and over- or underestimated measurement ranges of the investigated in-ear devices. For this, limits of agreement were set to 95%. Maximum and minimum pulse rates measured by means of the in-ear devices were compared with the ECG results using one-way repeated-measures ANOVA. An alpha of 0.05 was used to determine statistical significance. In addition, the agreement of maximum rate between the ECG and the tested devices was defined by means of the Intra-Class Correlation Coefficient (ICC) according to Liu et al. [37]. Excellent, good, moderate, and low agreement thresholds were defined as ICC values of ≥0.90; 0.75–0.90; 0.60–0.75; and ≤0.60, suggested by Fokkema et al. [35].

3. Results

3.1. Preliminary Analysis

The Kolmogorov–Smirnov test as well as visual data plotting of the criterion measure (Bodyguard 2), Cosinuss°One, and the Dash Pro revealed that the overall rates among all participants were significantly different from a normal distribution (resting conditions: $D(2376) = 0.066$, $p < 0.001$ for ECG and $D(2376) = 0.080$, $p < 0.001$ for Cosinuss°One and $D(2376) = 0.081$, $p < 0.001$; stress conditions: $D(2547) = 0.079$, $p < 0.001$ for ECG and $D(2547) = 0.075$, $p < 0.001$ for Cosinuss°One and $D(2547) = 0.073$, $p < 0.001$ for Dash Pro). To account for the differences between criterion measure and alternative method, Bland and Altman [38] suggest to investigate the variances for normal distribution, too. The preliminary applied Kolmogorov–Smirnov test on differences between criterion measure and alternative method did significantly deviate from a normal distribution. However, visual inspection indicated mostly normally distributed data (resting conditions: $D(2376) = 0.172$, $p < 0.001$ for Cosinuss°One and $D(2376) = 0.192$, $p < 0.001$ for Dash Pro; stress conditions: $D(2547) = 0.280$, $p < 0.001$ for Cosinuss°One and $D(2547) = 0.216$, $p < 0.001$ for Dash Pro). Hence, the procedure suggested by Bland and Altman [38,39] was implemented.

3.2. Resting Heart/Pulse Rate and Heart/Pulse Rate ≤90 bpm

The differences between the resting rates and the rates ≤90 bpm of the investigated in-ear devices and the ECG are provided in Table 2.

Table 2. Comparison among different devices for resting heart/pulse rate and heart/pulse rate ≤90 bpm. Values are mean ± standard deviation (SD), intra-class correlation coefficient (ICC), mean absolute error (MAE) ± standard deviation (SD), and mean absolute percentage error (MAPE).

	Resting Heart/Pulse Rate		Heart/Pulse Rate ≤90 bpm	
	Mean ± SD (bpm)	**ICC**	**MAE ± SD (bpm)**	**MAPE (%)**
Cosinuss°One	53.6 ± 8.3	0.94	1.5 ± 1.8	2.5
Dash Pro	55.0 ± 9.7	0.98	2.0 ± 2.5	3.2
ECG	54.9 ± 10.1			

On average, the participants achieved a resting heart rate of 54.9 ± 10.1 bpm in the ECG examinations. The average in-ear measured resting pulse rate of the Cosinuss°One and the Dash Pro is 53.6 ± 8.3 bpm and 55.0 ± 9.7 bpm, respectively.

Figure 4 is an exemplary presentation of the in-ear devices' pulse rate and the ECG's heart rate, recorded during the 10 min rest measurement in a lying position.

For the main analysis, one-way repeated-measures ANOVA was conducted. Mauchly's tests indicated that the assumption of sphericity had not been violated, $X^2(2) = 4.27$, $p > 0.05$, therefore non-corrected tests are reported. The results revealed that the minimum rates were not significantly affected by the measurement device, $F(2, 38) = 3.17$, $p > 0.05$.

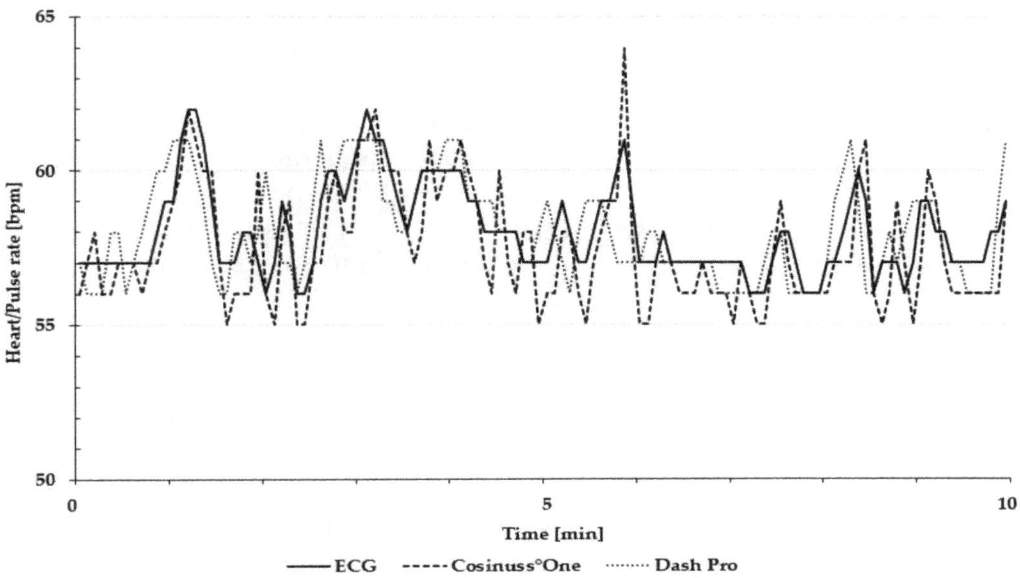

Figure 4. Exemplary presentation of pulse and heart rate during the 10 min rest measurement in a lying position. The heart rate of ECG is depicted as the solid line; the pulse rate of Cosinuss°One is depicted as the dashed line; and the pulse rate of Dash Pro is depicted as the dotted line.

Both in-ear devices are quite similar in terms of mean absolute error and MAPE, whereas the Dash Pro indicates higher values than the Cosinuss°One. In addition, the Cosinuss°One and the Dash Pro show excellent agreement in comparison to ECG, $R = 0.94$ for Cosinuss°One and $R = 0.98$ for Dash Pro.

Figure 5 shows Bland–Altman plots of the Cosinuss°One and the Dash Pro in-ear devices in comparison to the ECG with Bodyguard 2.

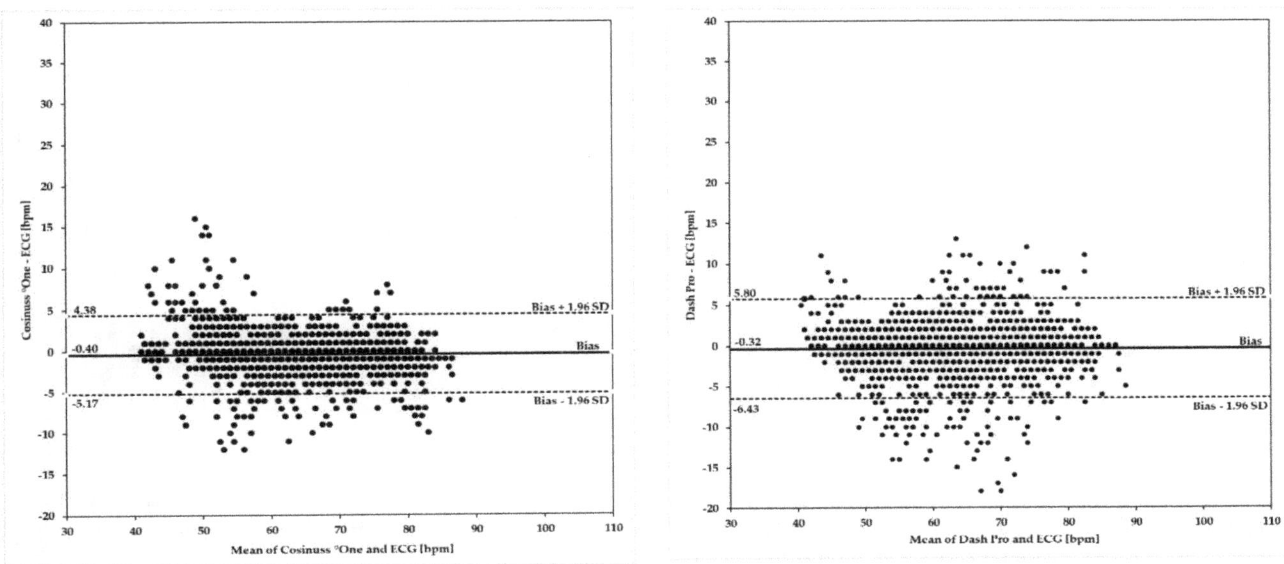

(a) (b)

Figure 5. Bland–Altman plots using heart/pulse rates ≤90 bpm. Investigated in-ear devices: (**a**) Cosinuss°One; (**b**) Dash Pro. Plots indicate differences of the rate values on the y-axis relative to the mean of the two methods (ECG and in-ear measurement) on the x-axis. Limits of agreement (LoA) were calculated as mean ± 1.96 × SD. Biases are depicted as a solid line; LoA are depicted as dashed lines.

Upper and lower limits of agreement (ULoA, LLoA) as well as the mean differences of the in-ear devices' PR ≤90 bpm compared to the ECG's HR are labeled in Figure 5a,b. Both in-ear devices show considerable deviations in scattering when compared to the ECG and tend to underestimate the heart rate by 0.40 bpm for Cosinuss°One and by 0.32 bpm for the Dash Pro. Bland–Altman analysis of the Cosinuss°One (Figure 5a) and the Dash Pro (Figure 5b) show that variability occurred across the spectrum of rates ≤90 bpm. The Cosinuss°One indicates more variability between 40 bpm and 60 bpm, while the Dash Pro shows higher variability across the midrange rates. In addition, the differences in variance are visualized. The Cosinuss°One (ULoA-LLoA: 9.55 bpm) shows lower scattering among its measurements when compared to the Dash Pro (ULoA-LLoA: 12.23 bpm). The Cosinuss°One had 95% of differences within +4.38 bpm and −5.17 bpm of the ECG, while the Dash Pro had 95% of differences within +5.80 bpm and −6.43 bpm.

3.3. Heart/Pulse Rate ≥100 bpm

The mean absolute error and the MAPE of the investigated in-ear devices' pulse rate ≥100 bpm are provided in Table 3.

Table 3. Comparison among in-ear devices for pulse rates ≥100 bpm. Values are mean absolute error (MAE) ± standard deviation (SD), mean absolute percentage error (MAPE).

	Pulse Rate ≥ 100 bpm	
	MAE ± SD (bpm)	**MAPE (%)**
Cosinuss°One	1.8 ± 2.8	1.3
Dash Pro	1.8 ± 2.8	1.4

Both in-ear devices are quite similar in terms of mean absolute error and MAPE. Figure 6a is an exemplary presentation of the in-ear devices' pulse rate and the ECG's heart rate, recorded during the stress protocol to the individual exhaustion. Figure 6b illustrates high differences between ECG and the in-ear devices around 100 bpm.

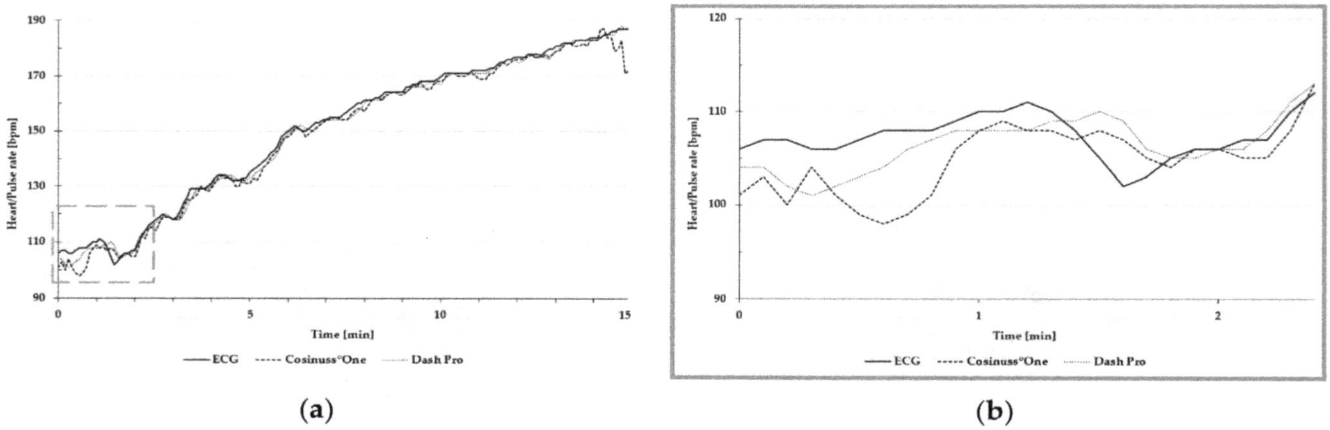

Figure 6. Exemplary presentation of pulse and heart rate (**a**) during the entire stress protocol; (**b**) around 100 bpm. The heart rate of ECG is depicted as the solid line; the pulse rate of Cosinuss°One is depicted as the dashed line; and the pulse rate of Dash Pro is depicted as the dotted line.

Figure 7 shows Bland–Altman plots of the Cosinuss°One and the Dash Pro in-ear devices in comparison to the ECG with Bodyguard 2.

Upper and lower limits of agreement (ULoA, LLoA) as well as the mean differences of the in-ear devices' PR ≥100 bpm compared to the ECG's HR are labeled in Figure 7a,b. Both in-ear devices show considerable deviations in scattering when compared to the ECG and tend to underestimate heart rate by 1.60 bpm for Cosinuss°One and by 0.51 bpm for the Dash Pro. Bland–Altman analysis of the Cosinuss°One (Figure 7a) and the Dash Pro (Figure 7b) shows that variability occurred across the spectrum of rates ≥100 bpm. The Cosinuss°One indicates more variability between 100 bpm and

150 bpm, while the Dash Pro shows higher variability between 100 bpm and 115 bpm. In addition, the differences in variance are visualized. The Cosinuss°One (ULoA-LLoA: 11.48 bpm) shows lower scattering among its measurements when compared to the Dash Pro (ULoA-LLoA: 12.67 bpm). The Cosinuss°One had 95% of differences within +4.14 bpm and −7.34 bpm of the ECG, while the Dash Pro had 95% of differences within +5.82 bpm and −6.85 bpm.

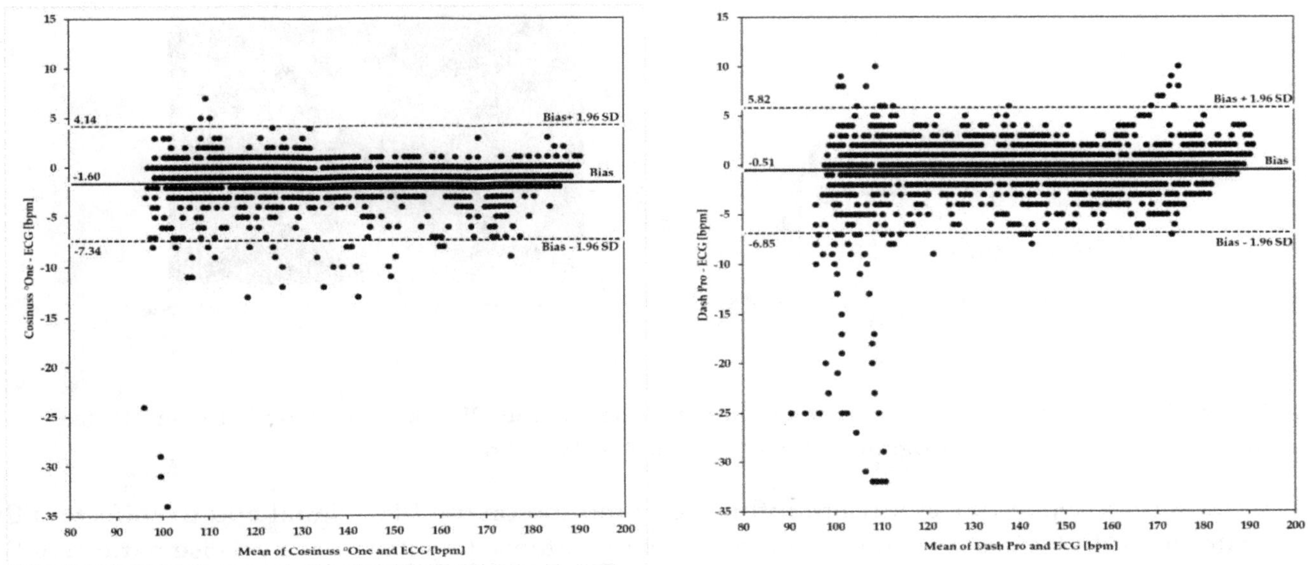

(a) (b)

Figure 7. Bland–Altman plots using heart/pulse rate ≥100 bpm. Investigated in-ear devices: (**a**) Cosinuss°One; (**b**) Dash Pro. Plots indicate differences of the rate values on the y-axis relative to the mean of the two methods (ECG and in-ear measurement) on the x-axis. Limits of agreement (LoA) were calculated as mean ± 1.96 × SD. Biases are depicted as a solid line; LoA are depicted as dashed lines.

3.4. Maximum Heart/Pulse Rate

The differences between the maximum heart/pulse rate of the investigated in-ear devices and the ECG are provided in Table 4.

Table 4. Comparison among different devices for maximum heart/pulse rate. Values are mean ± standard deviation (SD), intra-class correlation coefficient (ICC).

	Maximum Heart/Pulse Rate	
	Mean ± SD (bpm)	**ICC**
Cosinuss°One	181.6 ± 6.4	0.84
Dash Pro	183.7 ± 4.8	0.83
ECG	183.0 ± 5.1	

On average, participants achieved a HR_{max} of 183.0 ± 5.1 bpm in the ECG examinations. The average in-ear measured PR_{max} of the Cosinuss°One and the Dash Pro is 181.6 ± 6.4 bpm and 183.7 ± 4.8 bpm, respectively.

For the main analysis, one-way repeated-measures ANOVA was conducted. Mauchly's test indicated that the assumption of sphericity had not been violated, $X^2(2) = 3.66$, $p > 0.05$, therefore non-corrected tests are reported. In addition, the results revealed that the maximum rates were significantly affected by the measurement device, $F(2, 38) = 3.80$, $p \leq 0.05$. In addition, the Cosinuss°One and the Dash Pro show good agreement in comparison to ECG, $R = 0.84$ for Cosinuss°One and $R = 0.83$ for Dash Pro.

3.5. Motion Artefacts

To illustrate the influence of jaw movements on the PPG signal, one participant was asked to chew chewing gum as well as to talk throughout the data recording. The effects on the PPG signal and the pulse rate can be clearly seen in Figure 8a,b. Figure 8a illustrates the pulse rate of the Cosinuss°One, Figure 8b shows the spectrogram of the PPG signal of the Dash Pro.

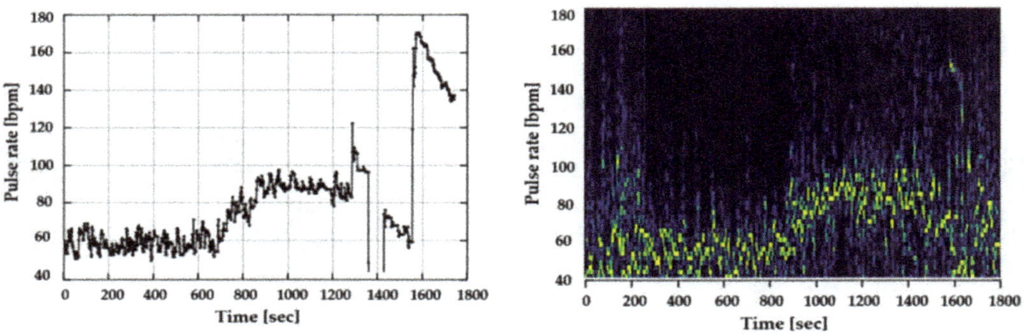

(a) (b)

Figure 8. Influence of jaw movements and talking on the PPG signal of both in-ear devices: (**a**) Cosinuss°One; (**b**) spectrogram of PPG signal of the Dash Pro.

Both figures depict the significant influence of motion on the PPG signal and the effect on the pulse rate. In both devices, signal interference was too intense to determine a precise pattern of the pulse rate.

4. Discussion

The present study examined the accuracy and precision of two ear-worn pulse rate measurement devices using PPG technology.

Systematic differences should be assessed using the MAPE. According to Nelson et al. [40], wearable devices should not exceed a MAPE threshold of ≤10% in order to be considered accurate. Fokkema et al. [35] suggest a threshold of ≤5%. In the present study, both devices indicated smaller MAPE scores at rates ≥100 bpm than at rates ≤90 bpm, but not exceeding the threshold of 5%. Thus, both in-ear devices can be classified as accurate almost completely within heart rates of 60–190 bpm, even according to Fokkema et al. [35].

To investigate the level of agreement between the in-ear devices and the criterion measure ECG, Bland–Altman plots were prepared according to Bland and Altman [36]. In resting condition as well as within the range of pulse rates ≥100 bpm, the Cosinuss°One revealed a narrower 95% limit of agreement than the Dash Pro. Both devices tended to slightly underestimate heart rate values within 60–190 bpm and showed high deviations from the ECG around 100 bpm. Although the limits of agreement might seem pretty narrow, these results have to be considered carefully. Heart and pulse rate data are a very sensitive source, e.g., for app-based training programs, and therefore imprecise and inaccurate raw data can lead to fatal results.

To determine the level of agreement, the ICC values of resting heart and pulse rates as well as maximum heart and pulse rates were examined. Under resting conditions, the Dash Pro and the Cosinuss°One show excellent agreement in comparison to ECG, whereas at maximum heart rates, a decrease to good agreement of both devices could be observed. Despite not exceeding the MAPE threshold of ≤5% and good to excellent levels of agreement, the results revealed that the maximum rates were significantly affected by the measurement device.

From a scientific point of view, there is only one commercial in-ear device, Bose Sound Sport (BSS; Bose Corporation, Framingham, MA, USA), which has been validated with respect to PPG pulse rate measurement to date. This underlines the lack of scientific validation studies. Pulse rate is a physiological parameter used for training control in sports or for monitoring the general state of health. Consumers must be protected, especially if activity trackers are to be used increasingly in the health and fitness sector. However, this access can only be defended or considered responsible if the current lack of transparency of the activity trackers industry is remedied through high-quality research, which can also help define general standards for these devices. The present study contributes to fill this gap. It shows the potential and the weaknesses of two commercially available in-ear devices in terms of measuring pulse rate.

Boudreaux et al. [41] conducted a study very similar to the present research. It is the first and, so far, the only study that investigated the accuracy and precision for pulse rate sensors in commercial headphones. The difference of this to the present study is the measurement site of PPG pulse rate detection. The measurement site of the Bose Sound Sport is the auricle. Both in-ear PPG devices validated in the present study use the external auditory canal for pulse rate measurement. Considering the measurement site and the consumer market, it should be noted that the present study is the first one to validate commercially available pulse rate monitors using PPG in the external auditory canal.

In the study of Boudreaux et al. [41], eight wearable devices, including the ear-worn Bose Sound Sport PPG device, were compared to a six-channel ECG regarding heart rate and caloric expenditure measurements. In addition to other stress situations, the BSS was also validated during cycling. For this purpose, a graded stress protocol was used, starting at rest and ending at a maximum stress of 200 W. The BSS slightly overestimates heart rate during low cycling intensities and underestimates heart rate during higher intensities. The latter agrees with the results of the present study. On average, the MAPE of the BSS was 7.4%. Under resting conditions, the MAPE of the BSS was 3.2%, very close to the Dash Pro and the Cosinuss°One, with MAPE values of 3.2% and 2.5%, respectively.

Considering the level of agreement, Boudreaux et al. [41] observed decreasing ICC values with higher exercise intensity and higher heart rates, respectively. This is in line with the results of the present study. The Cosinuss°One and the Dash Pro indicate a decrease from excellent to good agreement.

On the basis of MAPE values ≤5% and excellent to good levels of agreement, it can be stated that both the Dash Pro and the Cosinuss°One deliver accurate pulse rate values. In addition to accuracy, precision must also be considered as key factor when testing the validity of wearable devices. Due to high variance measured over the entire spectrum of heart/pulse rates, both in-ear devices of the present study have to be considered too imprecise as to be used as an alternative to the ECG.

Other than the mentioned study of Boudreaux et al. [41] and the present research, where commercially available ear-worn PPG devices were tested, the studies of Tigges et al. [23], Budidha and Kyriacou [16], and Leboeuf et al. [42] investigated self-developed pulse rate measurement systems based on PPG-technology. These devices are not commercially available. Tigges et al. [23] built such a device for scientific purposes and tested the device in the spectrum of 50–125 bpm under resting conditions. The Bland–Altman analysis showed a bias of −0.03 bpm, with 95% of the data lying within the boundaries of +2.88 bpm and −2.94 bpm. The study of Leboeuf et al. [42] showed a bias of −0.2 bpm, with the sensor slightly underestimating heart rate data. Similar to these results, where the data showed excellent agreement up to 200 bpm within varying activities, Budidha and Kyriacou [16] also concluded that the ear canal might be a suitable site for pulse rate measurement conducted by PPG sensors.

In comparison to the in-ear pulse rate PPG devices, considerably more wrist-worn pulse rate devices were validated [7,43–53]. Both fitness trackers and sports watches were tested under different exercise conditions. In order to ensure comparability to the presented results of the in-ear devices, only the literature in which validation was conducted on both a bicycle ergometer and an ECG was used as criterion measure will be discussed further. Within the framework of these studies [43–46], the validity of the wrist-worn devices, e.g., Apple Watch, Fitbit Charge HR, Basis Peak, Samsung Gear S, Polar M600, was mostly examined at rest, low, and high intensities. All devices tended to underestimate the heart rate regardless of intensity under both resting and cycling conditions. For instance, Wallen et al. [43] and Horton et al. [46] indicated that increasing physical effort leads to decreasing accuracy of the heart rate measurement. The results of Wallen et al. [43] revealed that heart rate underestimation ranged from −0.52 bpm (Basis Peak) to −12.67 bpm (Fitbit Charge HR) at low intensities, and −7.42 bpm (Basis Peak) to −14.20 bpm (Fitbit Charge HR) at high intensities, depending on the wrist-worn device used. Horton et al. [46] compared the sports watch Polar M600 pulse rate with the ECG heart rate during rest and cycling. They demonstrated a heart rate underestimation of −0.1 bpm during rest and −1.9 bpm during cycling. These findings are in agreement with the present results that show heart rate underestimation ranged from −0.32 bpm (Dash Pro) to −0.40 bpm (Cosinuss°One) under resting conditions and from −0.51 bpm (Dash Pro) to −1.60 bpm (Cosinuss°One) under cycling conditions.

The results presented in this study suggest the weakness of the PPG pulse rate monitoring devices, both in-ear and the wrist-worn.

PPG is a low-cost medical technique applied to the skin that uses the transmission and reflection of light into the skin to measure changes in blood volume within a specific tissue [9]. Previous research [1,4,54] suggests that PPG devices may have limitations in measuring PR that arise from the continuous increase and decrease of compression of a wearable device's PR sensor on the skin. In addition to conditions of low blood circulation and movements of the sensor on the skin, ambient light, which falsifies the values of the receiving diode, can also be seen as a source of error in PPG heart rate measurement [55]. In-ear PPG pulse rate monitors were developed to solve these main problems. As Vogel et al. [21] were able to show, a PPG sensor in the auricle near the ear canal, which irradiates light into the skin by reflection measurement, is resistant to most of the above-mentioned interfering factors. Circulatory disturbances and ambient light were minimized by the placement inside the ear. The inner ear is supplied by the same artery as the brain, which is why the blood flow and thus the strength of the PPG signal received in the inner ear remains constant, in contrast to PPG sensors on the extremities [16].

Due to pulse transit time, differences between heart rate and pulse rate may occur in general. Time lag between the peak of R-wave on the ECG and the peak value of the corresponding pulse in the ear, measured by PPG, may be a reason for underestimating heart rate.

A main remaining weakness of PPG is an unreliable signal due to motion artefacts. For in-ear PPG pulse rate measurement, jaw movements are the most dominant artefact [21]. In the present study, the external auditory canal as an application site for commercially available PPG pulse rate measurements was therefore tested as an alternative to electrocardiographic heart rate measurement.

While it was shown that the external auditory canal is a limited alternative measurement site for pulse rate measurement, the specific conditions in this study have to be taken into consideration. The study was conducted under controlled testing conditions, as the subjects were instructed to reduce jaw movement, e.g., by talking as little as possible to deliberately minimize motion artefacts. In addition, motion artefacts, such as head movement and vibrations due to uneven terrain, were not taken into account in this study. Despite the instruction to cycle at a self-chosen number of rounds per minute (rpm), most of the participants cycled at 80–100 rpm. This frequency may have increased the deviation of both of the in-ear devices from the ECG at a heart rate around 100 bpm.

In his review article, Toshiyo Tamura [4] suggests various methods to eliminate motion artefacts.

A conclusion regarding the higher validity of PPG due to different wavelengths when comparing both devices in the present study could not be made. Even though the Cosinuss°One measures with green light while the Dash Pro uses infrared light, significant differences in the measurement accuracy and precision could not be shown, opposing the suggestion that the use of green LEDs allows a more accurate and precise detection of the pulse rate [9,29–31].

The subject group represents just a certain and small population. Due to the young age and the healthy condition of the subjects, conclusions that consider older or diseased people cannot be drawn. In addition, a gender-specific differentiation of the results cannot be made due to the unbalanced distribution of fourteen men and six women.

5. Conclusions

It can be concluded that PPG measurement in the ear is a promising technique in resting positions. For future improvement, however, motion artefacts should be significantly reduced in order to ensure accuracy and precision in in-ear PPG pulse rate measurement during activity. Therefore, extensive studies under real life conditions should be carried out for a better understanding of the interaction between measurement accuracy as well as precision and the effects of artefacts from motion. This requires a considerable contribution from the activity trackers industry. The existing lack of transparency, e.g., regarding the algorithms used, complicates the analysis of the problems and thus the development of solutions.

The results of this study give an insight into the validity of the PPG technology used in the ear. Particularly in consumer wearable devices, a device worn in the ear can have many advantages over chest- or wrist-worn devices, as sports-specific parameters could be broadcasted to the athlete without interfering with the current activity. The combination of hearing aids and their ability to measure pulse rate simultaneously, could be a future application of in-ear PPG technology to promote the safety of elders. For use in health care, general standards and guidelines, with respect to measurement accuracy and precision, have to be defined and introduced to the activity trackers industry.

Author Contributions: Conceptualization, S.P. and N.M.; methodology, S.P. and N.M.; formal analysis, S.P. and N.M.; investigation, S.P. and N.M.; writing—original draft preparation, S.P. and N.M.; writing—review and editing, S.P., N.M. and V.S.; visualization, S.P.; supervision, S.P. and V.S.

References

1. Achten, J.; Jeukendrup, A.E. Heart rate monitoring: Applications and limitations. *Sports Med.* **2003**, *33*, 517–538. [CrossRef]
2. Hertzman, A.B. The blood supply of various skin areas as estimated by the photoelectric plethysmograph. *Am. J. Physiol. Content* **1938**, *124*, 328–340. [CrossRef]
3. Sanders, J.; Wark, P.; Winfree, K.; Fallahzadeh, R.; Fernández, C.; Henriksen, A.; Mikalsen, M.H.; Woldaregay, A.Z.; Muzny, M.; Hartvigsen, G.; et al. Using Fitness Trackers and Smartwatches to Measure Physical Activity in Research: Analysis of Consumer Wrist-Worn Wearables. *J. Med. Internet Res.* **2018**, *20*, e110.
4. Tamura, T. Current progress of photoplethysmography and SPO_2 for health monitoring. *Biomed. Eng. Lett.* **2019**, *9*, 21–36. [CrossRef] [PubMed]
5. Jung, J.Y.; Lee, L.W. Zigbee device access control and reliable data transmission in Zigbee based health monitoring. In Proceedings of the 2008 10th International Conference on Advanced Communication Technology, Gangwon-Do, Korea, 17–20 February 2008; pp. 795–797.
6. Lee, Y.K.; Jo, J.; Shin, H.S. Development and Evaluation of a Wristwatch-Type Photoplethysmography Array Sensor Module. *IEEE Sens. J.* **2013**, *13*, 1459–1463. [CrossRef]
7. Cadmus-Bertram, L.; Gangnon, R.; Wirkus, E.J.; Thraen-Borowski, K.M.; Gorzelitz-Liebhauser, J. The Accuracy of Heart Rate Monitoring by Some Wrist-Worn Activity Trackers. *Ann. Intern. Med.* **2017**, *166*, 610–612. [CrossRef] [PubMed]
8. Maeda, Y.; Sekine, M.; Tamura, T. Relationship between measurement site and motion artifacts in wearable reflected photoplethysmography. *J. Med. Syst.* **2011**, *35*, 969–976. [CrossRef]
9. Maeda, Y.; Sekine, M.; Tamura, T. The Advantages of Wearable Green Reflected Photoplethysmography. *J. Med. Syst.* **2011**, *35*, 829–834. [CrossRef]
10. Maguire, M.; Ward, T. *The Design and Clinical Use of a Reflective Brachial Photoplethysmograph*; Maynooth University: Kildare, Ireland, 2002.
11. Rhee, S.; Yang, B.-H.; Asada, H. Artifact-resistant power-efficient design of finger-ring plethysmographic sensors. *IEEE Trans. Biomed. Eng.* **2001**, *48*, 795–805. [CrossRef] [PubMed]

12. Kyriacou, P.A.; Moye, A.R.; Gregg, A.; Choi, D.M.A.; Langford, R.M.; Jones, D.P.; Kyriacou, P. A system for investigating oesophageal photoplethysmographic signals in anaesthetised patients. *Med. Biol. Eng.* **1999**, *37*, 639–643. [CrossRef]
13. Mendelson, Y.; Pujary, C. Measurement site and photodetector size considerations in optimizing power consumption of a wearable reflectance pulse oximeter. In Proceedings of the 25th Annual International Conference of the IEEE Engineering in Medicine and Biology Society, Cancún, Mexico, 17–21 September 2003; pp. 3016–3019.
14. Dassel, A.C.M.; Graaff, R.; Sikkema, M.; Meijer, A.; Zijlstra, W.G.; Aarnoudse, J.G. Reflectance pulse oximetry at the forehead improves by pressure on the probe. *J. Clin. Monit.* **1995**, *11*, 237–244. [CrossRef] [PubMed]
15. Poh, M.-Z.; Swenson, N.C.; Picard, R.W. Motion-tolerant magnetic earring sensor and wireless earpiece for wearable photoplethysmography. *IEEE Trans. Inf. Technol. Biomed.* **2010**, *14*, 786–794. [CrossRef] [PubMed]
16. Budidha, K.; Kyriacou, P.A. The human ear canal: Investigation of its suitability for monitoring photoplethysmographs and arterial oxygen saturation. *Physiol. Meas.* **2014**, *35*, 111–128. [CrossRef] [PubMed]
17. Poh, M.-Z.; Kim, K.; Goessling, A.; Swenson, N.; Picard, R. Cardiovascular Monitoring Using Earphones and a Mobile Device. *IEEE Pervasive Comput.* **2012**, *11*, 18–26. [CrossRef]
18. Patterson, J.A.C.; McIlwraith, D.C.; Yang, G.-Z. A Flexible, Low Noise Reflective PPG Sensor Platform for Ear-Worn Heart Rate Monitoring. In Proceedings of the 2009 Sixth International Workshop on Wearable and Implantable Body Sensor Networks, Berkeley, CA, USA, 3–5 June 2009; pp. 286–291.
19. Wang, C.-Z.; Zheng, Y.-P. Home-Telecare of the Elderly Living Alone Using an New Designed Ear-wearable Sensor. In Proceedings of the 5th International Workshop on Wearable and Implantable Body Sensor Networks, Hong Kong, China, 1–3 June 2008; pp. 71–74.
20. Wang, L.; Lo, B.P.L.; Yang, G.-Z. Multichannel Reflective PPG Earpiece Sensor with Passive Motion Cancellation. *IEEE Trans. Biomed. Circuits Syst.* **2007**, *1*, 235–241. [CrossRef] [PubMed]
21. Vogel, S.; Hülsbusch, M.; Hennig, T.; Blazek, V.; Leonhardt, S. In-ear vital signs monitoring using a novel microoptic reflective sensor. *IEEE Trans. Inf. Technol. Biomed.* **2009**, *13*, 882–889. [CrossRef] [PubMed]
22. Goverdovsky, V.; Von Rosenberg, W.C.; Nakamura, T.; Looney, D.; Sharp, D.J.; Papavassiliou, C.; Morrell, M.J.; Mandic, D.P. Hearables: Multimodal physiological in-ear sensing. *Sci. Rep.* **2017**, *7*, 6948. [CrossRef] [PubMed]
23. Tigges, T.; Büchler, T.; Pielmuş, A.; Klum, M.; Feldheiser, A.; Hunsicker, O.; Orglmeister, R. Assessment of In-ear Photoplethysmography as a Surrogate for Electrocardiography in Heart Rate Variability Analysis. In *World Congress on Medical Physics and Biomedical Engineering 2018*; Lhotska, L., Sukupova, L., Lacković, I., Ibbott, G.S., Eds.; Springer: Singapore, 2019; pp. 293–297.
24. Shin, K.; Kim, Y.; Bae, S.; Park, K.; Kim, S. A Novel Headset with a Transmissive PPG Sensor for Heart Rate Measurement. In Proceedings of the 13th International Conference on Biomedical Engineering, Singapore, 3–6 December 2008; Lim, C.T., Goh, J.C.H., Eds.; Springer: Berlin/Heidelberg, Germany, 2009; pp. 519–522.
25. Agashe, G.S.; Coakley, J.; Mannheimer, P.D. Forehead pulse oximetry: Headband use helps alleviate false low readings likely related to venous pulsation artifact. *Anesthesiology* **2006**, *105*, 1111–1116. [CrossRef]
26. Mendelson, Y.; Ochs, B.D. Noninvasive pulse oximetry utilizing skin reflectance photoplethysmography. *IEEE Trans. Biomed. Eng.* **1988**, *35*, 798–805. [CrossRef]
27. Anderson, R.R.; Parrish, J.A. The Optics of Human Skin. *J. Investig. Dermatol.* **1981**, *77*, 13–19. [CrossRef] [PubMed]
28. Allen, J. Photoplethysmography and its application in clinical physiological measurement. *Physiol. Meas.* **2007**, *28*, R1–R39. [CrossRef]
29. Delgado-Gonzalo, R.; Parák, J.; Tarniceriu, A.; Renevey, P.; Bertschi, M.; Korhonen, I. Evaluation of accuracy and reliability of PulseOn optical heart rate monitoring device. In Proceedings of the 2015 37th Annual International Conference of the IEEE Engineering in Medicine and Biology Society (EMBC), Milan, Italy, 25–29 August 2015; pp. 430–433.
30. Lee, S.; Shin, H.; Hahm, C. Effective PPG sensor placement for reflected red and green light, and infrared wristband-type photoplethysmography. In Proceedings of the 2016 18th International Conference on Advanced Communication Technology (ICACT), Pyeongchang, Korea, 31 January–3 February 2016.
31. Spierer, D.K.; Rosen, Z.; Litman, L.L.; Fujii, K. Validation of photoplethysmography as a method to detect heart rate during rest and exercise. *J. Med. Eng. Technol.* **2015**, *39*, 264–271. [CrossRef] [PubMed]

32. European Union. Regulation (EU) 2016/679 of the European Parliament and the Council of 27 April 2016 on the protection of natural persons with regard to the processing of personal data and on the free movement of such data, and repealing Directive 95/46/EC (General Data Protection Regulation). *Off. J. Eur. Union* **2016**, *59*, 1–88.
33. European Union. Corrigendum to Regulation (EU) 2016/679 of the European Parliament and the Council of 27 April 2016 on the protection of natural persons with regard to the processing of personal data and on the free movement of such data, and repealing Directive 95/46/EC (General Data Protection Regulation). *Off. J. Eur. Union* **2018**, *61*, 2–5.
34. Parak, J. Accuracy of Firstbeat Bodyguard 2 Beat-To-Beat Heart Rate Monitor; (whitepaper). 2013. Available online: https://assets.firstbeat.com/firstbeat/uploads/2015/11/white_paper_bodyguard2_final.pdf (accessed on 20 August 2019).
35. Fokkema, T.; Kooiman, T.J.M.; Krijnen, W.P.; Van der Schans, C.P.; Groot, M. Reliability and Validity of Ten Consumer Activity Trackers Depend on Wlaking Speed. *Med. Sci. Sports Exerc.* **2017**, *49*, 793–800. [CrossRef] [PubMed]
36. Bland, J.M.; Altman, D. Statistical methods for assessing agreement between two methods of clinical measurement. *Lancet* **1986**, *327*, 307–310. [CrossRef]
37. Liu, J.; Tang, W.; Chen, G.; Lu, Y.; Feng, C.; Tu, X.M. Correlation and agreement: Overview and clarification of competing concepts and measures. *Shanghai Arch Psychiatry* **2016**, *28*, 115–120.
38. Bland, J.M.; Altman, D.G. Applying the right statistics: Analyses of measurement studies. *Ultrasound Obstet. Gynecol.* **2003**, *22*, 85–93. [CrossRef]
39. Bland, J.M.; Altman, D.G. Measuring agreement in method comparison studies. *Stat. Methods Med. Res.* **1999**, *8*, 135–160. [CrossRef]
40. Nelson, M.B.; Kaminsky, L.A.; Dickin, D.C.; Montoye, A.H. Validity of Consumer-Based Physical Activity Monitors for Specific Activity Types. *Med. Sci. Sports Exerc.* **2016**, *48*, 1619–1628. [CrossRef]
41. Boudreaux, B.D.; Hebert, E.P.; Hollander, D.B.; Williams, B.M.; Cormier, C.L.; Naquin, M.R.; Gillan, W.W.; Gusew, E.E.; Kraemer, R.R. Validity of Wearable Activity Monitors during Cycling and Resistance Exercise. *Med. Sci. Sports Exerc.* **2018**, *50*, 624–633. [CrossRef] [PubMed]
42. Leboeuf, S.F.; Aumer, M.E.; Kraus, W.E.; Johnson, J.L.; Duscha, B. Earbud-based sensor for the assessment of energy expenditure, HR, and VO2max. *Med. Sci. Sports Exerc.* **2014**, *46*, 1046–1052. [CrossRef] [PubMed]
43. Wallen, M.P.; Gomersall, S.R.; Keating, S.E.; Wisløff, U.; Coombes, J.S. Accuracy of Heart Rate Watches: Implications for Weight Management. *PLoS ONE* **2016**, *11*, e0154420. [CrossRef] [PubMed]
44. Jo, E.; Lewis, K.; Directo, D.; Kim, M.J.; Dolezal, B.A. Validation of Biofeedback Wearables for Photoplethysmographic Heart Rate Tracking. *J. Sports Sci. Med.* **2016**, *15*, 540–547. [PubMed]
45. Benedetto, S.; Caldato, C.; Bazzan, E.; Greenwood, D.C.; Pensabene, V.; Actis, P. Assessment of the Fitbit Charge 2 for monitoring heart rate. *PLoS ONE* **2018**, *13*, e0192691. [CrossRef] [PubMed]
46. Horton, J.F.; Stergiou, P.; Katz, L.; Fung, T.S. Comparison of Polar M600 Optical Heart Rate and ECG Heart Rate during Exercise. *Med. Sci. Sports Exerc.* **2017**, *49*, 2600–2607. [CrossRef] [PubMed]
47. Abt, G.; Bray, J.; Benson, A.C. The validity and inter-device variability of the Apple Watch™ for measuring maximal heart rate. *J. Sports Sci.* **2018**, *36*, 1447–1452. [CrossRef]
48. Støve, M.P.; Haucke, E.; Nymann, M.L.; Sigurdsson, T.; Larsen, B.T. Accuracy of the wearable activity tracker Garmin Forerunner 235 for the assessment of heart rate during rest and activity. *J. Sports Sci.* **2019**, *37*, 895–901. [CrossRef]
49. Wang, R.; Blackburn, G.; Desai, M.; Phelan, D.; Gillinov, L.; Houghtaling, P. Accuracy of Wrist-Worn Heart Rate Monitors. *JAMA Cardiol.* **2017**, *2*, 104–106. [CrossRef]
50. Stahl, S.E.; An, H.-S.; Dinkel, D.M.; Noble, J.M.; Lee, J.-M. How accurate are the wrist-based heart rate monitors during walking and running activities? Are they accurate enough? *BMJ Open Sport Exerc. Med.* **2016**, *2*, e000106. [CrossRef]
51. Reddy, R.K.; Pooni, R.; Zaharieva, D.P.; Senf, B.; El Youssef, J.; Dassau, E.; Doyle Iii, F.J.; Clements, M.A.; Rickels, M.R.; Patton, S.R.; et al. Accuracy of Wrist-Worn Activity Monitors During Common Daily Physical Activities and Types of Structured Exercise: Evaluation Study. *JMIR mHealth uHealth* **2018**, *6*, e10338. [CrossRef] [PubMed]

52. Gillinov, S.; Etiwy, M.; Wang, R.; Blackburn, G.; Phelan, D.; Gillinov, A.M.; Houghtaling, P.; Javadikasgari, H.; Desai, M.Y. Variable Accuracy of Wearable Heart Rate Monitors during Aerobic Exercise. *Med. Sci. Sports Exerc.* **2017**, *49*, 1697–1703. [CrossRef] [PubMed]
53. Shcherbina, A.; Mattsson, C.M.; Waggott, D.; Salisbury, H.; Christle, J.W.; Hastie, T.; Wheeler, M.T.; Ashley, E.A. Accuracy in Wrist-Worn, Sensor-Based Measurements of Heart Rate and Energy Expenditure in a Diverse Cohort. *J. Pers. Med.* **2017**, *7*, 3. [CrossRef] [PubMed]
54. Tamura, T.; Maeda, Y.; Sekine, M.; Yoshida, M. Wearable Photoplethysmographic Sensors—Past and Present. *Electronics* **2014**, *3*, 282–302. [CrossRef]
55. Trivedi, N.S.; Ghouri, A.F.; Shah, N.K.; Lai, E.; Barker, S.J. Effects of motion, ambient light, and hypoperfusion on pulse oximeter function. *J. Clin. Anesth.* **1997**, *9*, 179–183. [CrossRef]

13

Analysis of the Impact of Interpolation Methods of Missing RR-Intervals Caused by Motion Artifacts on HRV Features Estimations

Davide Morelli [1,2,*], Alessio Rossi [3], Massimo Cairo [2] and David A. Clifton [1]

1 Institute of Biomedical Engineering, Department of Engineering Science, University of Oxford, Oxford OX2 6DP, UK
2 Biobeats Group LTD, 3 Fitzhardinge Street, London W1H 6EF, UK
3 Computer Science Department, University of Pisa, Largo Bruno Pontecorvo 3, 56127 Pisa, Italy
* Correspondence: davide.morelli@eng.ox.ac.uk

Abstract: Wearable physiological monitors have become increasingly popular, often worn during people's daily life, collecting data 24 hours a day, 7 days a week. In the last decade, these devices have attracted the attention of the scientific community as they allow us to automatically extract information about user physiology (e.g., heart rate, sleep quality and physical activity) enabling inference on their health. However, the biggest issue about the data recorded by wearable devices is the missing values due to motion and mechanical artifacts induced by external stimuli during data acquisition. This missing data could negatively affect the assessment of heart rate (HR) response and estimation of heart rate variability (HRV), that could in turn provide misleading insights concerning the health status of the individual. In this study, we focus on healthy subjects with normal heart activity and investigate the effects of missing variation of the timing between beats (RR-intervals) caused by motion artifacts on HRV features estimation by randomly introducing missing values within a five min time windows of RR-intervals obtained from the nsr2db PhysioNet dataset by using Gilbert burst method. We then evaluate several strategies for estimating HRV in the presence of missing values by interpolating periods of missing values, covering the range of techniques often deployed in the literature, via linear, quadratic, cubic, and cubic spline functions. We thereby compare the HRV features obtained by handling missing data in RR-interval time series against HRV features obtained from the same data without missing values. Finally, we assess the difference between the use of interpolation methods on time (i.e., the timestamp when the heartbeats happen) and on duration (i.e., the duration of the heartbeats), in order to identify the best methodology to handle the missing RR-intervals. The main novel finding of this study is that the interpolation of missing data on time produces more reliable HRV estimations when compared to interpolation on duration. Hence, we can conclude that interpolation on duration modifies the power spectrum of the RR signal, negatively affecting the estimation of the HRV features as the amount of missing values increases. We can conclude that interpolation in time is the optimal method among those considered for handling data with large amounts of missing values, such as data from wearable sensors.

Keywords: heart rate; IoT wearable monitor; health

---

1. Introduction

In the last two decades, the interest in the variation of the timing between beats (RR-intervals) of the cardiac cycle, called heart rate variability (HRV), has widely increased in the psycho-physiological research field. Assessment of RR-intervals variability is possible through time and frequency domain analyses that provide parameters able to quantify the amount of fluctuations occurring between consecutive beats, giving therefore an indirect index of autonomic regulation. Actually, the parameters extracted from HRV analysis are useful to provide insight about sympathetic-parasympathetic balance of cardiac vagal tone that was found to be an indicator of cognitive, emotional, social and health status [1].

Thanks to the technological advancements of recent decades, it is now possible to continuously record heart activity during peoples' life via wrist-worn wearable devices equipped with heart rate sensors. This innovation might have a great impact on the medical field because of the low cost of the devices and the possibility to obtain continuous passive measurements performed in an ecological setting, gaining an overview of the users' health status by assessing HRV features during their daily life [2]. These wrist-worn wearable devices, however, produce several inconsistent RR-intervals produced not only by ectopic beats (e.g., atrial fibrillation and premature heart beat), but mainly by motion and mechanical artifacts induced by external stimuli. The number of abnormal RR-intervals increases from 1%—when heart beats are recorded with gold standard technology (i.e., electrocardiography)—[3] to more than 10%—when they are recorded with wrist-worn wearable devices. However, standard methods for calculating HRV features from the time-series of RR-intervals require accurate beat detection. Hence, handling the missing values became a fundamental aspect to correctly evaluate users' physiological response. As a matter of fact, these missing values affect the HRV analysis producing misleading results [4]. In previous studies, the inconsistent RR-interval data were handled by reconstructing the missing values using nearest-neighbour, linear, cubic spline and piecewise cubic Hermite interpolation methods [4,5]. However, these methods can also introduce changes in the reconstructed timeseries that could corrupt the signal spectrum [6], thus reducing the ability to estimate both time or frequency domains HRV features.

In this paper, we focus on healthy subjects with normal heart activity, and investigate the effects of interpolation on time (i.e., the timestamps when the heartbeats happen) and duration (i.e., the duration of the heartbeats) with an increasing amount of missing values (from 0% to 70%) in order to assess which interpolation strategy yields better results when estimating HRV features. In particular, in this paper we show that quadratic interpolation on time is the best approach to reconstruct the missing RR-intervals. Anyway, the main finding of this study is that the interpolation on time produce better HRV feature estimation that the interpolation on Duration suggested by all the previous studies.

1.1. Paper Contribution

To the best of our knowledge, this work is one of the first studies investigating the effect of high percentage of missing values (i.e., 30%, 50% and 70%) on HRV analysis. In previous studies, the inconsistency of RR-intervals was due to a small number of ectopic beats, while wrist-worn wearable devices introduce motion and mechanical artifacts that produce a huge quantity of abnormal heart beats.

Moreover, to the best of our knowledge, this is the first study to analyse the effect on HRV features of interpolation on time versus interpolation on duration. We show the difference among interpolation methods (i.e., no-interpolation, nearest neighbor, linear, quadratic and cubic spline) on both time and duration timeseries in order to detect which interpolation method yields lower error in HRV features estimations. This analysis permits to provide insight about how the interpolation methods work in quantifying the noise introduced into the timeseries.

We conclude by showing that interpolation on time is the best choice for preprocessing RR timeseries with missing values, contradicting the approach traditionally followed, based on durations timeseries.

1.2. Related Work

During the day, approximately 1% of beats are to be expected to be ectopic [3] when they are recorded by using gold standard instrument (i.e., Electrocardiography). An ectopic beat is a disturbance of the cardiac rhythm that induces premature ventricular or atrial contraction. The physiological artifact producing inconsistent beat seriously affects the HRV spectrum, and could result in erroneous results during HRV analysis by introducing non-existing frequencies into the spectrum [7]. In addition to physiological artifact, motion and mechanical artifacts induced by external stimuli introduce a large amount of inconsistent beats when the data are recorded by using wrist-worn wearable device [4–6]. This work is one of the firsts studies that investigate the effect of huge quantities of inconsistent beats that are not only derived from ectopic beats. Since missing data are common in the RR-interval timeseries derived from wrist-worn wearable device, they could complicate the analysis of HRV features making it sometimes impossible. To make reliable HRV analysis, previous studies suggested several preprocessing methods for RR-intervals timeseries (e.g., deletion, interpolations and filtering). However, these preprocessing methods have their own distinct effect on HRV analysis yielding different results [7].

The simplest way of handling the inconsistent RR-intervals provided in literature is to delete them [8]. In this approach, the abnormal RR-intervals are removed and the normal RR-intervals list are merged together. A huge issue of the deletion approach is that it reduces the overall length of the HRV signal. This may significantly influence HRV spectrum [8]. Other interpolation methods maintain the original number of samples, but, by manipulating the duration of RR-intervals, they also change the overall duration by some amount. There are several interpolation approaches useful for handling inconsistent RR-intervals, i.e., zero degree, linear and cubic spline [9]. Zero degree replaces the inconsistent RR-intervals with the mean of the closest normal values. Differently, linear interpolation fits a straight line over the inconsistent RR-intervals to obtain normal values. Finally, the most popular interpolation approach is the spline of order three (i.e., cubic spline). It fits a third degree polynomial smooth curve through a number of data points to obtain new values. This latter approach is recommended when there is only small number of inconsistent RR-intervals [9].

Finally, it was found that the interpolation introduces low frequency components (LF) and reduces high-frequency components (HF) power [6]. This aspect affects frequency domain HRV features [5], while little effect was found in time domain HRV features [4].

We were not able to find any previous work studying the effect of interpolation missing values on the duration versus time, and the propagation of error to HRV features.

2. Materials and Methods

2.1. Dataset

In this paper, we used *nsr2db* (Normal Sinus Rhythm RR Interval Database) PhysioNet dataset [10]. This dataset contains beat annotations of 54 normal sinus rhythm subjects (30 men: 28–76 years; 24 women: 58–73 years) extracted from 23 h long electrocardiogram (ECG) recordings, digitized at 128 samples per second, and beat annotations obtained by automated analysis with manual review and correction.

In order to compute HRV features, the 23 h time series of ECG recording of each user were split into 5 min windows. Moreover, to investigate the effect of missing values on HRV analysis, artificial missing RR-intervals (i.e., 30%, 50% and 70% of missing values) were inserted into the 5 min windows.

The missing values were created in accordance with a burst Gilbert model that simulates burst-error with a two-state Markov chain (i.e., good as 0 and bed as 1) [11]. We define P as the probability of transition form state 0 to the state 1 and p the probability of transition from state 1 to 0. Moreover, Q and q give the probabilities of remaining in the same states 0 or 1 (see Figure 1). Using these parameters, it is possible to represent average bit-error rate P_e as showed in Equation (1) and the average burst length (L_{length}) is set at 10.

$$P_e = \frac{P}{p + P}. \tag{1}$$

Given these equation, we define P, p, Q and q as showed in Equations (2)–(5), respectively.

$$p = 1/L_{burst} \tag{2}$$

$$P = \frac{P_{change}}{1 - P_{change}} * p \tag{3}$$

$$q = 1 - p \tag{4}$$

$$Q = 1 - P, \tag{5}$$

where the P_{change} is set in accordance with the missing values percentage that we want to add in the time series (e.g., if we want 20% of missing values we set P_{change} as 0.3). The missing values were introduced in the time series when the state of the two-state Markov chain is equal to 1. Examples of 30%, 50% and 70% of missing values created by Gilbert model are provided in Figure 2.

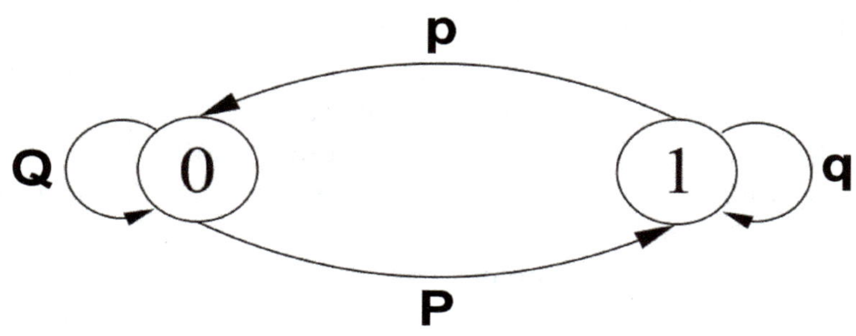

Figure 1. Gilbert model simulates burst-error with a two-state Markov chain (i.e., 0 and 1).

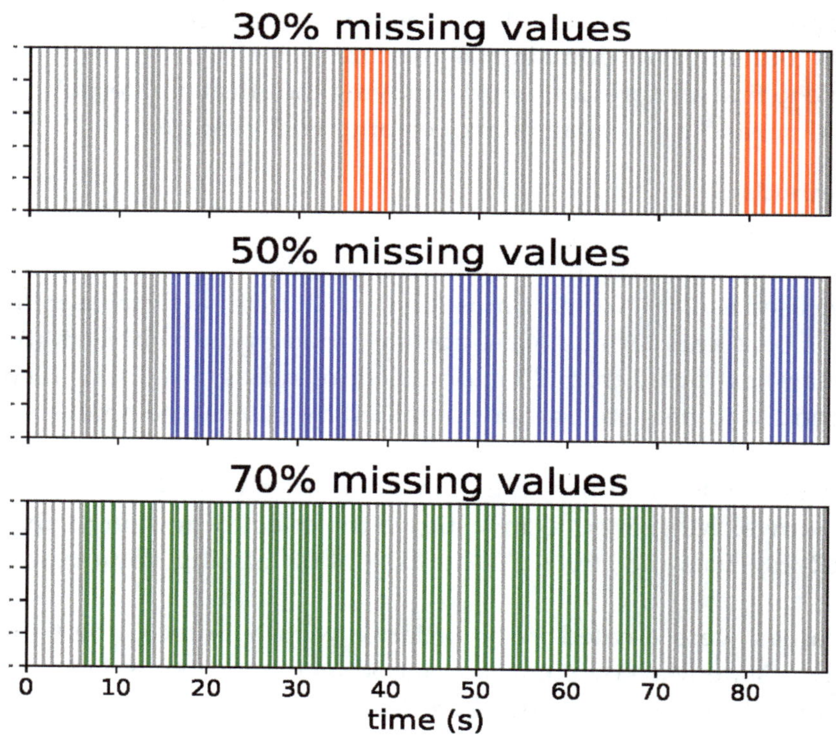

Figure 2. Examples of 30%, 50% and 70% of missing values created by Gilbert model. The colored lines refer to missing beats.

2.2. *Missing Values Interpolation*

The missing values were then handled with six different interpolation methods:

- No interpolation: this approach does not create interpolated values of missing RR-intervals. Differently to the Deletion method that remove missing values merging non-consecutive beats that induce in missing interpretation of HRV features, the no-interpolation method maintains the missing values into the RR-intervals time series.
- Nearest neighbor: the nearest neighbor or proximate interpolation is the easiest interpolation method [12]. This interpolation assigns the value of the closest known (existing) neighbor to the missing- value as shows in Equation (6).

$$X_i = \begin{cases} x_B & \text{if } i < \frac{a+b}{2} \\ x_A & \text{if } i \geq \frac{a+b}{2} \end{cases} \tag{6}$$

  where a and b are the indexes of x_A and x_B. Interpolated data by this method are discontinuous and it often yields the worst results [13]
- Linear: this method fits a straight line passing through points x_A and x_B [14]. Interpolated data by the linear model are bound between x_A and x_B as showed in Equation (7).

$$X_i = \frac{x_A - x_B}{a - b}(i - b) + x_B. \tag{7}$$

  Gaunck et al. [14] demonstrated that this method is efficient, and most of the time it is better than non-linear interpolations for predicting missing values in environmental phenomena with constant rates. In addition, they also found that in average this interpolation model underestimated the real values but it strongly depends on the distribution of the data.
- Quadratic: differently from the linear interpolation model, the quadratic function needs three points of interest to interpolate missing values in a time series as showed in Equation (8).

$$X_i = x_B \frac{(i-b)(x_C - x_A)}{2(b-a)} + \frac{(i-b)^2(x_A - 2x_B + x_C)}{2(b-a)^2}. \tag{8}$$

  Compared to the linear model, quadratic interpolation is found to be in general more accurate [13].
- Spline cubic: fitting datapoints using polynomials of degree higher than one leads to problems of oscillation outside the fitted points, known as Runge's phenomenon [15]. This problem can be avoided by using a spline, a function defined piecewise by polynomials, using datapoints as control points instead of forcing the fitted function to pass through the data points. Cubic spline is a spline composed of piecewise third-order polynomials. By using third degree polynomials is possible to ensure that the resulting curve is smooth [15], avoiding the problem of the straight polynomial interpolation that tends to induce distortions on the edges of the polynomials, given by the fact that, in general, the first and second derivative of the function defined by piecewise polynomials will not be continuous at the edges of polynomials. With cubic spline, it is possible to force the first and second derivatives of consecutive polynomials to be equal, ensuring smoothness of the resulting curve.

We applied each of the interpolation methods listed above to heartbeats expressed as a sequence of durations and as a sequence timestamps, then analyzed the error in HRV features estimations, in order to identify the best approach.

The on-duration approach is the one mostly used in literature to handle missing values. The data used as input to the interpolation methods was the sequence of durations of the heartbeats (the RR-intervals), obtained by subtracting the timestamp of each heartbeat from the timestamp of the subsequent heartbeat in the sequence of heartbeats.

Differently, we propose the the on-time approach whereby interpolation methods are applied to the sequence of timestamps of the heartbeats, postponing the differentiation preprocessing step that transforms timestamps into durations to after the interpolation step.

As shown in Figure 3 the difference between the on-time and on-duration approaches is the order of the processing steps: in the on-duration approach the timestamps are converted to durations as the first processing step; in the on-time approach this step is performed after interpolation is performed.

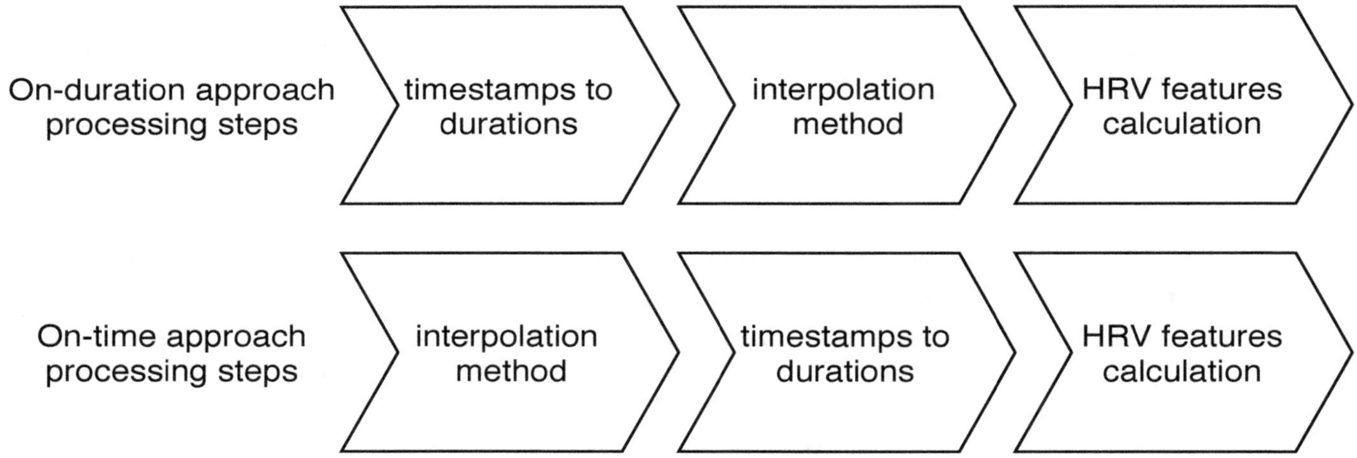

Figure 3. Processing steps in the on-time and in the on-duration approaches.

To better illustrate the differences between interpolation on time and duration, we simulated 100 heartbeats and then we randomly generated 10% of missing RR-intervals in this artificial timeseries by using Gilbert burst approach. The length of the RR-intervals timeseries changes when we interpolate the missing values on duration, while it remains the same when we interpolate on time (Table 1). This result suggests that the interpolation on duration moves beats away from their original position in time, introducing changes to the spectrum, while interpolation on time preserves the position on time of retained heartbeats. In particular, Table 1 shows that the low RR-intervals error (i.e., average difference between heartbeats duration) is obtained with linear interpolation on time. The nearest interpolation on time was not performed because interpolating with this approach is useless, as the interpolated values introduced into the timeseries would have the same time as the closest beat, creating physiologically impossible data.

Table 1. Difference between duration and time interpolation by using different approach (i.e., no-missing values, nearest neighbor, linear, quadratic, and cubic spline).

	Window Time (s)		**RMSE (s)**		**RE (%)**	
Interpolation	**Time**	**Duration**	**Time**	**Duration**	**Time**	**Duration**
No-missing values	90.11		—		—	
Nearest	—	91.95	—	0.096	—	5.11
Linear	90.11	91.83	0.075	0.090	3.70	4.86
Quadratic	90.11	92.13	0.084	0.107	4.35	5.83
Cubic spline	90.11	92.24	0.085	0.109	3.46	6.63

Figure 4 provide more detailed analyses of the difference between linear interpolation on both duration and time. The cumulative error when the missing values are interpolated on duration increases as the time series goes by because it creates RR-intervals in accordance with the closest interval values (i.e., the higher is the number of missing values, the higher is the cumulative error) depending on the interpolation type used (e.g., linear, quadratic and cubic spline). Differently, time interpolation did not introduce change in time series length due to the fact that this approach estimates intermediate values between the time when two observed beats happen in accordance with interpolation type.

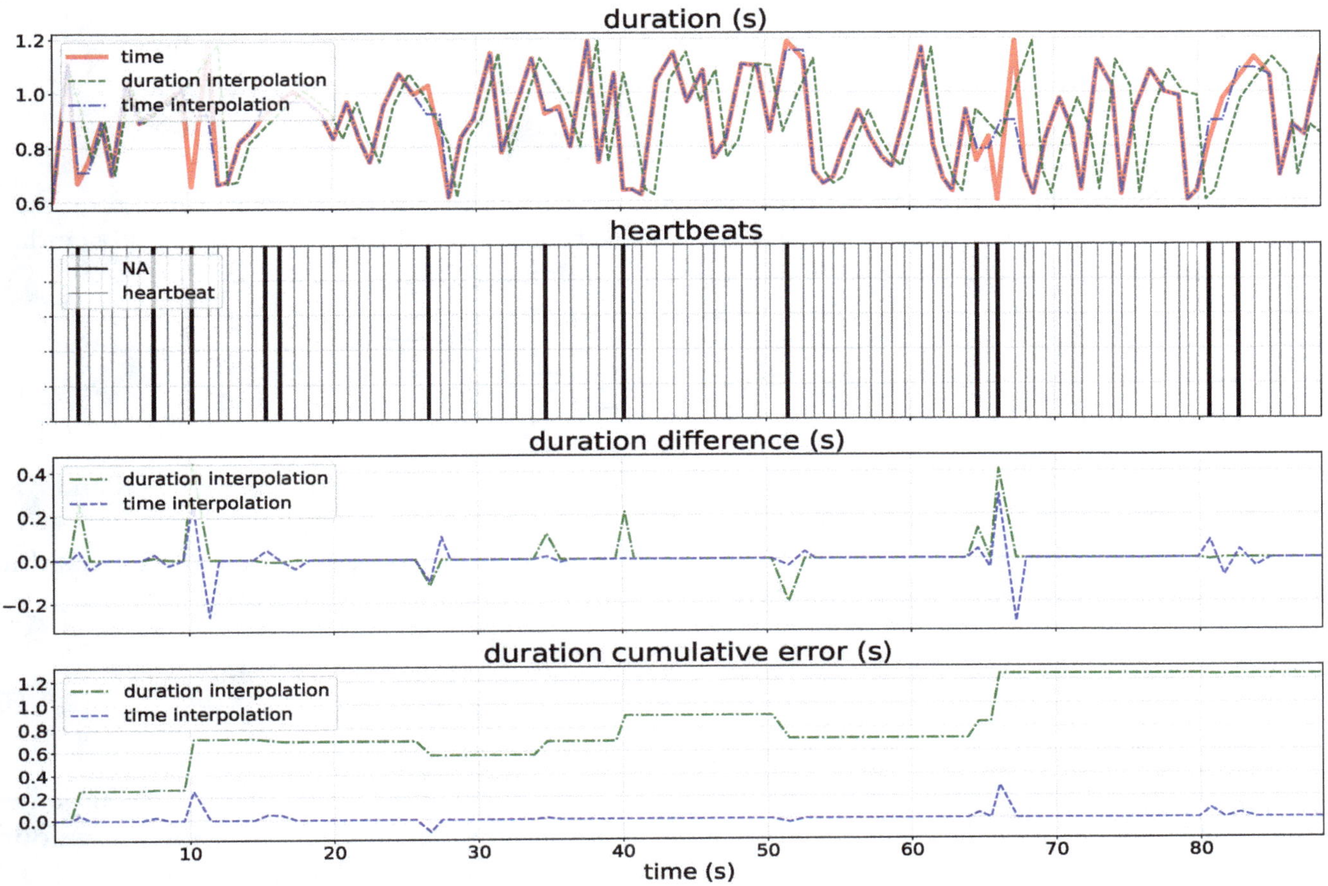

Figure 4. Difference between linear interpolation on time and duration. Red solid line refers to real variation of the timing between beats (RR-intervals) time series, green dashed line refers to the on-duration approach, and green dot dash line refers to the on-time approach.

2.3. Feature Engineering

To obtain HRV features, we analyzed real (i.e., without missing values values), non-interpolated, and interpolated (i.e., with different percentage of artificial missing values values) 5 min ECG time series. We analyze time domain HRV features, frequency, and non-linear domains. Time domain analysis usually contains various statistical variables of the duration time series. The frequency domain analysis investigates the power spectrum of RR-intervals time series in order to assess the cardiac autonomic balance (i.e., sympathetic and parasympathetic nervous systems activity). Additionally, non-linear HRV features try to capture the non-periodic behaviour of the HRV and the complexity that exists inside the RR-interval dynamics. The variables that we incude in our analysis, in both time and frequency domain, are defined as:

- Time domain:
  - HR mean: mean values of heart rate (HR) computed as showed in Equation (9).

$$HR_{mean} = \frac{1}{N-1} \sum_{i=1}^{N-1} 60/(R_{i+1} - R_i), \tag{9}$$

  where N is the number of beats and R is the time when the beats happened.
  - RMSSD: root mean square of the successive RR-intervals differences (Equation (10)) represents the strength of the autonomic nervous system (specifically the parasympathetic branch) at a given time.

$$RMSSD = \sqrt{\frac{1}{N-1}\sum_{i=1}^{N-1}[(R_{i+1}-R_i)-(R_i-R_{i-1})]^2}, \quad (10)$$

where N is the number of beats and R is the time when the beats happened.

- SDNN: standard deviation of RR-intervals (Equation (11)). It reflects the cyclic components responsible for variability in the RR-intervals time series. The SDNN is the "gold standard" for medical stratification of both morbidity and mortality [16].

$$SDNN = \sqrt{\frac{1}{N-1}\sum_{i=1}^{N}(RR_i-\overline{RR})^2}, \quad (11)$$

where N is the number of beats and RR is the intervals between two consecutive R and $\overline{RR}$ is the mean of RR-intervals in the time series.

- PNN50: the ratio between NN50 (i.e., number of pairs of successive RR intervals that differ by more than 50 ms) and the total number of RR-intervals (Equation (12)).

$$PNN50 = \frac{NN50_{count}}{N_{RR-intervals}} \quad (12)$$

- Frequency domain:
  - Power spectral density (PSD): describes the distribution of power into frequency components composing that signal. The Lomb–Scargle periodogram for PSD estimation was found to be the most appropriate method to analyze RR-interval data [5,6]. VLF (power in very-low-frequency ranges, i.e., $\leq$0.04 Hz), LF (power in low-frequency ranges, i.e., 0.04–0.15 Hz), HF (Power in high-frequency ranges, i.e., 0.15, 0.4 Hz), LF/HF ratio (ratio between LF and HF expressed as ms^2), and total power (Power in all the frequency ranges, i.e., $\leq$0.4) were obtained by the sum of the power in the relevant frequency range in the spectrum.
- Non-linear HRV features:
  - Poincaré plot: it is a type of recurrence plot used to quantify self-similarity in processes. A Poincaré plot is a graph of RR interval (RR_n) against the previous one ($RR_n - 1$). From this scatter plot, it is possible to quantitatively analyze the variance of two consecutive RR-intervals by fitting an ellipse to the plotted shape. $SD1$ is the standard deviation of Poincaré plot perpendicular to the line-of-identity, while $SD2$ is the standard deviation of the Poincaré plot along the line-of-identity.

2.4. Success Metrics

We assessed the difference of HRV variables computed on real time series and the ones with missing values by the root mean squared error (RMSE). Additionally, the relative errors (REs, see Equation (13)) were used to assess the effects of the missing data on the HRV features compared with the parameters calculated from the RR-intervals timeseries without missing data.

$$RE = \frac{|x_{real}-x_k|}{x_{real}} * 100, \quad (13)$$

where x_{real} refers to the HRV features computed from RR-intervals timeseries without missing values, while x_k refers to the values obtained from interpolated timeseries.

3. Results and Discussions

3.1. Results Summary

We analyzed 15,359 RR-intervals timeseries of 5 min in this study. Table 2 shows the descriptive statistic of the HRV features extracted from all users in the dataset. In particular, the users shows an average heart rate of about 75 $\pm$ 14 beats per minute.

Table 2. Descriptive statistic of hart rate variability (HRV) features. Mean and 95% coefficient intervals (CI) are provided for all the feature.

HRV Features	Mean	95% CI
IBI (s)	0.78	[0.54, 1.11]
PNN50 (n)	8	[4, 16]
RMSSD (s)	0.039	[0.017, 0.36]
SD1 (s)	0.027	[0.012, 0.26]
SD2 (s)	0.077	[0.040, 0.25]
SDNN (s)	0.059	[0.017, 0.25]
VLF (s^2)	0.87	[0.22, 4.15]
LF (s^2)	0.477	[0.12, 5.57]
HF (s^2)	0.28	[0.050, 3.024]
total power (s^2)	1.91	[0.53, 21.44]
LF/HF (s^2)	2.9	[1.2, 10.2]

Table 3 shows that the on-time approach (i.e., interpolation on the timestamp of heartbeats) produces more reliable HRV feature estimations compared to the on-duration approach (i.e., interpolation on interval duration between two consecutive heartbeats). In this table we provide the results of the best interpolation approach for each HRV feature and for all the percentages of missing values. The RE and RMSE values provided in this table refer to the error induced by missing values when we compare HRV features obtained from the real RR-intervals timeseries versus the ones obtained from interpolated timeseries. The best interpolation methods provided in Table 3 refer to the ones with lower RE. For all of the HRV features, the highest was the percentage of missing RR-intervals, and also the parameters estimation errors. This was due to the fact that the power spectrum of the RR-intervals signal changes with the number of missing values. The choice of the interpolation method also added different types of noise to the signal. As shown in Table 1, the interpolation on time, or not interpolation at all, produces more reliable HRV features compared to interpolating on duration.

Table 3. Best performing interpolation approach (i.e., with low RE) for each HRV feature in each percentage of missing values evaluated. The error in estimating HRV features is reported using RE and root mean squared error (RMSE).

Missing Values (%)	HRV	Interpolation How	Interpolation Method	RE (%)	RMSE
30	RMSSD (s)	No-interpolation		14.65	0.38
	SDNN (s)	Time	quadratic	9.42	0.34
	PNN50 (n)	No-interpolation		24.37	1.51
	SD1 (s)	No-interpolation		14.68	0.27
	SD2 (s)	Time	quadratic	8.57	0.47
	VLF (s^2)	Time	quadratic	14.50	0.82
	LF (s^2)	Time	quadratic	26.87	2.01
	HF (s^2)	Time	quadratic	32.18	4.48
	LF/HF (s^2)	Time	cubic	41.39	1.73
	total power (s^2)	Time	quadratic	17.16	6.26

Table 3. *Cont.*

Missing Values (%)	HRV	Interpolation How	Interpolation Method	RE (%)	RMSE
50	RMSSD (ms)	No-interpolation		23.13	0.76
	SDNN (s)	Time	quadratic	15.47	0.41
	PNN50 (n)	No-interpolation		39.01	2.35
	SD1 (s)	No-interpolation		23.18	0.54
	SD2 (s)	Time	quadratic	13.49	0.49
	VLF (s^2)	Time	quadratic	23.72	0.40
	LF (s^2)	Time	quadratic	42.42	1.12
	HF (s^2)	Time	quadratic	52.56	2.48
	LF/HF (s^2)	Time	cubic	58.07	2.26
	total power (s^2)	Time	quadratic	27.59	3.96
70	RMSSD (s)	No-interpolation		34.37	0.91
	SDNN (s)	Time	quadratic	22.76	0.47
	PNN50 (n)	Time	linear	63.90	3.88
	SD1 (s)	No-interpolation		34.46	0.59
	SD2 (s)	Time	quadratic	19.19	0.51
	VLF (s^2)	Time	quadratic	29.73	0.52
	LF (s^2)	Time	quadratic	56.41	1.45
	HF (s^2)	Time	quadratic	72.98	3.34
	LF/HF (s^2)	Time	cubic	72.07	2.80
	total power (s^2)	Time	quadratic	72.07	5.27

The lowest errors on HRV features estimation with missing RR-intervals are obtained using the no-interpolation or the interpolation on time approaches, while the interpolation on duration approach consistently yields the worst results (Table 3). Even if low timeseries difference were detected in simulated linear interpolation on time (Figure 4 and Table 1), Table 3 suggests that the best interpolation method depends of the HRV features that we want to assess. Moreover, this table also shows that, as suspected, the higher is the percentage of missing values, the higher is also the HRV feature estimation error (i.e., RE and RMSE).

3.2. HRV Features

3.2.1. Time Domain

RMSSD and PNN50 do not require any interpolation to obtain reliable estimations for all the percentages of missing values, while SDNN need quadratic interpolation on time (see Table 3). A possible explanation of this result is that RMSSD and PNN50 capture fast changes in heart activity, i.e., high spectrum frequencies, and SDNN captures slow changes, i.e., very low spectrum frequencies. Moreover, interpolation methods, especially interpolation on duration, act as low pass filters, affecting the signal measured by the HRV features (Figure 5). No interpolation changed the spectrum, but did not introduce fictuous durations, thus minimizing the impact on successive differences of durations, that were the first computation step of both RMSSD and PNN50.

3.2.2. Frequency Domain

Figure 5 shows the Lomb–Scargle spectral analysis for different percentages of missing values and for each interpolation method on both time and duration. This figure shows that different interpolation methods introduce different deformations in the resulting power spectra. It is interesting to notice that performing no interpolation results in a flatter spectrum, more similar to a white noise.

In the frequency domain, the interpolation method that produces the least error is the quadratic on time (see Table 3). This figure shows that, as the amount of missing values increases, the no-interpolation approach tends to flatten the HRV spectrum, making it similar to the spectrum of white noise. Figure 5 also shows that cubic spline interpolation on time tends to dampen low frequencies while enhancing high frequencies; that cubic spline interpolation on duration tends to dampen all frequencies; and that quadratic interpolation on duration tends to enhance all frequencies. Finally, Figure 5 also shows that linear and quadratic interpolations on time and that nearest neighbour and linear interpolation on duration have minimal impact on both low and high frequencies, with quadratic interpolation on time having the least effect on all frequencies.

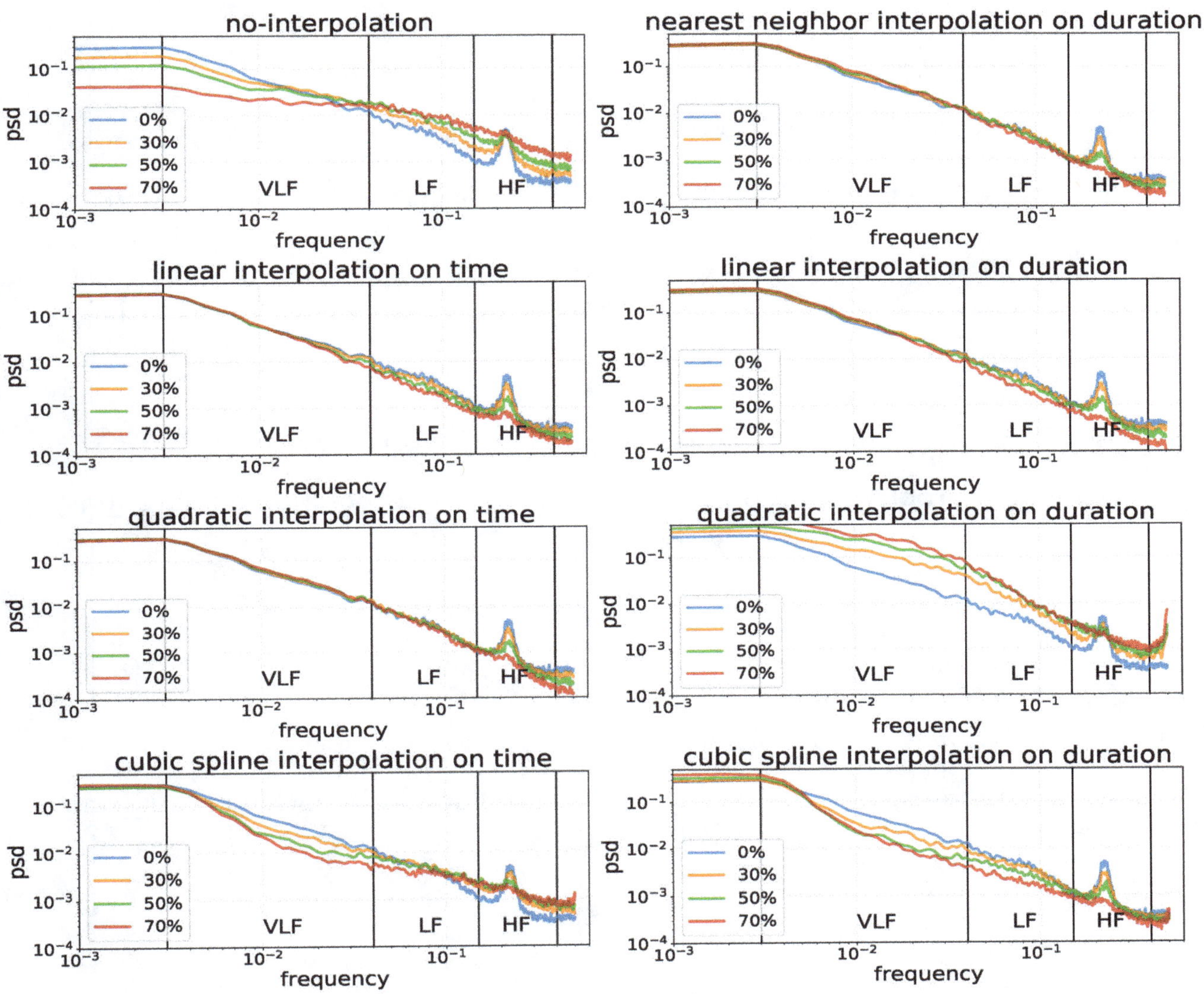

Figure 5. Frequency analysis of a user's RR-intervals timeseries recorded in 5 min with different percentages of missing values (i.e., 0%, 30%, 50% and 70%) handled with different interpolation methods (i.e., nearest neighbor, linear, quadratic and cubic spline) on both time and duration.

3.2.3. Non-Linear Domain

SD1 does not require any interpolation to handle missing values, while SD2 needs quadratic interpolation on time to obtain reliable result (see Table 3). To give an explanation of these results, in Figure 6 we provide an example of the relationship between $RR - interval_n$ and $RR - interval_{n+1}$ (i.e., Poincaré plot) where SD1 and SD2 are extracted. This figure shows Poincaré plots obtained after interpolating missing RR-intervals by using different interpolation method on both time and duration. This figure shows that when the missing values were interpolated on time, the variability of SD1 reduced as the percentage of missing values increased, while the SD2 remain constant. Differently, the interpolation on duration introduce error on both SD1 and SD2 increasing their variability as the missing values increase. Finally, in this figure it can be seen that no-interpolation and quadratic interpolation on time introduced less error compared to the other method on SD1 and SD2, respectively.

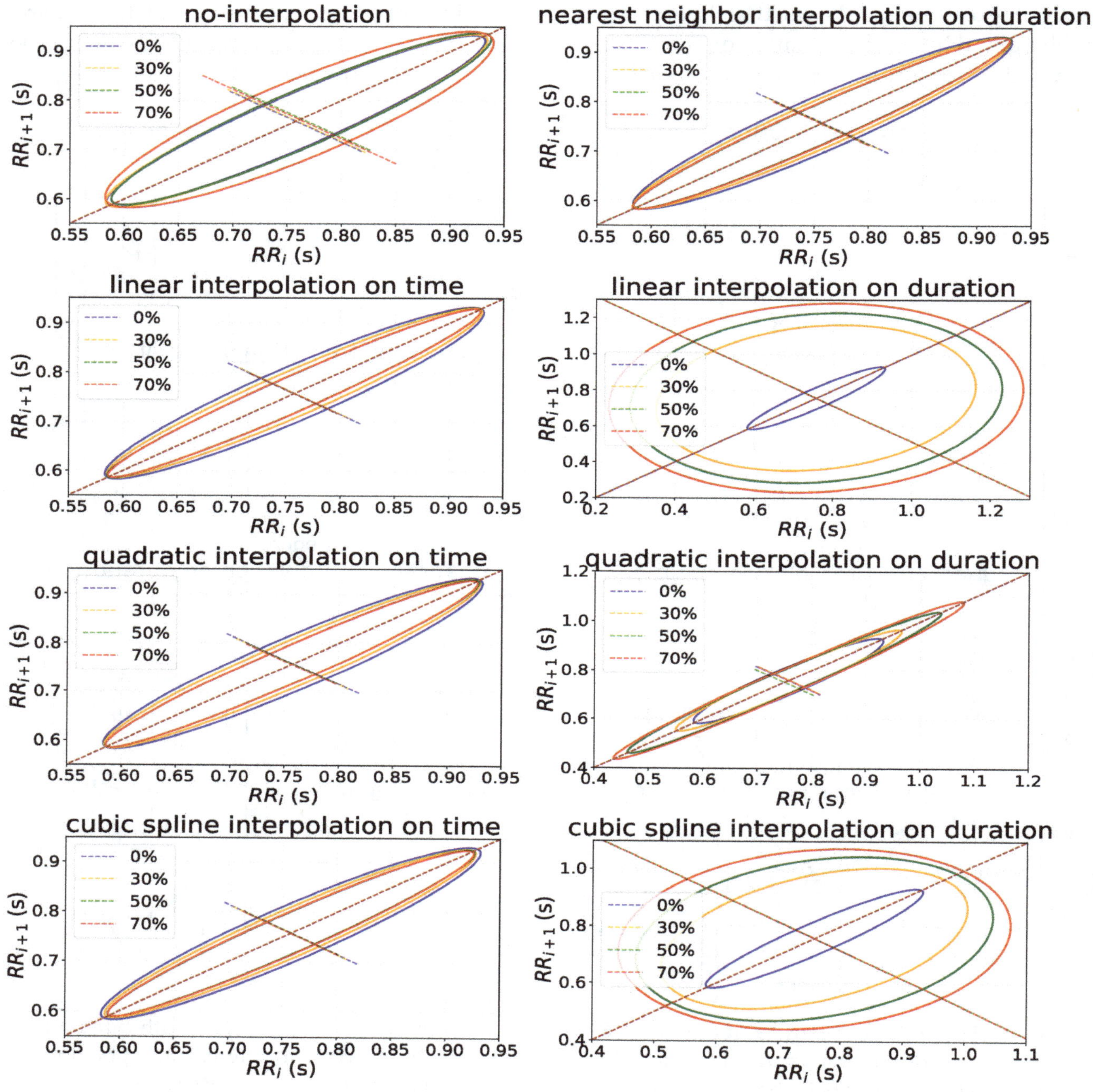

Figure 6. Poincaré plot of a user's RR-intervals timeseries recorded in 5 min with different percentage of missing values (i.e., 0%, 30%, 50% and 70%) handled with different interpolation methods (i.e., nearest neighbor, linear, quadratic and cubic spline) on both time and duration.

4. Conclusions

In this work we quantify the expected error propagation of missing values in RR-intervals timeseries to HRV features, as a function of preprocessing interpolation approach, and amount of missing data. The main findings of this study is that the interpolation of missing values in RR-intervals timeseries on time (i.e., the heartbeats timestamps) produces more reliable HRV features estimations compared to interpolation on duration.

By using this preprocessing approach, the quantification of the expected error on HRV features caused by a huge amount of missing values (e.g., motion artifacts on a wrist-worn wearable device) can support better estimations of users' well-being, by assessing their HRV features. This enables continuous passive monitoring of users' cardiovascular activity in a non-obtrusive way, collecting data during their daily activities that could enable further research on preventative health.

A limitation of this study is the fact that we limited our focus on healthy subjects with normal heart activity, limiting the analysis to large amounts of missing values induced by motion artifacts, ignoring physiological phenomena such as ectopic beats.

Future studies will be useful for researcher and companies, which give insight into heart rate variability recorded by wrist worn IoT wearable devices, in order to better understand the potentiality of the data extracted from these devices to make inference about people heath status. Future work is needed to assess the influence of missing values simulated in accordance with motion and mechanical artifacts induced by external stimuli during data acquisition by using wrist worn IoT wearable devices. Finally, future works will also include the investigating the influence of missing values on HRV features on short timeseries (e.g., 2 min, 1 min and 30 s) and the identification of the shortest time required to obtain accurate estimation of users' HRV features.

Author Contributions: Conceptualization, D.M., A.R. and M.C.; methodology, D.M., A.R. and M.C.; validation, D.M., A.R. and M.C.; formal analysis, D.M., A.R. and M.C.; investigation, D.M., A.R. and M.C.; writing—original draft preparation, D.M., A.R., M.C. and D.A.C.; writing—review and editing, D.M., A.R., M.C. and D.A.C.; visualization, A.R. and M.C.; supervision, D.M. and D.A.C.; project administration, D.M. and D.A.C.; funding acquisition, D.M. and D.A.C.

References

1. Laborde, S.; Mosley, E.; Thayer, J.F. Heart Rate Variability and Cardiac Vagal Tone in Psychophysiological Research—Recommendations for Experiment Planning, Data Analysis, and Data Reporting. *Front. Psychol.* **2017**, *8*, 213. [CrossRef] [PubMed]
2. Haghi, M.; Thurow, K.; Stoll, R. Wearable Devices in Medical Internet of Things: Scientific Research and Commercially Available Devices. *Healthc. Inform. Res.* **2017**, *23*, 4–15. [CrossRef] [PubMed]
3. Karlsson, M.; Hörnsten, R.; Rydberg, A.; Wiklund, U. Automatic filtering of outliers in RR intervals before analysis of heart rate variability in Holter recordings: A comparison with carefully edited data. *Biomed. Eng.* **2012**, *11*, 2. [CrossRef] [PubMed]
4. Kim, K.K.; Lim, Y.G.; Kim, J.S.; Park, K.S. Effect of missing RR-interval data on heart rate variability analysis in the time domain. *Physiol. Meas.* **2007**, *28*, 1485–1494. [CrossRef] [PubMed]
5. Kim, K.K.; Kim, J.S.; Lim, Y.G.; Park, K.S. The effect of missing RR-interval data on heart rate variability analysis in the frequency domain. *Physiol. Meas.* **2009**, *30*, 1039–1050. [CrossRef] [PubMed]
6. Clifford, G.D.; Tarassenko, L. Quantifying errors in spectral estimates of HRV due to beat replacement and resampling. *IEEE Trans. Biomed. Eng.* **2005**, *52*, 630–638. [CrossRef] [PubMed]
7. Peltola, M.A. Role of editing of R–R intervals in the analysis of heart rate variability. *Front. Physiol.* **2012**, *3*, 148. [CrossRef] [PubMed]
8. Salo, M.; Huikuri, H.; Seppänen, T. Ectopic beats in heart rate variability analysis: Effects of editing on time and frequency domain measures. *Ann. Noninvasive Electrocardiol.* **2001**, *6*, 5–17. [CrossRef] [PubMed]
9. Kamath, M.V.; Fallen, E.L. Correction of the heart rate variability signal for ectopics and missing beats. In *Heart Rate Variability*; Futura Publishing Company: Armonk, NY, USA, 2001; pp. 75–85.
10. Normal Sinus Rhythm RR Interval Database, doi:10.13026/C2S881. Available online: https://physionet.org/physiobank/database/nsr2db/ (accessed on 1 June 2019)
11. Hideki, I. *Essentials of Error-Control Coding Techniques*; Academic Press: Cambridge, MA, USA, 1990.
12. Sibson, R. A brief description of natural neighbor interpolation. In *Interpreting Multivariate Data*; John Wiley & Sons: Sheffield, UK, 1980; pp. 24–27, ISBN 978-0-471-28039-2.
13. Lepot, M.; Aubin, J.B.; Clemens, F.H.L.R. Interpolation in Time Series: An Introductive Overview of Existing Methods, Their Performance Criteria and Uncertainty Assessment. *Water* **2017**, *9*, 796. [CrossRef]

14. Gnauck, A. Interpolation and approximation of water quality time series and process identification. *Anal. Bioanal. Chem.* **2004**, *380*, 484–492. [CrossRef] [PubMed]
15. De Boor, C. *A Practical Guide to Splines*; Springer: Berlin, Germany, 1978.
16. Shaffer, F.; Ginsberg, J.P. An Overview of Heart Rate Variability Metrics and Norms. *Front. Public Health* **2017**, *5*, 258. [CrossRef] [PubMed]

14

Comparison of Different Sets of Features for Human Activity Recognition by Wearable Sensors

Samanta Rosati *, Gabriella Balestra and Marco Knaflitz

Department of Electronics and Telecommunications, Politecnico di Torino, 10129 Torino, Italy; gabriella.balestra@polito.it (G.B.); marco.knaflitz@polito.it (M.K.)

* Correspondence: samanta.rosati@polito.it

Abstract: Human Activity Recognition (HAR) refers to an emerging area of interest for medical, military, and security applications. However, the identification of the features to be used for activity classification and recognition is still an open point. The aim of this study was to compare two different feature sets for HAR. Particularly, we compared a set including time, frequency, and time-frequency domain features widely used in literature (*FeatSet_A*) with a set of time-domain features derived by considering the physical meaning of the acquired signals (*FeatSet_B*). The comparison of the two sets were based on the performances obtained using four machine learning classifiers. Sixty-one healthy subjects were asked to perform seven different daily activities wearing a MIMU-based device. Each signal was segmented using a 5-s window and for each window, 222 and 221 variables were extracted for the *FeatSet_A* and *FeatSet_B* respectively. Each set was reduced using a Genetic Algorithm (GA) simultaneously performing feature selection and classifier optimization. Our results showed that Support Vector Machine achieved the highest performances using both sets (97.1% and 96.7% for *FeatSet_A* and *FeatSet_B* respectively). However, *FeatSet_B* allows to better understand alterations of the biomechanical behavior in more complex situations, such as when applied to pathological subjects.

Keywords: human activity recognition; wearable sensors; MIMU; genetic algorithm; feature selection; classifier optimization; machine learning

1. Introduction

Human Activity Recognition (HAR) is a growing research field of great interest for medical, military, and security applications. Focusing on the healthcare domain, HAR was successfully applied for monitoring and observation of the elderly [1], remote detection and classification of falls [2], medical diagnosis [3], rehabilitation and physical therapy [4].

A HAR system is usually made up of two components: (1) a wearable device, equipped with a set of sensors (i.e., accelerometers, gyroscopes, magnetometers, ...) suitable for capturing human movements during daily life, and (2) a processing tool that recognizes the activity performed in a given instant by the subject. The most common systems employed for HAR are miniature magnetic and inertial measurement units (MIMUs) that work only as a data logger, performing the signal acquisition and storage, while an external system (pc, tablet, smartphone) is needed to process signals and recognize the activities. However, for all those applications in which a real-time feedback is required, it is important to create a stand-alone device able both to acquire several magnetic-inertial signals for long periods of time and to identify the performed activities as fast as possible. From this perspective, the desired device should be lightweight, small and easy to be worn from the subject, provided with a long-lasting battery, and equipped with a microcontroller having enough internal memory for signals and activities storage and able to support the implementation of a classifier for activity recognition. From the classifier point of view, it should be as fast as possible, in order to return a real-time feedback, with low storage requirements and easy to be realized on a microcontroller. In a previous work, we showed that a suitable machine learning classifier is Decision Tree (DT), that is also able to reduce the number of input variables, decreasing the computational time, even if its accuracy was lower than other methods [5].

Another challenging and still open aspect when dealing with HAR is the identification of the correct set of input variables (or features) for the classifier. Analyzing the literature, different approaches can be found. The most popular approach is based on time-domain features [6–8], that are usually of a statistical nature: mean value, median, variance, skewness, kurtosis, percentiles and interquartile range. Some studies use cross-correlation coefficients to quantify the similarity between signals coming from different axes [9,10], but other studies demonstrated the inefficiency of these features [11]. To give an idea of the energy and power contained in signals, frequency-domain features, such as signal power, root mean square value, auto-correlation coefficients, mean and median frequency, and spectral entropy, are commonly extracted [8,12]. Finally, some approaches based on the time-frequency domain can be found in the literature, in particular using the Discrete Wavelet Transform (DWT), that allows a decomposition of signals into several coefficients, each containing frequency data across temporal changes [13]. A detailed review of features used for HAR applications and belonging to time, frequency and time-frequency domains can be found in [14]. Although the great majority of applications use these kinds of features, three main problems must be addressed: (1) the extraction of frequency-domain and wavelet-domain features could result really hard for a microprocessor [15]; (2) the great majority of these features are not directly related to the acquired signals and, thus, they are difficult to attribute to physical quantities, complicating the interpretation of the results and the understanding of errors; (3) the number of variables proposed in the literature is huge and this is not always associated with high classification accuracy since some of them could be sources of noise [16].

Feature Selection (FS) is a fundamental step when dealing with high-dimensional data, allowing for eliminating those variables that are redundant or irrelevant for the system description. Moreover, it has been proven that FS increases the classification performance [17], due to the removal of those variables introducing noise during the classifier construction and application. Two main categories of FS algorithms have been proposed in the literature and successfully applied in the biomedical field for dataset [18], signal [19] and image [20] processing: filter and wrapper methods [21]. Filter methods perform FS independently of the learning algorithm: variables are examined individually to identify those more relevant for describing the inner structure of the analyzed dataset. Since each variable is considered independently during the selection procedure, groups of features having strong discriminatory power may be ignored. Conversely, in wrapper methods, the selection of the feature subset is performed simultaneously with the estimation of its goodness in the learning task. For this reason, this latter category of FS methods usually can reach better performances than filter methods [21], since it allows for exploring also feature dependencies. On the other hand, wrapper FS could be computationally very intensive and the obtained feature subset optimized only for the specific learning algorithm or classifier.

Moreover, once a feature subset is fixed, different classification results might be obtained changing the classifier parameters, since they strongly influence the classification performance [22]. Several approaches have been developed for parameters tuning, e.g., grid search, random search, heuristic search [23]. However, the simultaneous selection of the optimal feature subset and optimization of the classifier parameters is likely the only way assuring to reach the best performances. Since an exhaustive search of the best couple feature subset-classifier parameters is unfeasible in most real situations, heuristic search represents a convenient way to find a good compromise between reasonable computational time and sub-optimal solutions. In particular, genetic algorithms (GAs) have been applied for solving optimization problems connected to FS [17] and parameter tuning [22], but very scarce applications can be found for the simultaneous optimization of both aspects.

The aim of this study is to compare two sets of features for real-time HAR applications: *FeatSet_A* comprising time, frequency and time-frequency domain parameters presented in the literature and *FeatSet_B* consisting of variables belonging only to the time-domain and derived from the understanding of how a specific activity will affect the sensor signals. The most informative features for each set were identified using a GA that simultaneously performs feature selection and optimization of the classifier parameters. Then, the obtained feature subsets were compared analyzing the performances reached by four different machine learning classifiers.

The rest of the paper is divided as follows: Section 2 describes related works about HAR using wearable sensors. Section 3 presents the protocol and population involved in our experiment, the extracted features and the GA used for simultaneous FS and classifier optimization. Results are presented in Section 4 and discussed in Section 5. Section 6 concludes this study and proposes future directions in this context.

2. Related Work

A huge number of studies was proposed in the literature for HAR by means of wearable sensors. Although an exhaustive analysis of publications dealing with these aspects is beyond the scope of this paper (a recent review can be found in [24]), several aspects can be used to characterize and summarize these studies, such as acquired signals, extracted features and algorithms used for dimensionality reduction and activity recognition.

Accelerometric signals are common to all HAR applications. Some studies used this information alone [25–27], but more often accelerometers were combined with gyroscopes [12,28,29] and magnetometers [30,31]. In few cases other signals were taken into account such as quaternions [32], temperature [1], gravity [33] or data acquired from ambient sensors [1].

Once they were acquired, the raw signals were rarely employed as they are [33,34] but usually some kind of processing was applied to extract a set of informative features. In general, most of extracted features belongs to the time-domain (e.g., mean, standard deviation, minimum value, maximum value, range, . . .) and the frequency-domain (such as mean and median frequency, spectral entropy, signal power, entropy) [32,35,36]. However, other different variables can be found in literature, such as time-frequency domain variables used in the studies by Eyobu et al. [12] and Tian et al. [37], or the cepstral features proposed by San-Segundo et al. [26] and Vanrell et al. [38].

Regarding the dimensions of the obtained feature sets, three different approaches were followed in the literature. In some studies no dimensionality reduction was performed and, thus, the whole set of variables was used for the recognition phase [39,40]. The second approach achieves dimensionality reduction by means of a transformation of the original set of variables in a new one with lower dimensionality. The most common method belonging to this category is the principal component analysis (PCA), that was employed for example in ref. [41,42]. Finally, different FS methods were used to reduce the number of variables without any transformation, such as Minimum Redundancy Maximum Relevance [43], recursive feature elimination [34], Information Gain [25], or evolutionary algorithms [44].

Since the aim of a HAR application is to identify the performed activity, a proper learning algorithm must be applied as final step. The great majority of the studies in this fields was based on supervised learning algorithms, ranging from machine learning (support vector machine [33], decision tree [27], random forest [32], multilayer perceptron [44], . . .) to the emerging deep learning neural networks [45–47]. However, sporadic applications of unsupervised learning algorithms were proposed [48]. Ensemble learning, that combines different classifiers to improve the final performances, was proposed by Tian et al. [37] and Garcia-Ceja et al. [40].

3. Materials and Methods

3.1. Signal Acquisition and Experimental Setup

Signals were acquired using a MIMU-based device by Medical Technology (Torino, Italy). The sensor unit consisted of a tri-axial accelerometer, a tri-axial gyroscope and a tri-axial magnetometer allowing for acquiring acceleration, rate of turn, and Earth-magnetic field data, for a total of nine signals. The measurement range was $\pm$ 4 g for the accelerometers, $\pm$ 2000°/s for the gyroscopes and $\pm$ 4 G for the magnetometers. The sampling frequency of all signals was 80 Hz. An example of signals acquired during a walk of a healthy subject is shown in Figure 1. For the purpose of this study, signals were recorded in local data storage devices and transmitted to a laptop for the following analysis.

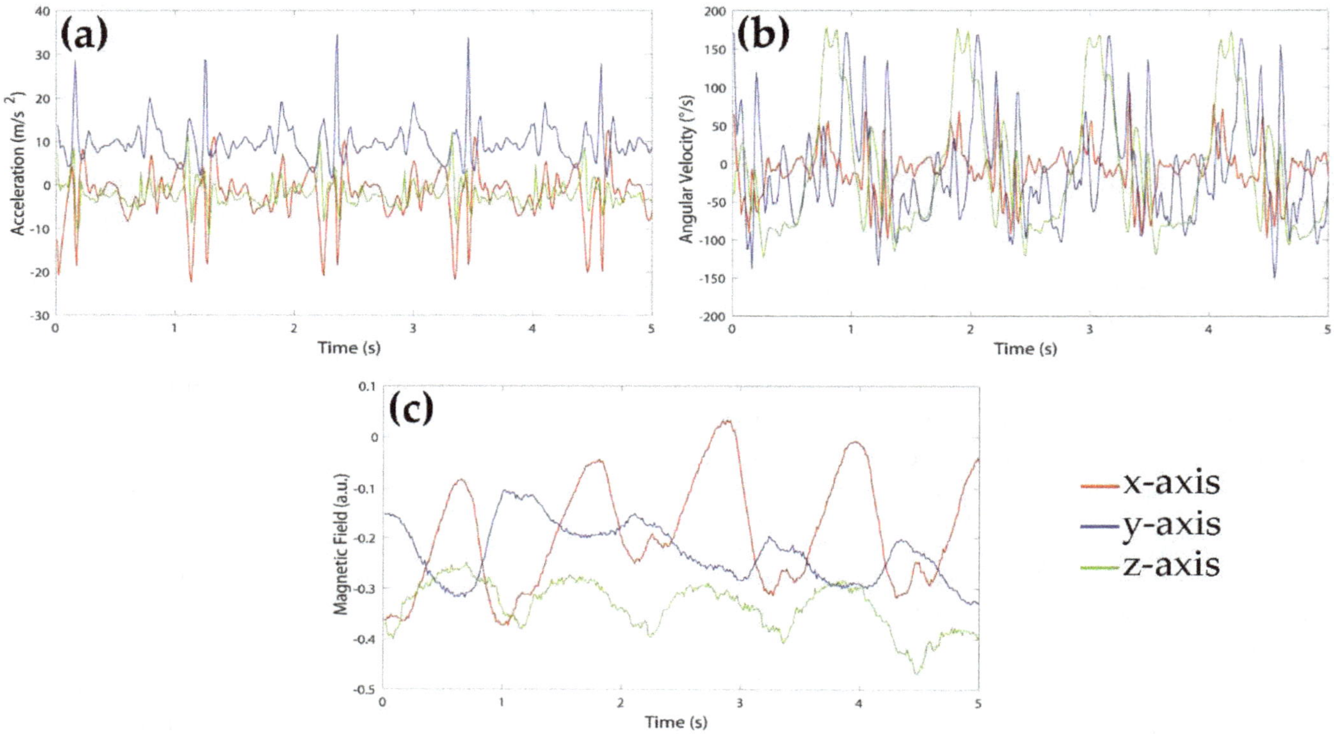

Figure 1. Example of signals acquired by (**a**) accelerometer, (**b**) gyroscope and (**c**) magnetometer during 5 s of walking of a healthy subject.

The MIMU sensor was located on the lateral side of the right thigh. The *y*-axis was oriented in down-top vertical direction, *x*-axis was aligned to the antero-posterior direction, and *z*-axis was aligned to the medio-lateral direction, pointing to lateral side. Sixty-one young and healthy subjects (28 males, 33 females; age: 22 $\pm$ 2 years; age range: 20–28 years; height: 169.9 $\pm$ 8.3 cm; weight: 64.3 $\pm$ 11.0 kg) with no history of physical disabilities or injuries were involved in this study. All subjects were asked to perform seven simple activities: resting (A_1, comprising sitting and laying), upright standing (A_2), level walking (A_3), ascending and descending stairs (A_4 and A_5), uphill and downhill walking (A_6 and A_7). All activities lasted 60 s and were repeated five times by each subject. Activities were executed in indoor and outdoor areas, following a default path, without any speed restriction and style of performing. Each subject signed an informed consent form. Since this was an observational study and subjects were not exposed to any harm, the study protocol was not submitted to an ethical committee nor to an institutional review board.

3.2. Dataset Construction and Feature Extraction

To avoid bias due to the magnetic direction of the performed activities during signals acquisition and magnetic disturbances on the magnetometer, only inertial information (i.e., accelerometer and gyroscope signals) was used for HAR. Each signal was segmented using a 5 s sliding window with an overlap of 3 s between subsequent windows. The total number of processed windows was included in the validation set while the training set was obtained by randomly selecting 10% of windows for each activity of each subject.

For every window, two sets of features were extracted: *FeatSet_A*, comprising features commonly used in literature, and *FeatSet_B*, containing only time-domain features derived from the analysis of the expected biomechanical effect of a given activity on the sensor signals. Since features included in the two sets had different ranges, the min-max scaling method was applied to the training sets to obtain variables between 0 and 1:

$$Var\_norm_i = \frac{Var_i - \min(Var_i)}{\max(Var_i) - \min(Var_i)} \tag{1}$$

where Var_i is the original value of the *i*-th variable.

Even if standardization using mean and variance of each variable is commonly used for machine learning purposes, it is suitable where close-to-Gaussian distribution could be assumed and might be inappropriate for very heterogeneous features [49]. In this study we used features belonging to very different domains, thus we preferred to use the min-max scaling that also preserves the original value distribution of each variable.

Finally, since all machine learning methods tested in this study were supervised methods, each window in the training and validation sets was labeled with the activity performed by the subject in that specific moment. In particular, an integer number was used to codify each activity, ranging from 1 to 7 for activities from A_1 to A_7, respectively.

3.2.1. *FeatSet_A*

FeatSet_A included 222 features belonging to different domains. In particular, for the six considered signals we calculated:

- 20 time-domain features [14,50,51] (mean value, variance, standard deviation, skewness, kurtosis, minimum and maximum values, 25th and 75th percentiles, interquartile range, 10 samples of the autocorrelation sequence);
- three frequency-domain features [14,50,51] (mean and median frequency of the power spectrum, Shannon spectral entropy);
- 14 time-frequency domain features [14] (norms of approximation and detail coefficients, considering seven levels of decomposition of the discrete wavelet transform).

3.2.2. *FeatSet_B*

A set of 221 features was extracted based on the time-domain analysis of the signals. First, we defined the positive and negative peaks as the maximum and the minimum values reached between two consecutive zero crossings, respectively. Then, we calculated the following 33 features for the six signals:

- number of zero crossing (one feature);
- number of positive and negative peaks (two features);
- mean value, standard deviation, maximum, minimum, and range of duration for positive, negative, and total peaks (15 features);
- mean value, standard deviation, maximum, minimum, and range of time-to-peak for positive, negative, and total peaks (15 features).

Moreover, we computed single and double integration of the acceleration in the antero-posterior and vertical directions, and the single integration of the rate of turn in medio-lateral direction. These signals represented the velocity and distance traveled by the limb in the corresponding directions. Other 23 features were extracted from these signals:

- mean of the single and double integration of vertical acceleration (two features);
- mean and RMS value of single integration of antero-posterior acceleration (two features);
- RMS value of double integration of antero-posterior acceleration (one feature);
- number of positive, negative and total peaks of the single integration of the rate of turn in medio-lateral direction (three features);
- mean value, standard deviation, maximum, minimum, and range of duration of positive, negative and total peaks of the single integration of the rate of turn in medio-lateral direction (15 features).

3.3. Recognition of Static Activities

Since static (resting and upright standing) and dynamic activities (level walking, ascending and descending stairs, uphill and downhill walking) showed very different types of behavior from the signal point of view, we decided to implement a first recognition step, based on a couple of rules, to discriminate these two classes of movements. Figure 2 shows an example of accelerometer and gyroscope signals acquired during upright standing (panels a and b) and walking (panels c and d) of a healthy subject.

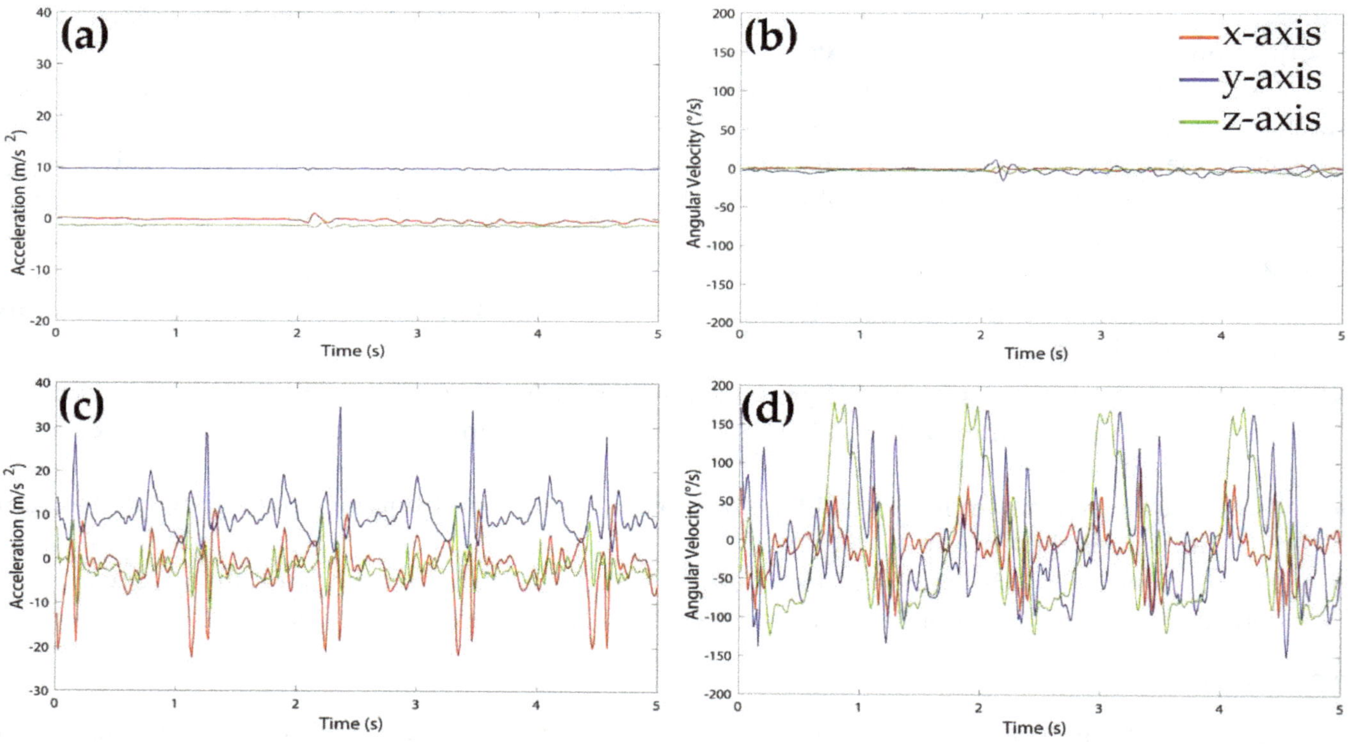

Figure 2. Example of signals acquired by accelerometer (**left panels**) and gyroscope (**right panels**) during 5 s of upright standing (panels (**a**,**b**)) and walking (panels (**c**,**d**)) of a healthy subject.

The following rule was used to separate windows representing static activities from those associated to dynamic activities:

if variance of gyroscope signal in z direction *is* below 600 deg$\cdot$s^{-1}, *then* window represents a static activity, *else* window represents a dynamic activity.

Windows recognized as static activities were further separated between resting and standing windows according to the following rule:

if mean of accelerometer signal in y direction *is* below 8.5 m$\cdot$s^{-2}, *then* the window is classified as resting, *else* the window is classified as standing.

All windows recognized as dynamic activities were pooled together and used for the following step of HAR based on GA and machine learning classifiers.

3.4. Genetic Algorithm for Simultaneous Feature Selection and Classifier Optimization

GA [52] is a well-known optimization algorithm belonging to the class of metaheuristics, i.e., algorithms designed to search for optimal solutions of a given optimization problem in a reasonable time. A GA is inspired to the Darwin's theory of evolution and, as such, it evolves a population of possible solutions (or individuals) toward better solutions, using the genetic operators of mutation and crossover. The main steps of a generic GA can be summarized as follows:

(1) Generation of an initial population: a random pool of individuals is generated by the algorithm, where an individual is represented by a binary vector, and the fitness value for all of them is calculated. The fitness function is a mathematical function that measures the goodness of a specific individual to solve the optimization problem.
(2) Parents' selection: a subset of individuals is selected to be parents of a new generation of solutions by means of a selection operator. The most used operator is the roulette wheel.
(3) Application of genetic operators: a new generation of individuals is obtained by applying mutation and crossover to the parents. Mutation produces a change in one or more bits of a solution and it is used for maintaining genetic diversity from one generation to the next. The bits to be mutated are randomly selected according to a mutation probability (usually very low, from 0.1 to 0.2). By mutation, a "1" bit in the original solution becomes a "0" bit and vice-versa. Crossover is applied to a couple of individuals with the aim of combining their genetic information. The two individuals are cut in correspondence of one or more random cut-points and the produced substrings are exchanged between them. Each individual has a crossover probability (usually higher than 0.8) to be part of at least one couple.
(4) Termination: if the stopping condition is not reached, a new population of individuals is selected among children and parents and the algorithm restarts from Step 2. The stopping condition is usually based on a given number of iterations or to a plateau in the fitness values of the new generations.

In this study we developed an ad-hoc GA for searching the optimal feature subset and classifier parameters, simultaneously. Four classifiers belonging to machine learning were tested and optimized: K-Nearest Neighbors (KNN), Feedforward Neural Network (FNN), Support Vector Machine (SVM) and Decision Tree (DT). Since all couples classifier-feature set were optimized, a total of 8 GAs were implemented (four classifiers $\times$ two feature sets).

Each solution was represented by a binary vector made up of two concatenated substrings: a first substring used for the selection of the most informative features to be input in the classifier and a second substring codifying the classifier parameters. For the first substring, we associated one bit to each available feature, obtaining a number of bits equal to the total number of features included in the considered feature set (*FeatSet_A* or *FeatSet_B*). A bit assuming value equal to "1" identified a feature included in the subset and used by the classifier, while a "0" labelled a not-used feature. The number of bits constituting the second substring was defined for each specific classifier, according to the number of parameters to be optimized and the values we wanted to explore. The details of the codification scheme used for the second substring can be found in the following sections for each classifier tested in this study.

The initial population of possible solutions comprised 400 individuals. The fitness function of each solution was measured according to the following equation:

$$fitness = 1 - acc + 0.3 \times \left(\max_{\forall activity} (acc_{activity}) - \min_{\forall activity} (acc_{activity}) \right) \tag{2}$$

where the total accuracy (*acc*) and the accuracy for the *i*-th activity ($acc_{activity}$) were calculated on the validation set for each specific classifier and were expressed in percentage between 0 and 1. The classifiers were trained using the training set, fed with the feature subset defined by the first substring and set up with the parameters codified in the second substring. In Equation (2), the first part of the formula aims at maximizing the classifier performances and the second part is a penalty term introduced to balance the performances among the different classes. Lower fitness values are associated with better solutions.

The parents' selection was based on the roulette wheel algorithm [52], in which the probability of each individual to be selected as parent is proportional to its fitness: individuals with better fitness values have higher probability to become parents of the new generation.

Crossover was implemented with four random cut-points and probability equal to 1. The mutation probability was set to 0.2. Two stopping conditions were implemented: maximum number of iterations (experimentally established as 30) and a plateau in the best fitness value for 15 consecutive iterations. All GAs and classifiers were implemented in Matlab2018a® (The MathWorks, Natick, MA, USA) environment.

3.4.1. K-Nearest Neighbors

KNN algorithm is a simple classification algorithm based on the calculation of the distance (usually the Euclidean distance) between the new element to be classified and the elements in the training set. Firstly, the training elements are sorted in descending order according to their distance from the new element. Then, the most frequent class of the first K elements (called neighbors) is associated to the new element.

For this kind of classifier, only the value of the K neighbors must be decided. A common starting value for K is $K_{in} = \sqrt{N}$ [53], where N was the number of elements in the training set. Beginning from this consideration, we decided to analyze 32 values around K_{in} and, thus, we used five bits for the second substring of each GA solution ($2^5 = 32$): each possible value assumed by the second substring was associated to a specific K value to be set in the classifier.

3.4.2. Feedforward Neural Network

A FNN is made up of a set of neurons, connected by weighted arcs, that process the input information according to the McCulloch and Pitts model [54]:

$$y = f\left(\sum_i w_i \cdot x_i\right) \tag{3}$$

where y is the output of the neuron, w_i are weights of the incoming connections, x_i are inputs to the neuron, and f is called transfer function and should be selected according to the classification problem.

Neurons in a FNN are organized in layers: in the input layer, one neuron for each input variable is required; the number of neurons in the output layer is decided according to the number of classes to be recognized and the selected transfer function; between input and output layers a certain number of hidden layers can be inserted, whose dimensions are usually decided testing different configurations.

In this study we fixed a basic network structure with input layer and first hidden layer both including one neuron for each feature selected according to the first substring of the GA solution, and an output layer made up of one neuron returning the recognized activity. Then, the number of hidden layers was increased according to the second substring of each solution: three bits were used for adding from one to eight further hidden layers to the basic structure. Each new hidden layer included 1/2 of the previous layer neurons.

The sigmoid transfer function was used for all hidden layers and the linear transfer function was set for the output neuron. Since the output neuron retuned a real value for each classified element, the round operator was applied to the FNN output and used to assign the final class.

3.4.3. Support Vector Machine

A SVM is a binary classifier (meaning that it is able to distinguish between two classes) that projects the input elements in a new multidimensional space, usually with higher dimensionality than the original one, in which the elements belonging to the two classes are linearly separable. The mapping from the original to the new space is accomplished by means of a function called kernel function, that could be linear or non-linear according to the problem complexity. In the new space, the separation between the classes is obtained with a hyperplane that maximizes its distance from the so-called support vectors. These are the elements of the two classes nearest to the hyperplane and their distance from the hyperplane is called margin.

For this kind of classifier, two different parameters must be set: the kernel function and the penalty term C, that regulates the tradeoff between large margins and small misclassification errors. Thus, we codified in the second substring both information, using two bits for choosing the kernel function and 4 bits for selecting the C value. For the kernel, we examined four different functions: linear, Gaussian, polynomial of order 2 and polynomial of order 3. For the penalty term, the value was set according to the following equation:

$$C = \begin{cases} 0.5 & if\ C_{dec} = 0 \\ 1 & if\ C_{dec} = 1 \\ (C_{dec} - 1) \times 10 & otherwise \end{cases} \tag{4}$$

where C_{dec} is the decimal value of the 4 bits codifying the C term. Using Equation (4) we were able to explore values between 0.5 and 140.

Since the SVM is a binary classifier and, in this study, we would like to identify seven different activities, we implemented a multiclass model for SVM. It combined 21 SVMs using the one vs one strategy in which, for each classifier, only two classes were evaluated, and the rest was ignored. In this way all possible combinations of class pairs were evaluated. The final classification is then obtained using the majority voting.

3.4.4. Decision Tree

A DT is a tree-like classifier belonging to machine learning methods. In general, the tree is constructed top-down by recursively dividing the training set into partitions according to a given splitting rule in the form of *"if variable*$_i$ *< threshold then partition1, else partition2"*. For each splitting rule, a new node is created in the tree. The best splitting rule is identified as that producing two partitions as pure as possible, where pure means that all the elements into a given partition belong to the same class. The construction of a branch stops when the obtained partition is pure or if no more variables can be used for partitioning: in case of pure partitions, the class of the elements is assigned to the leaf node, while in case of no pure partitions, the corresponding leaf node is labeled with the most represented class in the partition. During DT construction it could happen that not all available variables are used, thus a selection of the most discriminant features could be obtained as byproduct of this classifier. Once the tree has been constructed, a new element is classified iteratively applying the splitting rules and following the corresponding branch until a leaf node is reached: the class of the leaf is automatically associated to the new element.

Although several algorithms have been proposed for the tree construction and the identification of the best splitting rule for each node, the CART algorithm [55] and the Gini index [55] are commonly used for the these purposes, respectively, and applied in this study. Once these methods have been selected, no other parameters must be set for DT construction and running. For this reason, in our GA the optimization of the DT did not require bits associated to the second substring.

3.5. Post-Processing

Each couple feature subset-classifier parameters identified by GAs was used for classifying all dynamic windows in the validation set. Furthermore, a post-processing algorithm based on majority voting was implemented on the outputs of each classifier, to reduce isolated classification errors: considering 5 subsequent windows, the most frequently recognized activity was assigned to the entire group of 5 overlapping windows.

3.6. Performance Evaluation

The performances of the eight couples feature subset-classifier parameters were evaluated in terms of accuracy reached for each dynamic activity in every subject involved in the study, after post-processing. The results obtained for *FeatSet_A* and *FeatSet_B* across the 61 subjects were also compared by means of a Student t-test (paired, 2-tail, significance level: $\alpha = 0.05$), for each activity separately. Moreover, the *F1-score* [56] was calculated for each classifier as:

$$F1 - score = \frac{2 \times precision \times recal}{precision + recall} \quad (5)$$

where *recall* measures the ratio between the number of true positive elements and the total number of positive elements and *precision* measures the ratio between the number of true positive elements and the total number of elements classified as positive.

4. Results

A total of 59780 windows were included in the validation set (61 subjects × 140 windows × 7 activities).

The separation of static activity windows from dynamic activity windows based on rules was able to correctly detect 100% of resting windows and 100% of upright standing windows. Thus, for GA implementation and performance evaluation, 42,700 dynamic windows were used as validation set and 4270 windows were randomly included in the training set.

Table 1 summarizes the GA results for each classifier and for the two feature sets. The following information, related to the best solution found by GAs, are reported: number of features selected by the first substring, classifier parameters codified in the second substring, accuracy obtained on the training set used for the classifier construction, and accuracy reached on the validation set comprising all dynamic windows.

Table 1. GA results for each classifier and for the two feature sets.

Classifier	# of Selected Features		Classifier Parameters		Accuracy on Training Set		Accuracy on Validation Set	
	FeatSet_A	*FeatSet_B*	*FeatSet_A*	*FeatSet_B*	*FeatSet_A*	*FeatSet_B*	*FeatSet_A*	*FeatSet_B*
KNN	106	132	*K* = 55	*K* = 55	87.7%	86.6%	87.7%	86.1%
FNN	114	138	*#hidden layers* = 6 *#hidden neurons* = [114, 57, 29, 15, 8, 4]	*#hidden layers* = 6 *#hidden neurons* = [138, 69, 35, 18, 9, 5]	91.7%	49.7%	89.7%	48.5%
SVM	118	133	*kernel* = gaussian *scale* = 20	*kernel* = gaussian *scale* = 10	100.0%	99.9%	98.5%	96.4%
DT	151	103	None	None	97.7%	97.1%	85.9%	82.7%

As it emerges from the table, the GA allowed a substantial reduction of the number of features that was almost halved for both feature sets. Except for DT, a higher number of variables were selected from *FeatSet_B* with respect to *FeatSet_A*, even if this was not associated to substantial differences in the classifiers parameters and this did not produce better performances, neither on training nor on validation set.

Figure 3 shows, for each optimized couple feature subset-classifier parameters, the mean accuracy and the standard error across the 61 subjects involved in the study after post-processing.

Analyzing the behavior of the four classifiers, it emerges that the SVM reached the best performances, allowing to correctly recognize more than 95% of windows for all dynamic activities and for both feature subsets. Comparing the two feature subsets, no significant differences were observed for every dynamic activity using SVM and DT, while FNN fed with *FeatSet_B* was not able to reach acceptable results. This behavior is also evident in Figure 4, where the mean accuracy and F1-score across all seven activities (both static and dynamic) examined in this study is showed for each classifier. Overall, the highest accuracy achieved by the SVM is 97.1% and 96.7% for *FeatSet_A* and *FeatSet_B* respectively, while the worst mean accuracy was 65.5% obtained using FNN fed with *FeatSet_B*. The same behavior can be observed for the F1-score (Figure 4 panel b): the SVM had a score equal to 0.971 and 0.967 for the two sets, meaning that very high values of recall and precision were reached in both cases.

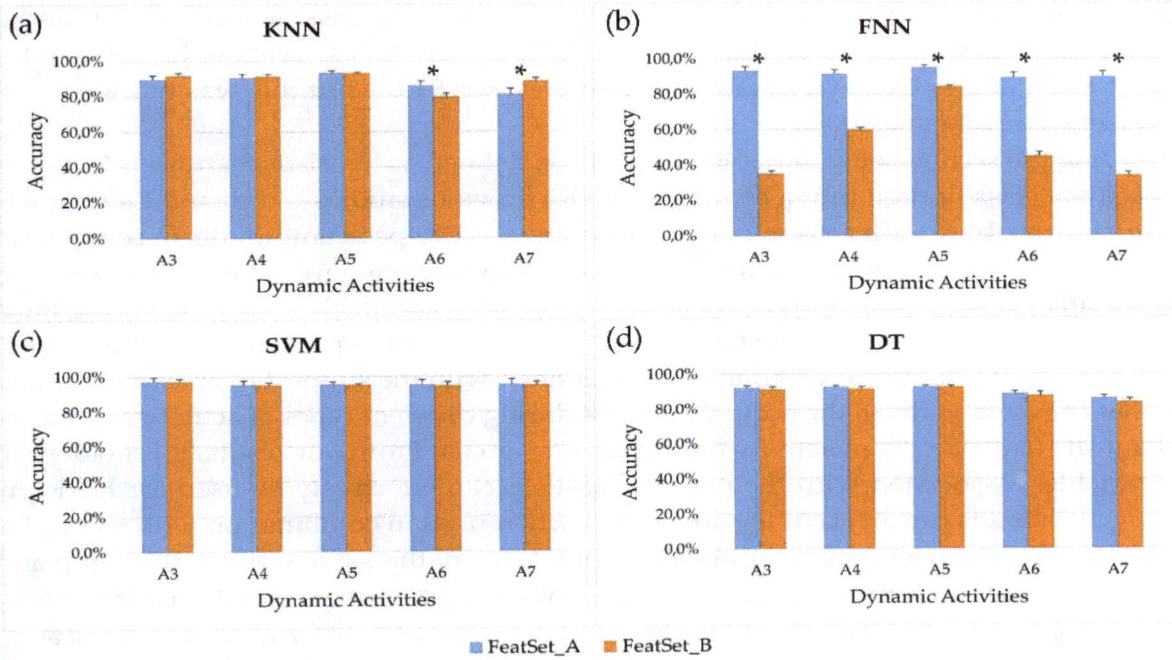

Figure 3. Mean accuracy (bar) and standard error (whisker) across the 61 subjects involved in the study for each dynamic activity (level walking (A_3), ascending and descending stairs (A_4 and A_5), uphill and downhill walking (A_6 and A_7)), after post-processing. Four classifiers are analyzed: (**a**) K-Nearest Neighbors; (**b**) Feedforward Neural Networks; (**c**) Support Vector Machine; (**d**) Decision Tree. Asterisks (*) mark significant differences between accuracies reached by *FeatSet_A* and *FeatSet_B* (p-value < 0.05).

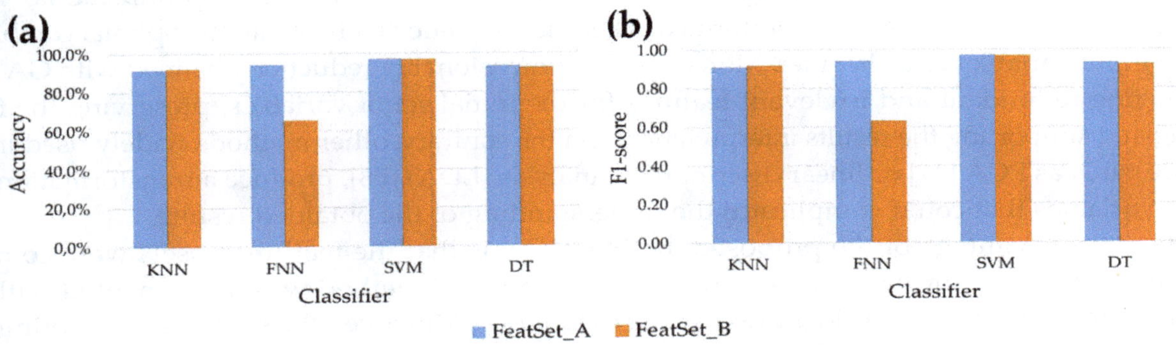

Figure 4. Mean accuracy (panel (**a**)) and F1-score (panel (**b**)) of the four classifiers across the seven activities (both static and dynamic activities), after post-processing, for the two sets of features.

5. Discussion

In this work we compared two sets of features for HAR applications, one comprising features widely used in literature for similar purposes [24] and the second set including variables connected to the expected biomechanical meaning of a given activity on the sensor signals.

With respect to the *FeatSet_A*, our results are in accordance with or better than those obtained by other similar studies. In a recent study by Yurtman et al. [41], the authors compared seven machine learning classifiers using only time- and frequency-domain features. Their results showed that, considering both static and dynamic activities, the best classifier was the SVM, that allowed them to recognize the 86.4% of activities. Similarly, in our study the best results were achieved by the SVM, although our mean accuracy across the seven examined activities was 97.1%. Moreover, our methodology allowed to correctly recognize all windows related to static activities (accuracy = 100%), whereas in ref. [41] better performances were obtained for non-stationary activities with respect to stationary ones (accuracy of 90.7% and 70.6% respectively). Attal et al. [8] analyzed the total accuracy across static and dynamic activities of different classifiers and they found that the best method for HAR was the KNN, that reached 99.3% of correct classification. In our case, the mean accuracy of KNN across the seven examined activities was 91.6% but this was our worst result for *FeatSet_A* (see Figure 4 panel a).

Regarding the second set of variables, sometimes defined as heuristic features [14], it was rarely used for activity classification thus a comparison with previous studies is difficult. Reference [1] used some heuristic variables, such as zero crossing rate and peak-to-peak amplitude, in combination with other time-domain and frequency-domain features. The gyroscope signal integration was used in the study by Najafi et al. [57] for identifying postural transactions and further processed using the discrete wavelet transform. However, to the best of our knowledge, no studies proposed an entire set of features context-based. In our study, these variables were defined with the support of an expert in movement analysis that analyzed in detail the acquired signals during different types of activity and the expected biomechanical effect of a given activity on the sensor signals. From our results it is evident that this kind of variables, associated with the proper classifier, can effectively be used for HAR purposes with very good results (mean accuracy above 96% when used in combination with SVM). From the implementation point of view, the computational complexity of this set of features is lower than the one required by frequency and time-frequency domain features [15], since no transformation of the signals is needed and features are extracted only in time-domain. Moreover, having a direct physical meaning, heuristic features can be useful for supporting the interpretation of results in more complex situations, for example in the monitoring of pathological subjects. In fact, in presence of pathological conditions, the acquired MIMU signals could be altered and consequently some of the extracted features could differ from a "standard" condition. In this case, using *FeatSet_B* and analyzing the physical meaning of these "altered" variables, it could be possible to understand which biomechanical aspect is mostly compromised by a given pathology.

Finally, our study is the first in the HAR field in which the simultaneous optimization of feature subset and classifier parameters was performed. This allows to effectively obtain the optimal combination between input variables and classifier. Moreover, the dimensionality reduction obtained with GA allows for removing redundant and irrelevant features for the initial set of variables, preserving the feature meaning and supporting the results interpretation. On the contrary, other methods widely used in HAR literature, such as PCA [41] or linear discriminant analysis (LDA) [58], produce a transformation of the original variables that could complicates the understanding of the obtained results.

The main advantage of the proposed methodology is that the feature subsets were compared to the best of their performances. In fact, since a wrapper FS method was implemented with GAs, the optimal reduced subset was identified in both situations. Moreover, the simultaneous optimization of the classifiers allowed to find the proper set of parameters suitable for that specific input features.

One limitation of this study lies in the fact that only healthy subjects were involved in our experiment. However, our aim was to compare the two sets of features, thus the most basic and common situation was used, with no introduction of gait variability due to pathological conditions. Nevertheless, we are planning to enlarge our protocol to other neurological pathologies such as Parkinson disease. Moreover, we are implementing the HAR directly on a wearable device composed of three MIMU sensors (accelerometer, gyroscope and magnetometer) and a 32-bit microprocessor equipped with floating point processing unit. The optimized version of the SVM associated with the selected *FeatSet_B* variables was chosen to be implemented on this new device version.

6. Conclusions

This study focused on the emerging field of HAR and aimed at comparing a set of variables commonly used in literature with a completely new one, comprising only time-domain variables associated with the biomechanical meaning of acquired signals. Moreover, we used a methodology for simultaneous feature selection and classifier parameter optimization, based on GA and never used before in similar contexts. From our results it emerged that the two sets of features can both reach very high recognition accuracy, above 96%, if associated with the SVM classifier. However, the newly-proposed set of variables can be easier to be interpreted and their biomechanical meaning could be employed to better understand alterations of the biomechanical behavior in more complex situations, such as when applied to pathological subjects.

Author Contributions: Investigation, S.R.; Methodology, S.R. and G.B.; Supervision, G.B. and M.K.; Writing—original draft, S.R.; Writing—review & editing, G.B. and M.K.

References

1. Wang, Y.; Cang, S.; Yu, H. A Data Fusion-Based Hybrid Sensory System for Older People's Daily Activity and Daily Routine Recognition. *IEEE Sens. J.* **2018**, *18*, 6874–6888. [CrossRef]
2. Tsinganos, P.; Skodras, A. On the Comparison of Wearable Sensor Data Fusion to a Single Sensor Machine Learning Technique in Fall Detection. *Sensors* **2018**, *18*, 592. [CrossRef] [PubMed]
3. González, S.; Sedano, J.; Villar, J.R.; Corchado, E.; Herrero, Á.; Baruque, B. Features and models for human activity recognition. *Neurocomputing* **2015**, *167*, 52–60. [CrossRef]
4. Roy, S.H.; Cheng, M.S.; Chang, S.-S.; Moore, J.; De Luca, G.; Nawab, S.H.; De Luca, C.J. A Combined sEMG and Accelerometer System for Monitoring Functional Activity in Stroke. *IEEE Trans. Neural Syst. Rehabil. Eng.* **2009**, *17*, 585–594. [CrossRef] [PubMed]
5. De Leonardis, G.; Rosati, S.; Balestra, G.; Agostini, V.; Panero, E.; Gastaldi, L.; Knaflitz, M. Human Activity Recognition by Wearable Sensors: Comparison of different classifiers for real-time applications. In Proceedings of the 2018 IEEE International Symposium on Medical Measurements and Applications (MeMeA), Rome, Italy, 11–13 June 2018; IEEE: Piscataway, NJ, USA, 2018; pp. 1–6.
6. Altun, K.; Barshan, B.; Tunçel, O. Comparative study on classifying human activities with miniature inertial and magnetic sensors. *Pattern Recognit.* **2010**, *43*, 3605–3620. [CrossRef]
7. Torres-Huitzil, C.; Nuno-Maganda, M. Robust smartphone-based human activity recognition using a tri-axial accelerometer. In Proceedings of the 2015 IEEE 6th Latin American Symposium on Circuits & Systems (LASCAS), Montevideo, Uruguay, 24–27 February 2015; IEEE: Piscataway, NJ, USA, 2015; pp. 1–4.
8. Attal, F.; Mohammed, S.; Dedabrishvili, M.; Chamroukhi, F.; Oukhellou, L.; Amirat, Y.; Attal, F.; Mohammed, S.; Dedabrishvili, M.; Chamroukhi, F.; et al. Physical Human Activity Recognition Using Wearable Sensors. *Sensors* **2015**, *15*, 31314–31338. [CrossRef] [PubMed]
9. Bao, L.; Intille, S. Activity recognition from user-annotated acceleration data. *Pervasive Comput.* **2004**, 1–17.
10. Aminian, K.; Rezakhanlou, K.; De Andres, E.; Fritsch, C.; Leyvraz, P.-F.; Robert, P. Temporal feature estimation during walking using miniature accelerometers: An analysis of gait improvement after hip arthroplasty. *Med. Biol. Eng. Comput.* **1999**, *37*, 686–691. [CrossRef] [PubMed]
11. Pirttikangas, S.; Fujinami, K.; Nakajima, T. Feature selection and activity recognition from wearable sensors. *UCS* **2006**, *6*, 516–527.

12. Steven Eyobu, O.; Han, D.; Steven Eyobu, O.; Han, D.S. Feature Representation and Data Augmentation for Human Activity Classification Based on Wearable IMU Sensor Data Using a Deep LSTM Neural Network. *Sensors* **2018**, *18*, 2892. [CrossRef] [PubMed]
13. Preece, S.J.; Goulermas, J.Y.; Kenney, L.P.J.; Howard, D. A Comparison of Feature Extraction Methods for the Classification of Dynamic Activities From Accelerometer Data. *IEEE Trans. Biomed. Eng.* **2009**, *56*, 871–879. [CrossRef] [PubMed]
14. Preece, S.J.; Goulermas, J.Y.; Kenney, L.P.J.; Howard, D.; Meijer, K.; Crompton, R. Activity identification using body-mounted sensors—A review of classification techniques. *Physiol. Meas.* **2009**, *30*, R1–R33. [CrossRef] [PubMed]
15. Figo, D.; Diniz, P.C.; Ferreira, D.R.; Cardoso, J.M.P. Preprocessing techniques for context recognition from accelerometer data. *Pers. Ubiquitous Comput.* **2010**, *14*, 645–662. [CrossRef]
16. Frawley, W.J.; Piatetsky-Shapiro, G.; Matheus, C.J. Knowledge discovery in databases: An overview. *AI Mag.* **1992**, *13*, 57–70. [CrossRef]
17. Giannini, V.; Rosati, S.; Castagneri, C.; Martincich, L.; Regge, D.; Balestra, G. Radiomics for pretreatment prediction of pathological response to neoadjuvant therapy using magnetic resonance imaging: Influence of feature selection. In Proceedings of the 2018 IEEE 15th International Symposium on Biomedical Imaging (ISBI 2018), Washington, DC, USA, 4–7 April 2018; IEEE: Piscataway, NJ, USA, 2018; pp. 285–288.
18. Zaccaria, G.M.; Rosati, S.; Castagneri, C.; Ferrero, S.; Ladetto, M.; Boccadoro, M.; Balestra, G. Data quality improvement of a multicenter clinical trial dataset. In Proceedings of the 39th Annual International Conference of the IEEE Engineering in Medicine and Biology Society (EMBC), Seogwipo, Korea, 11–15 July 2017; IEEE: Piscataway, NJ, USA, 2017; pp. 1190–1193.
19. Rosati, S.; Balestra, G.; Molinari, F. Feature Extraction by QuickReduct Algorithm: Assessment of Migraineurs Neurovascular Pattern. *J. Med. Imaging Heal. Inform.* **2011**, *1*, 184–192. [CrossRef]
20. Rosati, S.; Meiburger, K.M.; Balestra, G.; Acharya, U.R.; Molinari, F. Carotid wall measurement and assessment based on pixel-based and local texture descriptors. *J. Mech. Med. Biol.* **2016**. [CrossRef]
21. Li, J.; Cheng, K.; Wang, S.; Morstatter, F.; Trevino, R.P.; Tang, J.; Liu, H. Feature Selection: A Data Perspective. *ACM Comput. Surv.* **2017**, *50*, 1–45. [CrossRef]
22. Lessmann, S.; Stahlbock, R.; Crone, S.F. Genetic Algorithms for Support Vector Machine Model Selection. In Proceedings of the 2006 IEEE International Joint Conference on Neural Network Proceedings, Vancouver, BC, Canada, 16–21 July 2006; IEEE: Piscataway, NJ, USA, 2006; pp. 3063–3069.
23. Rojas-Dominguez, A.; Padierna, L.C.; Carpio Valadez, J.M.; Puga-Soberanes, H.J.; Fraire, H.J. Optimal Hyper-Parameter Tuning of SVM Classifiers With Application to Medical Diagnosis. *IEEE Access* **2018**, *6*, 7164–7176. [CrossRef]
24. Nweke, H.F.; Teh, Y.W.; Mujtaba, G.; Al-garadi, M.A. Data fusion and multiple classifier systems for human activity detection and health monitoring: Review and open research directions. *Inf. Fusion* **2019**, *46*, 147–170. [CrossRef]
25. Saha, J.; Chowdhury, C.; Biswas, S. Two phase ensemble classifier for smartphone based human activity recognition independent of hardware configuration and usage behaviour. *Microsyst. Technol.* **2018**, *24*, 2737–2752. [CrossRef]
26. San-Segundo, R.; Blunck, H.; Moreno-Pimentel, J.; Stisen, A.; Gil-Martín, M. Robust Human Activity Recognition using smartwatches and smartphones. *Eng. Appl. Artif. Intell.* **2018**, *72*, 190–202. [CrossRef]
27. Yang, F.; Zhang, L. Real-time human activity classification by accelerometer embedded wearable devices. In Proceedings of the 2017 4th International Conference on Systems and Informatics (ICSAI), Hangzhou, China, 11–13 November 2017; IEEE: Piscataway, NJ, USA, 2017; pp. 469–473.
28. Hassan, M.M.; Uddin, M.Z.; Mohamed, A.; Almogren, A. A robust human activity recognition system using smartphone sensors and deep learning. *Futur. Gener. Comput. Syst.* **2018**, *81*, 307–313. [CrossRef]
29. Wang, A.; Chen, G.; Wu, X.; Liu, L.; An, N.; Chang, C.-Y.; Wang, A.; Chen, G.; Wu, X.; Liu, L.; et al. Towards Human Activity Recognition: A Hierarchical Feature Selection Framework. *Sensors* **2018**, *18*, 3629. [CrossRef] [PubMed]
30. Baldominos, A.; Saez, Y.; Isasi, P. Evolutionary Design of Convolutional Neural Networks for Human Activity Recognition in Sensor-Rich Environments. *Sensors* **2018**, *18*, 1288. [CrossRef] [PubMed]

31. Li, F.; Shirahama, K.; Nisar, M.; Köping, L.; Grzegorzek, M.; Li, F.; Shirahama, K.; Nisar, M.A.; Köping, L.; Grzegorzek, M. Comparison of Feature Learning Methods for Human Activity Recognition Using Wearable Sensors. *Sensors* **2018**, *18*, 679. [CrossRef] [PubMed]
32. Zhu, J.; San-Segundo, R.; Pardo, J.M. Feature extraction for robust physical activity recognition. *Human-Centric Comput. Inf. Sci.* **2017**, *7*, 16. [CrossRef]
33. Köping, L.; Shirahama, K.; Grzegorzek, M. A general framework for sensor-based human activity recognition. *Comput. Biol. Med.* **2018**. [CrossRef] [PubMed]
34. Ponce, H.; Martínez-Villaseñor, M.; Miralles-Pechuán, L.; Ponce, H.; Martínez-Villaseñor, M.D.L.; Miralles-Pechuán, L. A Novel Wearable Sensor-Based Human Activity Recognition Approach Using Artificial Hydrocarbon Networks. *Sensors* **2016**, *16*, 1033. [CrossRef] [PubMed]
35. Jansi, R.; Amutha, R. Sparse representation based classification scheme for human activity recognition using smartphones. *Multimed. Tools Appl.* **2018**, 1–19. [CrossRef]
36. Jansi, R.; Amutha, R. A novel chaotic map based compressive classification scheme for human activity recognition using a tri-axial accelerometer. *Multimed. Tools Appl.* **2018**, *77*, 31261–31280. [CrossRef]
37. Tian, Y.; Wang, X.; Chen, W.; Liu, Z.; Li, L. Adaptive multiple classifiers fusion for inertial sensor based human activity recognition. *Cluster Comput.* **2018**, 1–14. [CrossRef]
38. Vanrell, S.R.; Milone, D.H.; Rufiner, H.L. Assessment of Homomorphic Analysis for Human Activity Recognition from Acceleration Signals. *IEEE J. Biomed. Heal. Informatics* **2018**, *22*, 1001–1010. [CrossRef] [PubMed]
39. Cao, J.; Li, W.; Ma, C.; Tao, Z. Optimizing multi-sensor deployment via ensemble pruning for wearable activity recognition. *Inf. Fusion* **2018**, *41*, 68–79. [CrossRef]
40. Garcia-Ceja, E.; Galván-Tejada, C.E.; Brena, R. Multi-view stacking for activity recognition with sound and accelerometer data. *Inf. Fusion* **2018**, *40*, 45–56. [CrossRef]
41. Yurtman, A.; Barshan, B.; Fidan, B.; Yurtman, A.; Barshan, B.; Fidan, B. Activity Recognition Invariant to Wearable Sensor Unit Orientation Using Differential Rotational Transformations Represented by Quaternions. *Sensors* **2018**, *18*, 2725. [CrossRef] [PubMed]
42. Ponce, H.; Miralles-Pechuán, L.; Martínez-Villaseñor, M.; Ponce, H.; Miralles-Pechuán, L.; Martínez-Villaseñor, M.D.L. A Flexible Approach for Human Activity Recognition Using Artificial Hydrocarbon Networks. *Sensors* **2016**, *16*, 1715. [CrossRef] [PubMed]
43. Doewes, A.; Swasono, S.E.; Harjito, B. Feature selection on Human Activity Recognition dataset using Minimum Redundancy Maximum Relevance. In Proceedings of the 2017 IEEE International Conference on Consumer Electronics—Taiwan (ICCE-TW), Taipei, Taiwan, 12–14 June 2017; IEEE: Piscataway, NJ, USA, 2017; pp. 171–172.
44. Wang, H.; Ke, R.; Li, J.; An, Y.; Wang, K.; Yu, L. A correlation-based binary particle swarm optimization method for feature selection in human activity recognition. *Int. J. Distrib. Sens. Networks* **2018**, *14*. [CrossRef]
45. Ignatov, A. Real-time human activity recognition from accelerometer data using Convolutional Neural Networks. *Appl. Soft Comput.* **2018**, *62*, 915–922. [CrossRef]
46. Hassan, M.M.; Huda, S.; Uddin, M.Z.; Almogren, A.; Alrubaian, M. Human Activity Recognition from Body Sensor Data using Deep Learning. *J. Med. Syst.* **2018**, *42*, 99. [CrossRef] [PubMed]
47. Jordao, A.; Torres, L.A.B.; Schwartz, W.R. Novel approaches to human activity recognition based on accelerometer data. *Signal Image Video Process.* **2018**, *12*, 1387–1394. [CrossRef]
48. He, H.; Tan, Y.; Huang, J. Unsupervised classification of smartphone activities signals using wavelet packet transform and half-cosine fuzzy clustering. In Proceedings of the 2017 IEEE International Conference on Fuzzy Systems (FUZZ-IEEE), Naples, Italy, 9–12 July 2017; IEEE: Piscataway, NJ, USA, 2017; pp. 1–6.
49. Stolcke, A.; Kajarekar, S.; Ferrer, L. Nonparametric feature normalization for SVM-based speaker verification. In Proceedings of the 2008 IEEE International Conference on Acoustics, Speech and Signal Processing, Las Vegas, NV, USA, 31 March–4 April 2008; IEEE: Piscataway, NJ, USA, 2008; pp. 1577–1580.
50. Janidarmian, M.; Roshan Fekr, A.; Radecka, K.; Zilic, Z. A Comprehensive Analysis on Wearable Acceleration Sensors in Human Activity Recognition. *Sensors* **2017**, *17*, 529. [CrossRef] [PubMed]
51. Altun, K.; Barshan, B. Human activity recognition using inertial/magnetic sensor units. In Proceedings of the International Workshop on Human Behavior Understanding, Istanbul, Turkey, 22 August 2010; pp. 38–51.
52. Engelbrecht, A.P. *Computational Intelligence: An Introduction*; Wiley Publishing: Hoboken, NJ, USA, 2007; ISBN 0470035617.

53. Rencher, A.C. *Methods of Multivariate Analysis*; J. Wiley: Hoboken, NJ, USA, 2002; ISBN 0471418897.
54. McCulloch, W.S.; Pitts, W. A logical calculus of the ideas immanent in nervous activity. *Bull. Math. Biophys.* **1943**, *5*, 115–133. [CrossRef]
55. Han, J.; Kamber, M.; Pei, J. *(Computer scientist) Data Mining: Concepts and Techniques*; Elsevier/Morgan Kaufmann: Amsterdam, The Netherlands, 2012; ISBN 9780123814791.
56. Sokolova, M.; Lapalme, G. A systematic analysis of performance measures for classification tasks. *Inf. Process. Manag.* **2009**, *45*, 427–437. [CrossRef]
57. Najafi, B.; Aminian, K.; Paraschiv-Ionescu, A.; Loew, F.; Bula, C.J.; Robert, P. Ambulatory system for human motion analysis using a kinematic sensor: Monitoring of daily physical activity in the elderly. *IEEE Trans. Biomed. Eng.* **2003**, *50*, 711–723. [CrossRef] [PubMed]
58. Chen, B.; Zheng, E.; Wang, Q. A locomotion intent prediction system based on multi-sensor fusion. *Sensors (Basel)* **2014**, *14*, 12349–12369. [CrossRef] [PubMed]

15

Analyzing Spinal Shape Changes During Posture Training Using a Wearable Device

Katharina Stollenwerk [1,*], Jonas Müller [2], André Hinkenjann [1] and Björn Krüger [2]

1 Hochschule Bonn-Rhein Sieg, Institute of Visual Computing, 53757 Sankt Augustin, Germany
2 Gokhale Method Institute, Stanford, CA 94305, USA
* Correspondence: katharina.stollenwerk@h-brs.de

Abstract: Lower back pain is one of the most prevalent diseases in Western societies. A large percentage of European and American populations suffer from back pain at some point in their lives. One successful approach to address lower back pain is postural training, which can be supported by wearable devices, providing real-time feedback about the user's posture. In this work, we analyze the changes in posture induced by postural training. To this end, we compare snapshots before and after training, as measured by the Gokhale *SpineTracker*™. Considering pairs of before and after snapshots in different positions (standing, sitting, and bending), we introduce a feature space, that allows for unsupervised clustering. We show that resulting clusters represent certain groups of postural changes, which are meaningful to professional posture trainers.

Keywords: posture analysis; spinal posture; accelerometer; wearable sensor

---

1. Introduction

Back pain is experienced by a large percentage of the world's population. Approximately 70% of the world's population experience lower back pain, contributing to the worldwide burden of disease. Levels of intensity and disability vary [1]:

- Grade I: low-intensity, low disability symptoms are experienced by 49%.
- Grade II: high-intensity, low disability symptoms are experienced by 12%.
- Grade III/IV: high-intensity, high disability symptoms are experienced by 11%.

In the U.S., 28% of the American workforce experiences lower back pain of various intensities at any given time, and during any given year 8% of the working population will be disabled due to low back pain [2,3]. According to Rubin and Devon [4], a majority of the population will suffer from a back problem at some point in their lives. This makes back pain the largest factor in the decline in productivity of workers, resulting in estimated economic costs ranging from $200 billion to $600 billion per year in the United States [5].

There is a wide range of treatments for back pain in use. This includes invasive methods, medication, exercise, supportive clothing, and postural change. The crowd-sourcing platform healthoutcome.org collects patients' ratings about all available treatments. In total more then 160,000 patient ratings have been collected for back pain, so far. Peleg et al. [6] report that results from this platform correspond to findings of randomized control trials. According to the crowd-sourcing platform itself, postural modifications are the highest-ranked interventions in terms of positive success. Posture training can be supported by wearable devices [7,8] to provide both, the user and the trainer, with real-time feedback about the student's posture.

In their review of works in the field of wearable technology for spine movement assessment [9], Papi et al. point out that the majority of articles in that field reported on the validity of their system with relatively few works making use of real-world data. They additionally state that the systems used were usually rather cumbersome. While their systematic review focussed on dynamic task performance only including papers themed in this direction, they excluded only three papers from their original compilation of 1610 qualifying papers (1566 of these were excluded based on their title or abstract) because the paper did not focus on *dynamic* task performance. This leads us to the valid assumption that real-world data is generally not widely used in dynamic or non-dynamic movement assessment of the spine.

Methods for analyzing changes in spine shape or posture [10–14] usually need a predefined 'normal' state to compare to or prevalently use statistical test to attempt differentiation between two defined groups. Section 2 on related work goes into detail on the aforementioned works.

We aim to address these gaps by systematically analyzing geometric changes in posture as a result of postural training by a Gokhale Method teacher and captured by the *SpineTracker*™ wearable (http://spinetracker.com, accessed 31 July 2019). To this end, we compare snapshots of the measured spine curve before training and the most recent target set by the teacher during or at the end of posture training. Our analysis does not rely on the definition of a global 'normal' spine shape.

The main contributions of this paper are:

1. The analysis of postural change in a large real-world data base of posture data, recorded using the SpineTracker wearable, by
    - devising a medium dimensional feature set from the spine curve data, well suited for further analysis and
    - showing how these data can be embedded into a two-dimensional feature space using a combination of standard dimensionality reduction techniques.
2. The demonstration that simple unsupervised clustering in the defined feature space results in a data separation which is geometrically and semantically meaningful.

The novelty of our approach lies in the fact that (a) works making use of real-world data to assess spinal movement, especially with wearables, are very rare, and that (b) we do not rely on any predefined 'normal' state to compare to.

Throughout this document we make use of the following terms: we use position to describe a passive, static state, e.g., standing, sitting. The realization of such a state by a person is called posture, emphasizing its execution as a multi-factor dynamic (active) process of both, skeletal alignment and muscle activation. When looking at a temporal sequence of motion data (here posture data), snapshot refers to a single element in that sequence.

The remainder of this work is organized as follows: We give an overview of related works in Section 2. A detailed description of the used materials and methods is given in Section 3. We present the results of our approach in Section 4 and discuss our findings in Section 5. Finally, the paper is concluded in Section 6.

2. Related Work

Human motion capturing refers to the recording of human movement and transforming them into a digital 3D representation. Full-body motion capture systems include optical and non-optical systems. Optical systems generally rely on imaging sensors and computer vision algorithms to capture a person with or without a set of passive or active markers attached to their body. Non-optical systems include motion capturing based on e.g., exoskeletons and inertial measurement unit (IMU) based systems. Optical systems generally suffer from being restricted to a capturing volume. Using inertial systems is one way to lift such restrictions.

2.1. IMU-Based Full-Body Motion Capture and Reconstruction

Roetenberg et al. [15] describe the Xsens (https://www.xsens.com, accessed 31 July 2019) IMU-based full-body human motion capturing relying on biomechanical models and sensor fusion algorithms. The system uses a set of 17 sensors. Earlier, Tautges et al. [16] enabled full-body animation through four 3D accelerometers attached to wrists and ankles in combination with a large database of motion clips recorded with a marker-based optical motion capture system. Extending on the aforementioned work, Riaz et al. [17] use accelerometer data of wrists and the lower trunk together with ground contact information (computed from trunk sensor) for data-driven motion reconstruction.

2.2. Capturing of Body Parts, Specifically the Shape of the Spine

Sometimes it is desirable to only capture data from specific body parts in order to capture these in finer detail. Examples include capturing of the face [18,19], arms [20], legs [21], hands [22,23], and spine [7,10,12,24–30].

There have been different technologies for measuring the curvature of the spine reaching from image-based surface reconstruction methods (e.g., static and dynamic rasterstereography [24,25], CT scans [10], laser-triangulation [26]) over a ribbon of (eight) fibre-optic sensors, e.g., Williams et al. [27], strips of (twelve) strain-gauge elements, e.g., Consmüller et al. [28], and accelerometers, e.g., Stollenwerk et al. [7], to inertial sensors, e.g., Wong and Wong [12], Cajamarca et al. [29], and Voinea et al. [30].

Wong and Wong [12] developed a smart garment with three inertial sensors (3D accelerometer, three 1D gyroscopes) for posture training. Sensors were mounted between T1 and T2, between T11 and L1, and on S1 (The human spine [31] is divided into four segments (from top to bottom): cervical spine (neck region), thoracic spine (mid-back), lumbar spine (lower back), and sacrum (base of the spine). Each of these regions consists of several vertebrae (here listed from top to bottom). The cervical spine consists of seven vertebrae, abbreviated C1 through C7. The following twelve vertebrae belong to the thoracic spine and are abbreviated T1 through T12. Beneath the thoracic spine are the five lumbar vertebrae, L1–L5. The sacrum is a triangular-shaped bone located below L5. It consists of five fused sacral vertebrae S1–S5). The authors estimated inclination angles in the sagittal and coronal plane of thoracic and lumbar spine and measured posture change as a change in inclination between pairs of neighboring sensors. They also included a small study on the garment's posture feedback system concluding that it helped participants to avoid poor postures.

Cajamarca et al. [29] built StraightenUp+, a low-cost wearable device for monitoring posture explicitly designed for older persons. StraightenUp+ is a backpack-shaped waist-adjustable harness vest in which three inertial sensors (3D gyroscopes and 3D accelerometers), along with other necessary hardware, are attached to the vertical rear strap. Sensors are distributed equidistantly along the vertical strap covering approximately the full length of the back. They use the sensor data to identify a fixed set of eight physical activities.

Voinea et al. [30] and Stollenwerk et al. [7] describe a 2D reconstruction model for the shape of the human spine based on inertial sensors and plain accelerometers. Although Voinea et al.'s sensors are capable of outputting 3D orientations, they only use a single angle for spine shape reconstruction. In their setup, the five sensors are distributed equidistantly between C7 and L4 vertebrae. While from a reconstruction image their model looks a lot like the one used in [7], Voinea et al.'s models are designed to explicitly represent a C-shaped spine (kyphosis) and an S-shaped spine (normal), the authors of [7] do not make that assumption. Another difference is that [7] puts the first sensor on the L4 vertebra but distributes the following sensors equidistantly over a fixed-length segment independent of the person's spine length.

An overview of commonly used technologies for spine movement assessment along with respective spine outcomes is reported in the Papi et al. review of works in the field of wearable technology for spine movement assessment [9]. As explained in detail in the introduction (Section 1), this work gave rise to our assumption that in general, real-world data is rarely used in the movement assessment of the spine, neither in dynamic nor in non-dynamic settings.

2.3. Methods for Data Analysis

Hay et al. [10] compare spine curves extracted from CT images to a model spine curve computed from multiple individuals without spinal disorders and a history of back pain. Aiming at the detection and quantification of pathologies, the comparison is based on the amount of curve deviation from the model, the deviation of the curvature as well as the torsion along the curve.

In their paper, Brink et al. [11] evaluate the amount of postural change in adolescent computer users after a period of twelve months in order to understand associations between postural change and upper quadrant musculoskeletal pain. For this purpose, different sitting postural angles were recorded and individually analyzed with respect to magnitude and orientational change using univariate and multivariate linear regression models. Sitting postural angles considered were head flexion, neck flexion, craniocervical angle, and trunk flexion. These angles mainly target the upper spinal region. In a small three-day posture feedback study (first day without feedback, second and third day with feedback) Wong and Wong [12] compare average trunk angles between days with and without feedback as well as between days with feedback.

Franklin and Conner-Kerr [13] investigated the relationship of postural changes during pregnancy and back pain. They measured and compared means and standard deviations as well as state analysis of variance (ANOVA) results for a total of nine postural variables (seven postural angles and head and shoulder displacements) of women in the first and third trimesters of pregnancy. Gonzáles-Sanchez et al. [14] compare thoracolumbar curvature angles between two groups (normal weighted and obese persons) using Student's t-test (parametric test for independent data) and Wilcoxon's test (non-parametric tests) in order to find out if there are statistically significant differences between the two groups.

As stated before (Section 1), methods summarized here either rely on a predefined 'normal' state to compare to or use statistical tests to compare two defined groups. In contrast to this, we aim at an analysis of changes in spinal shape essentially comparing two arbitrary spine curves of one person at two points in time, one before (unguided) and one after posture training (guided). To the best of our knowledge, there is no method for the geometric analysis of that change.

3. Materials and Methods

In this section we describe the system used for data recording in Section 3.1, the data we worked with (Section 3.2) as well as the derived feature space (Section 3.3) and dimensionality reduction techniques in Sections 3.4 and 3.5. The following Section 3.6 contains information on minimum spanning trees and how they can be used for clustering. We detail our processing pipeline in Section 3.7 and conclude with an explanation of visualization methods used to present results (Section 3.8).

3.1. Wearable

The system used for capturing the spinal shape is the *SpineTracker* developed by Gokhale Method Enterprises, Stanford, CA, USA. It consists of five individual accelerometer-based sensors (Figure 1a) which are attached to the lower back of the user as shown in Figure 1b,c. In contrast to single-device posture wearables, the five-sensor approach enables the capture of more detailed spinal curvature information also covering a larger portion of the spine.

All five sensor units were technically identical. The sensors connected and streamed data wirelessly to one host via bluetooth; currently this may be an iOS device or a computer. The sensors support sample rates of up to 50 Hz, thus allowing for a variety of applications, ranging from slow-motion measurements, e.g., sitting, to faster movements such as brisk walking.

More detailed technical information on the wearable as well as the model used for reconstruction of a spine shape from the accelerometer readings and the systematic evaluation of the system's accuracy (sensors and reconstruction method) can be found in [7].

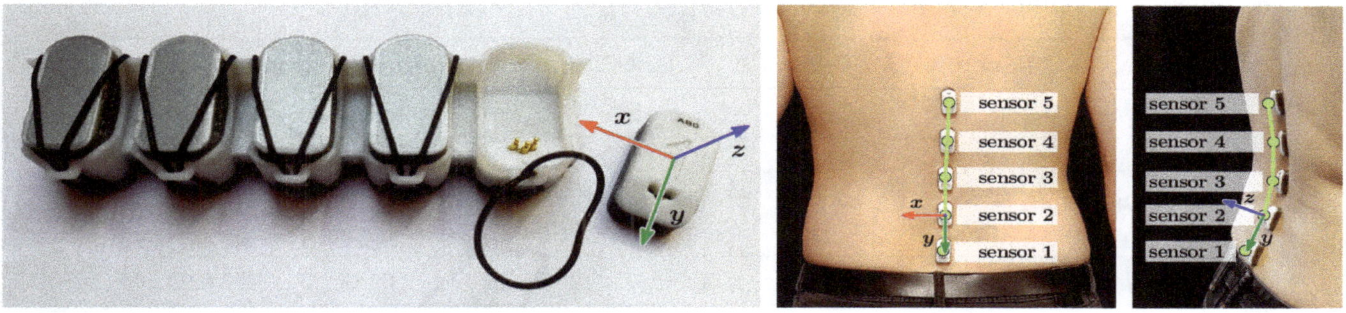

(a) (b) (c)

Figure 1. Photos of the *SpineTracker* sensor system. (**a**) Four of the five sensors are sitting in the charger. The sensor outside the charger is shown with its local coordinate system. A single sensor has the dimensions 33 mm × 16 mm × 10 mm. Each sensor is attached to a person's lumbar spine with double sided tape. (**b**,**c**) Back and side view of sensor positioning on the lumbar spine including directions of the sensor coordinate system. Sensors are overlayed with a reconstructed spine curve (green dots and line).

3.2. Data

The data representing the shape of the spine is usually either a set of angles or a set of 2D positions: when streaming data from the sensors, spine shape information is stored as a sequence of forward tilts $\tau_{\text{acc},i}, i = 1, \ldots, 5$ of the five *SpineTracker* sensors ordered by sensor ID. Using the spine curve model described in [7], these five angles are transformed into a 2D spine curve consisting of six 2D points P_j (a base point P_0 and five sensor positions $P_i, i = 1, \ldots, 5$) and arc segments connecting these points. For consistent visualization, the spine curve is positioned in space in a way that the first sensor lies in the origin, $P_1 = (0, 0)$.

The *SpineTracker* sensor system can also capture single frames ("snapshots") from the data stream that will represent the shape of the spine at that point in time. We used a database of such snapshots of three distinct positions: standing, sitting, and (hip) hinging. Snapshots can be unguided or guided. In an unguided snapshot, a person assumed one of the positions on their own and without a trainer's intervention or support. A guided snapshot was taken when the position was assumed under the guidance of a posture trainer. Each single snapshot in this database was labelled either "guided" or "unguided".

From this database, we considered per-user snapshot pairs. These pairs consist of one unguided posture and one teacher-guided posture in which the highest amount of change is to be expected. i.e., for the unguided postures, we extracted the respective initial posture snapshot of a position (t_0 snapshot). For the guided postures, we used the latest guided snapshot (t_1 snapshot) available. The t_0 *snapshots* hence represent the most unlearned realizations of the position and the t_1 *snapshots* contain the current best imitation of the position the user aims for at the moment of capture. As a consequence, we use exactly one pair per user and position even if more snapshots of that user are available for a specific position. For ethical reasons all data was anonymized. Table 1 gives details on the size of the database used, split by position, as well as overall. It additionally shows statistics on the time passed between unguided and guided snapshots.

In order to show that there was a significant difference in angles between the t_0 and t_1 snapshot pairs in one or more sensors, indicating plausibility of further analysis, we considered each sensor individually and conducted a paired samples Wilcoxon test (also called the Wilcoxon signed-rank test) [32].

Table 1. General statistics of the data basis used for our analysis. The column labelled # samples contains information on the number of snapshot pairs per position. The # users states how many different users recorded such pairs. The last four columns state the minimum, average, median, and maximum time passed between the snapshots in each pair. Time is displayed as a tuple of days (d), hours (hh), minutes (mm), and seconds (ss).

	# Samples	# Users	Time Difference, Format: "d hh:mm:ss"			
			Minimum	Mean	Median	Maximum
standing	393	393	0 00:30:07	30 01:34:18	2 00:39:43	443 03:38:05
sitting	386	386	0 00:30:13	23 23:03:02	2 01:16:43	399 00:23:05
hip hinging	362	362	0 00:37:44	24 11:23:42	2 00:54:51	385 21:39:54
full	1141	425	0 00:30:07	26 05:26:02	2 01:08:07	443 03:38:05

The database of (t_0, t_1) posture pairs used in this work is publicly available at https://skylab.vc.h-brs.de/kstoll2m/PosturePairsDB19/ (Supplementary Materials).

3.3. Feature Extraction

For each pair of snapshots in the database of position-posture-pairs we compute a feature vector F. F is composed of the normalized difference d_j of the sensor positions in the t_0 and t_1 snapshots and the length l_j of the difference

$$l_j = \left\| P_{j|t_1} - P_{j|t_0} \right\|_2 \tag{1}$$

$$d_j = \frac{P_{j|t_1} - P_{j|t_0}}{l_j}, \tag{2}$$

where $P_{j|t_0}$ ($P_{j|t_1}$) is the j-th 2D spine curve point in snapshot t_0 (t_1). This way, spinal shape change is expressed by the 2D directional change between the two snapshots and the 1D amount of change. This results in a 15 dimensional feature vector, five 2D directions d_j and five 1D lengths l_j, $j \in \{0, 2, 3, 4, 5\}$, for each snapshot pair. We only considered five of the six spine curve points leaving out the sensor positioned in zero (P_1). For general statistics we continue to use the sensor angle data $\tau_{acc,i|t}$, $i = 1, \ldots, 5$, $t \in \{t_0, t_1\}$.

3.4. Principal Component Analysis

Principal component analysis (PCA) [33] is one of the oldest and most widely used linear dimensionality reduction techniques. It is based on the eigendecomposition of the data's covariance matrix. Its eigenvectors are sorted by their respective eigenvalue forming the new orthogonal coordinate axes (principal component) of the underlying data set. The directions of the new coordinate axes coincide with the directions of maximum variation of the original data points. Geometrically spoken, PCA rotates the Cartesian coordinate system of a high dimensional point set in a way that maximizes the variance of the data along each axis. After the transform, axes are sorted by descending variance. Dimensionality reduction is achieved by retaining only the first n principal components.

3.5. T-Stochastic Neighbor Embedding

T-stochastic neighbor embedding (t-SNE) [34] is a more recent non-linear dimensionality reduction technique for mapping high-dimensional data to a low-dimensional space (often called a map). It is based on the following:

- A fix data similarity matrix of conditional distances between pairs of data points in the original high-dimensional space. Conditional distances are computed based on a combination of the pairwise Euclidean distances and a point-specific Gaussian distribution.

- A similar point-wise neighborhood estimation in the low-dimensional target space (map similarity matrix), exchanging the Gaussian distribution with a one degree-of-freedom Student's t-distribution.

The goal is to iteratively adapt the map similarity matrix to best fit the data similarity matrix. This is achieved by minimization of the Kullback–Leibler divergence [35] of the two probability distributions underlying the two similarity matrices.

3.6. Minimum Spanning Tree and Clustering

A minimum spanning tree (MST) is a graph theory concept fulfilling the following criteria: given an undirected graph $G = (V, E)$ of vertices V and weighted edges E, an MST is a tree $(V, E' \subseteq E)$ including all vertices of G using a minimum number of edges E' such that the total weight of the edges is minimal. The MST is unique if all edge weights are distinct, which is a reasonable assumption for real-world scenarios.

MSTs can be used for clustering. Let $G = (V, E)$ be a fully connected graph of the data points (V) of a data set. Let the weight of each edge $e = \{v, w\} \in E$ be defined as e.g., the Euclidean distance between the data points v and w it connects. This graph is used to construct an MST which is then used for clustering: Subsequent cutting of edges with highest weight increases the number of connected components in this graph. Connected components represent clusters.

3.7. Processing Pipeline

An overview of our processing pipeline is given in Figure 2. For each pair of snapshots in our database, we compute each posture's 2D spine curve and extract one feature vector per snapshot pair as described above (Section 3.3). We perform PCA to the set of extracted features to reduce the dimensionality of the data while retaining over 95% of the feature data's variance. We additionally use t-SNE to further reduce the dimensionality to two dimensions. PCA, as well as other linear dimensionality reduction techniques, preserves the global structure of the data. This preservation of global structure results from maintaining a high variability in the data which in turn translates in a separation of dissimilar data points. The non-linear dimensionality reduction t-SNE tries both, keep similar data points close together and dissimilar data points far apart. This is particularly interesting for finding clusters of data points in higher dimensional space.

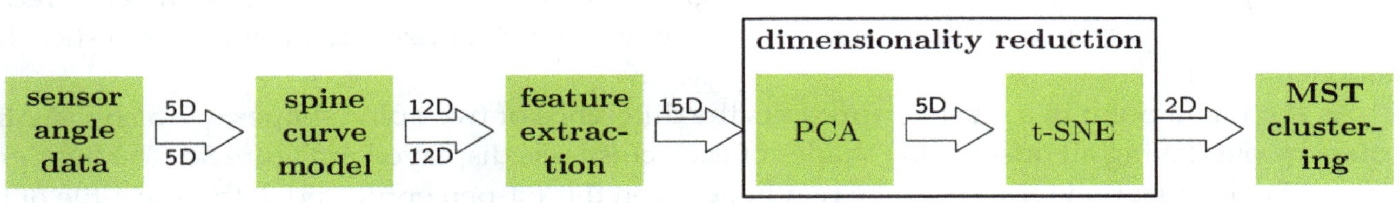

Figure 2. Overview of the processing pipeline used. Individual steps are marked by boxes, arrows indicate the direction of the pipeline. Each arrow is annotated with dimensionality of the data output by the preceding step. Two dimension labels indicate that the data from the two postures in each posture pair is not yet combined.

Clustering generally groups data points sharing a set of properties. Even though postural training is a highly individual process, we assume that the recorded data will exhibit certain differences and commonalities. This in turn will allow us to combine posture pairs into distinct clusters. We apply MST-clustering to the two-dimensional t-SNE map of the chosen feature space, as there is no prior knowledge on the general structure of clusters in the 2D t-SNE map. We compute the Euclidean distance between all pairs of t-SNE map points, which results in a similarity matrix of the map. The MST is constructed on this similarity matrix. Using MST-clustering is a reasonable choice due to the following properties:

1. The t-SNE map equalizes the density of neighboring data points in the higher dimensionality evening out distances between neighboring points in the map. As a consequence condensed clusters are spread and spread clusters are contracted.
2. In MST-clustering, data points are grouped together by proximity and need neither be separable by a regular geometric curve nor grouped around a centroid.

3.8. Visualization of Results

We visualize clustering results using the 2D t-SNE map of the data coloring each point by its cluster ID. We compute the angle difference between the t_1 and t_0 snapshots, $\tau_{\mathrm{acc},i|t_1} - \tau_{\mathrm{acc},i|t_0}$, $i = 1, \ldots, 5$. This set of difference angles was used to reconstruct an *offset spine shape*. The resulting offset base position $P_{\mathrm{offset},0}$ and offset sensor positions $P_{\mathrm{offset},i}$, $i = 1, \ldots, 5$, ordered by increasing y-coordinate, represent the computed differences as offset from a vertical line. Figure 3b shows an example of such an *offset spine shape*. The underlying two reconstructed spine shapes are illustrated in Figure 3a.

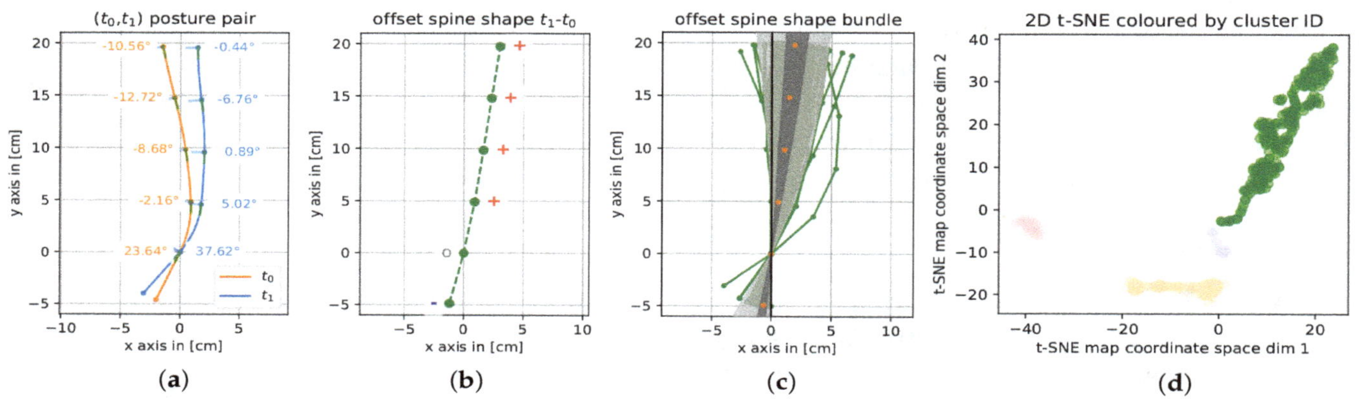

Figure 3. (**a**) Two spine shapes reconstructed from the t_0 and t_1 input angles and (**b**) resulting *offset spine shape*. (**c**) Offset spine shape bundle representing a data cluster in the feature set's T-stochastic neighbor embedding (t-SNE) map (**d**), colored by cluster ID.

Spine shapes are annotated with the sensor angle data they were constructed from and an indication to which side the person is looking: the line in each sensor position points away from the person's back.

Offset spine shapes are annotated with the sign of each offset position's x-coordinate. A red '+' stands for positive, a grey 'o' for zero, and a blue '-' for a negative horizontal offset from a vertical line positioned in zero.

As each data point in a cluster represents the difference of two spine shapes, we also visualize clusters by overlaying all offset spine shapes of each cluster as displayed in Figure 3c. The light grey area in this visualization represents the region between the 1st-percentile and 99th-percentile of the horizontal distribution of the data. Covering the central 50% of the horizontal extent of the offset spine shapes (at each point level), the dark grey area shows the region between the 25th-percentile and the 75th-percentile. Orange dots mark the median of the horizontal extent of the data. This overlay serves as visualization of the main orientation of the offset spine shapes in a specific cluster.

4. Results

In the following, we first list the results of the angle data analysis (Section 4.1) and motivate why this analysis is relevant. We then describe the behavior of the clustering under variation of the t-SNE parameter perplexity in Section 4.2. For this section, too, we state reasons for analyzing results from this variation. The last Section 4.3 presents and analyzes the results of the clustering of the posture data divided by position based on their geometry.

4.1. Analysis of the Angle Data

As normality test (Shapiro-Wilk [36], Anderson-Darling [37], Q-Q Plot [38]) indicated that the data is not normally distributed, we use the non-parametric paired samples Wilcoxon test (also called the Wilcoxon signed-rank test) [39] to check whether there was a difference in posture for the unguided and guided snapshots already on a single sensor level. We could confirm that for all positions, there was at least one sensor in which the median change in angle between the unguided t_0 snapshots and the guided t_1 snapshot pairs was significantly different from zero.

For standing, there was a significant difference in angle between the t_0 and t_1 snapshot pairs for all sensors ($p < \varepsilon = 10^{-6}$). For sitting the difference between the two snapshots is significant for only the first sensor ($p < \varepsilon$). Finally, the angle difference between t_0 and t_1 snapshot pairs is below the standard significance threshold $\alpha = 0.05$ for all but one sensor for hip hinging ($p < \varepsilon$ for four out of five sensors).

Descriptive statistics of both snapshots for all positions and sensors are listed in Table 2. The last column of the table marks the previously reported sensors for which $p < \alpha$. Figure 4 provides additional information on the distribution of the five sensors' angle data for each position.

Table 2. Mean, standard deviation (sd), minimum (min), maximum (max), and median (med) values as well as the interquartile range (IQR) of all five sensor's angle data for t_0 and t_1 snapshots. A star in the last column stands for a rejected null hypothesis of the Wilcoxon signed-rank test ($p < 0.05$).

	t_0 Snapshots					t_1 Snapshots					
	Mean (SD)	**Min**	**Max**	**Med**	**IQR**	**Mean (SD)**	**Min**	**Max**	**Med**	**IQR**	
standing											
sensor 1	19.6 (10.3)	−24.6	57.8	19.4	11.8	22.5 (8.0)	−4.5	48.2	22.7	10.2	*
sensor 2	10.1 (10.7)	−19.8	54.1	10.0	13.0	13.8 (9.2)	−14.4	51.4	13.3	12.4	*
sensor 3	−4.1 (10.3)	−40.4	53.8	−4.5	11.1	−0.1 (9.0)	−27.9	54.1	−0.9	10.4	*
sensor 4	−12.3 (8.9)	−29.6	82.0	−13.1	8.5	−8.2 (6.6)	−30.1	45.3	−8.3	7.0	*
sensor 5	−12.0 (9.5)	−28.2	115.7	−12.8	8.3	−7.6 (7.3)	−24.9	77.2	−7.7	7.5	*
sitting											
sensor 1	12.0 (10.0)	−34.1	45.2	11.8	13.4	16.7 (10.2)	−22.3	56.1	16.2	11.4	*
sensor 2	6.0 (9.4)	−21.6	35.1	5.6	12.3	6.3 (8.5)	−16.0	43.2	5.9	9.8	
sensor 3	−0.6 (8.7)	−26.9	37.1	−0.7	10.6	−1.0 (7.1)	−25.1	35.3	−0.9	7.8	
sensor 4	−6.8 (7.4)	−32.5	32.0	−6.7	9.9	−6.9 (6.9)	−30.3	40.6	−6.6	8.2	
sensor 5	−6.9 (8.2)	−84.7	36.8	−7.3	9.1	−6.7 (5.9)	−20.5	22.0	−6.8	7.7	
hip hinging											
sensor 1	75.5 (18.1)	2.7	114.8	77.7	22.7	81.8 (14.5)	21.9	116.9	83.7	19.1	*
sensor 2	77.4 (18.8)	−9.7	121.0	80.1	22.8	79.9 (14.5)	33.1	116.3	81.0	19.8	
sensor 3	79.1 (20.1)	−16.9	128.1	81.7	23.6	75.1 (15.1)	27.7	111.4	75.7	20.4	*
sensor 4	82.1 (21.6)	−22.2	128.5	85.2	24.9	69.3 (15.1)	20.2	109.1	71.2	19.5	*
sensor 5	87.8 (22.6)	−26.3	142.0	90.7	25.3	69.1 (14.6)	9.4	111.8	70.5	17.8	*

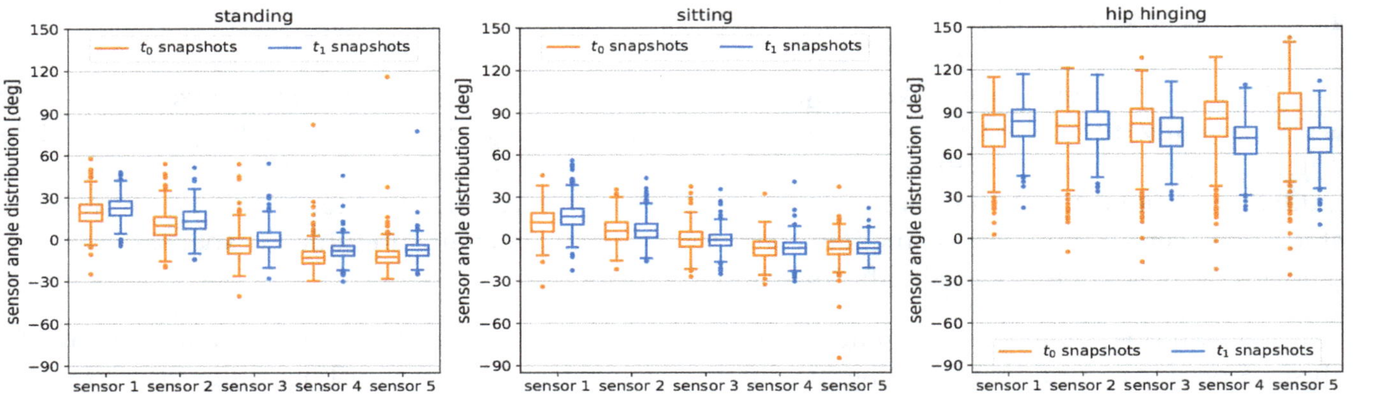

Figure 4. Boxplots of the angle distribution of the t_0 and t_1 snapshots grouped by sensor. The box frames the lower (Q_1) to upper (Q_3) quartile values of the data. The horizontal line inside each box marks the data's median. Whiskers include data between $Q_1 - 1.5$ IQR and $Q_3 + 1.5$ IQR, where IQR $= Q_3 - Q_1$ abbreviates the interquartile range. Outliers outside the whisker range are marked with dots.

4.2. Clustering under Varying t-SNE Perplexity

The t-SNE parameter *perplexity* reflects the number of neighbors expected in its distance optimization process. In their paper [34] van der Maaten and Hinton state that variation of perplexity has little influence on the performance of t-SNE. In order to assert clustering of our data is prevalently consistent under variation of perplexity, we show the results of clustering the 2D t-SNE map into four (six for hip hinging) clusters for perplexity values ranging from 25 to 40 in steps of five in Figure 5.

As Figure 5 shows, most of the time the general size of the clusters were approximately identical under variation of perplexity. This was also true for the data represented by these clusters. The only noteworthy exception is observed in *sitting* when using a perplexity value of 40, also see Figure 6a,b in comparison to Figure 6c, which is drawn using a perplexity value of 25 but is the same for 30 and 35. While the general shape of the t-SNE map superficially appears unchanged, distances between groups of data points slightly shift. The three segments of cluster 1 were pulled apart and partially moved closer to cluster 0, thus changing the split position of clusters 0 and 1 and associating about 25 data points more (less) to cluster ID 0 (1) than for lower perplexity values.

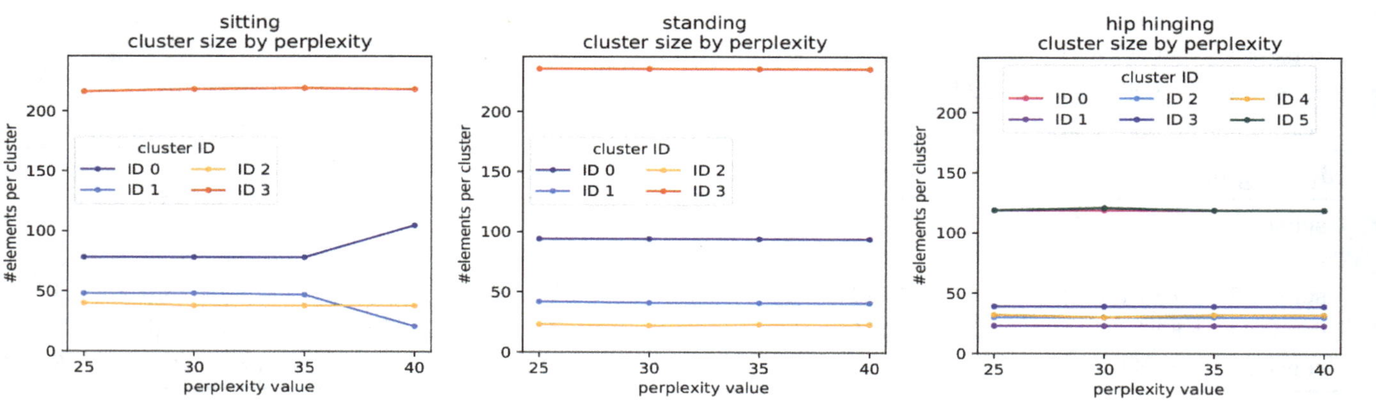

Figure 5. The number of elements per cluster under variation of the perplexity value, plotted by cluster ID.

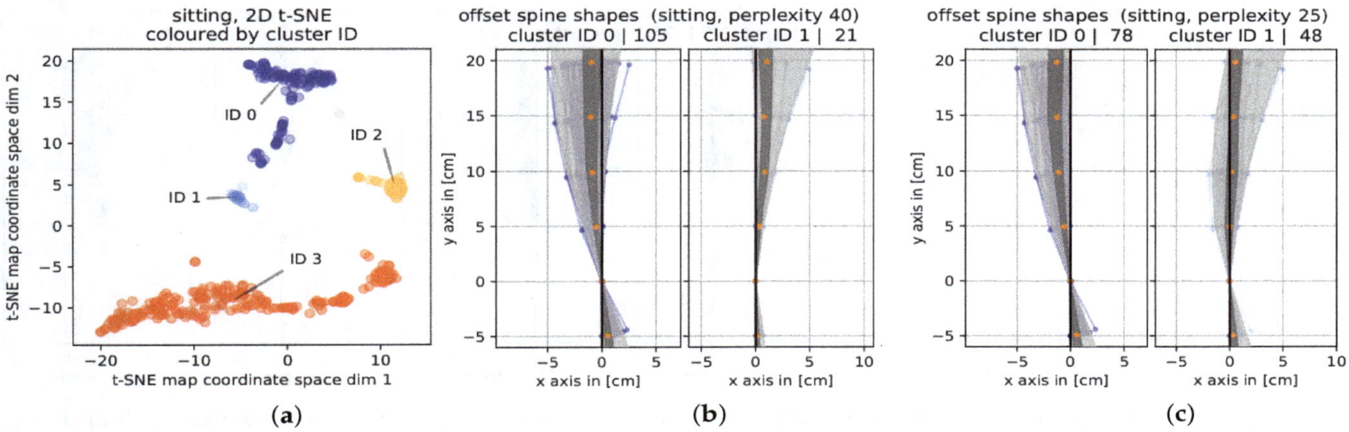

Figure 6. Visual comparison of changes in clustering when varying perplexity. (**a**) A 2D t-SNE map and (**b**) offset spine shape bundles per cluster for a perplexity value of 40. (**c**) offset spine shape bundles per cluster for a perplexity value of 25. The offset spine shape bundles displayed represent the only two clusters that changed for a perplexity value of 40. All axis titles of the offset spine shape bundles contain information of the cluster ID and the number of elements in that cluster.

Inspecting the data (offset spine shape bundles) more closely, we see that with a perplexity value of 40, almost all offset spine shapes in cluster ID 1 havd a positive x-coordinate, while this was not the case for lower perplexity values. For lower values, these two clusters are predominantly split based on the horizontal offset from zero in the base position P_0 and the topmost position P_5. The data in the other clusters remain identical throughout parameter variation.

Choice of Parameters for Cluster Analysis

Throughout the results presented in this paper we used the following parameters. The number of PCA components was chosen such that the resulting lower dimensional space still captures over 95% of the feature data variance. For the computation of the 2D t-SNE map, we fixed the cost parameter perplexity to 30, which is approximately the centre of achieving repeatedly stable results for clustering (see Figure 5). Optimization parameters of t-SNE are left to the implementation defaults [40] as these in general only affect the rate of convergence [41]. Upon initial inspection of the data, and after confirming that clusters would be stable when varying parameters in repeated computations, we set the number of clusters to four for standing and sitting and to six for hip hinging.

4.3. *Analysis of Clusters per Position*

The following three sections analyze results from clustering from a geometric point of view, assigning a geometric meaning to each cluster. The analysis is separated into the three positions: standing Section 4.3.1, sitting Section 4.3.2, and hip hinging Section 4.3.3.

4.3.1. Standing

Figure 7 illustrates the results of clustering the data from posture pairs of *standing* into four components in form of their 2D t-SNE map and in form of offset spine shape bundles. For the visualization of cluster representatives (t_0 and t_1 posture pairs and $t_1 - t_0$ offset spine shapes), please see Figure A2 in the Appendix A.

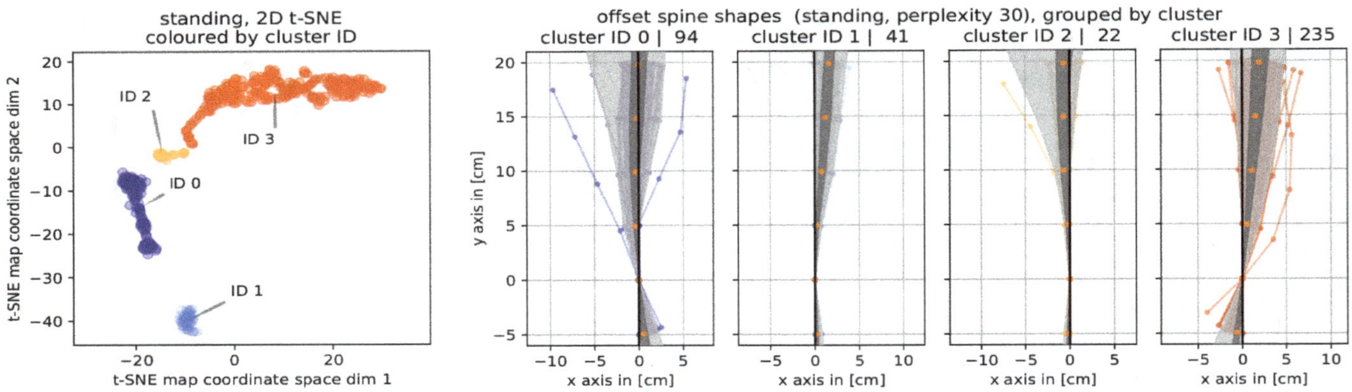

Figure 7. Results for clustering posture pairs of *standing*. **(left)** The T-SNE map labelled with and colored by cluster ID. **(right)** Corresponding cluster bundles of *offset spine shapes* including information about the cluster ID and the number of elements in that cluster in each axis title.

Geometrically, the four clusters were separated mainly based on the position of the offset spine shapes' base points and further by the orientation of the upper part. For the first and second cluster (IDs 0 and 1), the offset spine shapes all had positive base point x-coordinates while these were negative for the third and fourth cluster (IDs 2 and 3). The first and second cluster differ in the position representing the second sensor ($P_{\text{offset},2}$), for ID 0 its x-coordinate is always negative while it was always positive for ID 1). The upper part of the offset spine shape bundle of cluster ID 0 shared no particular orientation, this part is clearly leaning in positive x direction. This pattern was repeated for the third and fourth cluster (IDs 2 and 3), in which the third cluster tends to negative values and the fourth cluster leans to positive values. Again a clear geometric separation can only be seen for the offsets in $P_{\text{offset},2}$.

4.3.2. Sitting

Figure 8 shows the results of clustering the data from sitting posture pairs into four components using the 2D t-SNE map and the offset spine shape bundles per cluster. Again, we show representative spine curve shapes and offset spine curve shapes for each cluster in the Appendix A, Figure A4.

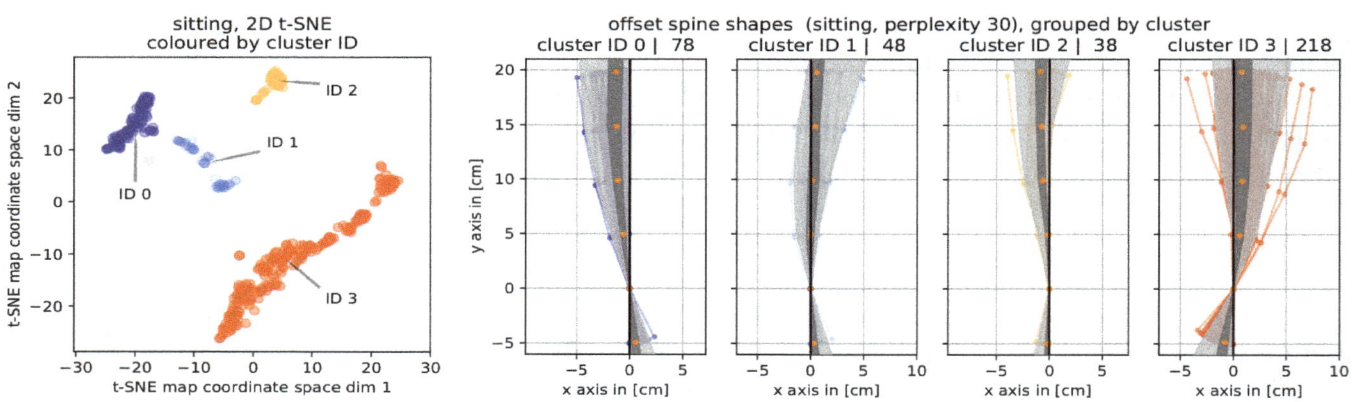

Figure 8. Results for clustering posture pairs of *sitting*. **(left)** The t-SNE map labelled with and colored by cluster ID. **(right)** Corresponding cluster bundles of *offset spine shapes* including information about the cluster ID and the number of elements in that cluster.

The geometric pattern observed in *standing* repeats for *sitting*: the four clusters are separated mainly based on the position of the offset spine shapes' base points and further by the orientation of the upper part: For the first and second cluster (IDs 0 and 1), the offset spine shapes all have positive base point x-coordinates while these are negative for the third and fourth cluster (IDs 2 and 3). The two groups can each be further separated into positive slanted clusters (IDs 1 and 3) and negative slanted clusters (IDs 0 and 2). While only sensor 1 shows a significant difference between the angular data of the unguided and guided snapshot pairs on a per sensor level (see Section 4.1 and Table 2), the combined information on all five sensors allows for a class separation into four clusters.

4.3.3. Hip Hinging

The results of clustering t_0 and t_1 posture pairs of the position hinging into six clusters are presented in Figure 9. As before, we show the 2D t-SNE map colored by cluster ID along with the corresponding offset spine shape bundles. For representative spine curves for each cluster, please refer to the Appendix A, Figure A6.

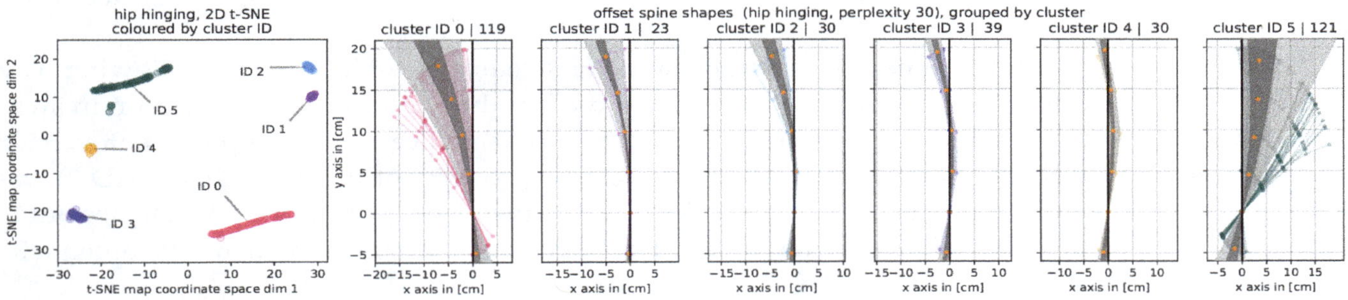

Figure 9. Results for clustering posture pairs of *hip hinging*. (**left**) The t-SNE map labelled with and colored by cluster ID. (**right**) Corresponding cluster bundles of *offset spine shapes*.

Here, the geometry of the offset spine shapes reveals a clear pattern. Again, an initial distinction between the clusters can be made based on the position of the base points. One cluster (ID 0) had only positive x-valued base points while this is purely negative for four of the five others (IDs 1–4) and almost purely negative (except for seven samples) for the last cluster (ID 5). In the upper part, all samples in the first cluster (ID 0) more or less strongly slanted to the left, all upper offset spine shape points having a negative x-coordinate. This was also the case for the upper part of the second cluster (ID 1). For the subsequent clusters (IDs 2–5) the position at which the offset spine shapes of that cluster cross the thought vertical line passing through $x = 0$ moved stepwise up. For cluster ID 1 there was no crossing. In cluster ID 1, the offset spine shapes cross that line between $P_{\text{offset},2}$ and $P_{\text{offset},3}$, i.e., the x-coordinate of all $P_{\text{offset},2}$ is > 0 and it is < 0 for all $P_{\text{offset},k}$, $k \in \{3, 4, 5\}$. For the next cluster (ID 2), the crossing is between $P_{\text{offset},3}$ and $P_{\text{offset},4}$. This progression continues up to the last cluster (ID 5) in which there is no crossing in the observed area, meaning that all offset spine curves slant in positive direction ($x > 0$ for $P_{\text{offset},k}$, $k \in \{2, 3, 4, 5\}$). These properties defines the separation of clusters with IDs 1–5.

5. Discussion

This section shortly summarizes results (Sections 5.1 and 5.2), puts this work in context with existing research (Section 5.3), and lists limitations in Section 5.4.

5.1. Summary of Results

For all three positions, sitting, standing, hip hinging, we found a significant change in posture between the sets of guided and unguided snapshot pairs. We used a Wilcoxon signed-rank test on the sensor angle data representation of the posture pairs. This results indicated that is is plausible to further analyze posture pairs in our data base with respect to postural change.

We confirmed that our clusters remain stable under variation of the t-SNE parameter perplexity.

In the geometric analysis of the clusters for each position, it turned out that clusters formed based on the position of offset spine shapes, the base points, and the direction of the upper part. This underlines the necessity of a multi-sensor system to achieve a meaningful separation into different clusters. The separation of the upper part was more fine-grained as there are six clusters for hip hinging.

Showing several samples per cluster to a professional posture trainer, the samples and clusters, that are based on our geometric feature, had a meaning for her. Her assessments are summarized in the following section.

5.2. Sample-Based Evaluation per Cluster by a Professional Posture Trainer

Several samples of unguided and guided posture pairs per cluster were shown to a professional posture teacher. She has experience in comparing such posture pairs and is able to understand how the change in posture within such a posture pair affects the shape of the spine as well as posture in general. This information is important to give semantic meaning to our clusters which formed based on geometric features.

A professional posture trainer interprets clusters for *standing* (see Figure 7) the following way: Cluster ID 0 represents a loss of pelvic anteversion and often (but not always) a reduction in sway. The second cluster (ID 1) stands for a group of users who have sacrificed a little in pelvic anteversion and very much straightened out a sway. The most notable property of the third cluster (ID 2) was a high reduction of sway. The second property which this cluster shares with the last cluster but to a smaller degree is an increased pelvic anteversion. The last cluster cluster could not be attributed with a definitive property describing the changes in the upper part.

From the perspective of a professional posture trainer, in *sitting* (see Figure 8), cluster ID 0 represents cases that have less curvature in the upper lumbar area and (possibly due to having reduced that curvature) reduced pelvic anteversion. The second cluster (ID 1) stands for sacrificing (a little) pelvic anteversion and straightening out a sway. Both remaining clusters (IDs 2 and 3) exhibit an increase in pelvic anteversion. Only cluster ID 2 could clearly be associated with a reduced sway while for the fourth cluster (ID 3) there was no clear attribution to a consistent change in posture valid throughout the cluster.

The posture trainer's assessments of the clustering for *hip hinging* (see Figure 9) was this: Cluster ID 0 in the guided t_1 snapshots did not go as far with the pelvis as in the unguided t_0 snapshot and learned to stop rounding the upper part of the back in order to reach deeper. People in cluster ID 1 go further down in t_1 than in t_0 or as deep as in t_0 in the lowest part of the pelvis and also stopped rounding the upper back. The next cluster (ID 2) represents students who stopped rounding in the upper lumbar area and who have increased their pelvic anteversion. Cluster four (ID 3) is a group with more anteversion in the pelvis and a straighter upper back. This general pattern repeats for cluster ID 4: rounding in t_0, not rounded any more in the t_1 snapshot and slightly more pelvic anteversion. In the last cluster (ID 5) the posture trainer sees students who use a sway to overcome their inability to tip their pelvis (alone), thus their pelvic tip increases but so does their sway.

5.3. Relation to Existing Research

Previous work on spine shape analysis has for a long time been majorly interesting in medicine. There, analysis is mainly driven by pathology quantification, by relation investigation, or by evaluation of a new technology. Pathology quantification (e.g., Hay et al. [10], 24 participants) is often tightly tied to a definition of a 'normal' spine shape, determining and assessing a given spine shape by its deviation from the 'normal' one. Relation driven investigations give answer to questions like *is there a relation between weight groups (normal, obese) and differences in spinal curvatures?* ([14], 39 participants), or *is there a relation of back pain and changes in spine curvature during pregnancy?* ([13], twelve participants), or *is upper back pain related to the amount of postural change in young computer users?* ([11], 153 participants). Relation driven questions are tested for significance and hypothesis confirmation using statistical tests, e.g., ANOVA, Student's t-test, or Wilcoxon's test.

Wearables have become an increasingly promising tool for posture monitoring and analysis. Posture change comparisons here are also often based on a 'neutral' or 'normal ' position: In an evaluation study, Wong and Wong [42] (three participants, three repetitions of each position) use accelerometers to measure postural change in terms of curvature variation from a *neutral sitting* position for three pre-defined modifications: sitting with left (right) lateral bending, and sitting while flexing forward. They computed curvature variation with respect to *neutral sitting*.

Without the notion of a 'normal' state for spine shape or posture and without pre-defined groups to put into relation to one another, we invert the process described above: Based on a database of spine shapes of unguided and guided posture pairs, we cluster changes in spinal shape. Clusters form based on the geometry of the change and represent a semantically meaningful separation of the data according to the assessment of a professional posture trainer.

5.4. Limitations

Our database did not have information on gender, age, height, or weight of the users. Therefore, we could not separate our analysis based on such criteria. However, these factors can have a considerable impact on the shape of the spine: Nachemson et al. [43] reported a minor tendency for the influence of age on increased stiffness of intervertebral discs. The authors also found that in bending, female motion segments are more flexible than male. According to Hay et al. [10], the BMI, which is based on weight and height, is related to thoracic sagittal kyophosis. Youdas et al. [44] found an association between BMI and pelvic inclination.

Another limitation of our presented work is the choice of the number of clusters. These were mainly based on observations in the 2D t-SNE map. Especially in light of the posture trainer's evaluation of the clusters, it is easily seen that the number of clusters suggested by the geometry does not necessarily reflect the number of clusters found by the posture trainer. Therefore it would be highly beneficial to include several posture trainer's knowledge on patterns in change into the clustering approach and maybe even into feature design.

We showed several samples per cluster to only one professional posture trainer for postural change evaluation. As this work aimed at describing a general methodology for analysis of changes in spine shape, we did not do a blind-test cross-validation with several posture trainers, removing any information relating a sample to a cluster and have several posture trainers assess the samples. However, this would make the evaluation of the postural change in the clusters independent and improve the reliability of the clusters that formed based on geometric features and the trainers' assessments.

6. Conclusions and Future Work

This work aimed at analyzing the change of the spinal shape under posture training in three different positions: sitting, standing, and hip hinging. In particular, it compared snapshots of an unguided-guided posture pair based on features computed from the 2D spine curve geometry. Clustering was used to group posture changes with common geometric characteristics. The results from clustering our spine-shape-geometry inspired features could be identified with specific changes in posture by a professional posture trainer. Our large data base consists of real-world spine curves of over 350 single-user posture pairs and is pathology-unrelated. Our analysis is independent from a definition of a global *normal* spine shape. Instead, it is a highly individual process based on each individual's spine shape before and after posture training. This makes the successful separation of change in spinal shape into geometrically and semantically meaningful clusters (second contribution stated in the introduction, see Section 1) both interesting and important. We believe that this is the first work in the field of wearable-sensor-based evaluation of spine curves that analyzes this many distinct data points based on geometric features without relying on the definition of a *normal* spine shape.

Future work includes blind-test cross-validation of multiple sample posture pairs per clusters by several posture trainers as well as a more detailed grouping of our data based on additional information about e.g., age and gender. Further research could also include comparison against pain ratings using standard questionnaires, e.g., the low back pain specific Roland Morris questionnaire, or targeting general health status measurement SF12 and SF36, and eventually associate pain levels or changes therein with certain groups of posture change.

Furthermore it will be interesting to integrate feedback based on common features in spinal shape change, represented by clusters, into posture training. This could e.g., be implemented by also categorising posture training exercises based on a student's progress and suggest exercises tailored to their group of shape change. Moving partially away from clustering postural change towards analysis of spinal shape change of an individual user could provide them with helpful instant feedback on which region they need improvement on and how to get there. This also could be realized using e.g., an exercise specifically designed to improve the identified region. It would need a previously taken guided snapshot to compare the current user snapshot to.

Author Contributions: conceptualization, B.K., K.S., J.M., A.H.; methodology, K.S., B.K.; software, K.S.; validation, K.S., B.K., J.M., A.H.; formal analysis, K.S.; resources, A.H., B.K., J.M.; data curation, K.S., B.K.; writing—original draft preparation, K.S., B.K.; writing—review and editing, J.M., K.S., B.K., A.H.; visualization, K.S.; supervision, B.K.; all authors critically revised the manuscript and approved the content of the submission.

Acknowledgments: We would like to extend our sincere thanks to Esther Gokhale who has gone through and assessed all posture samples we showed to her.

Appendix A. Sample Spine Curve of Posture Pairs per Cluster

On the following pages, we will show representative spine curve posture pairs for each cluster. For better overview and localization of presented sample (cluster representative), we re-plot the t-SNE map and corresponding cluster bundles from the results. Each cluster in the t-SNE maps is additionally annotated with the location of the cluster representatives. Figures A1 and A2 draw the results of clustering and sample posture pairs for *standing*. Clusters and representatives for the position *sitting* are displayed in Figures A3 and A4. Finally, Figures A5 and A6 depict clusters and cluster representatives for *hip hinging*.

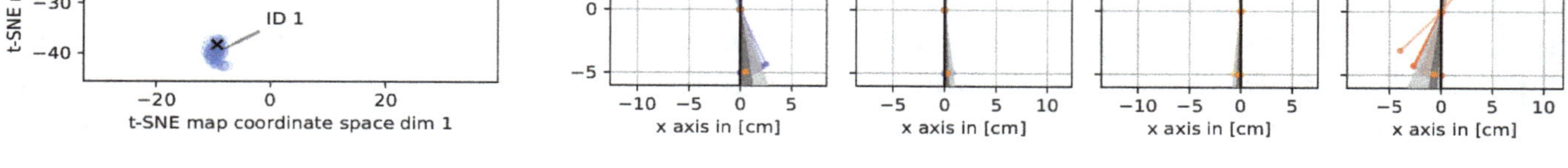

Figure A1. Results for clustering posture pairs of *standing*. (**left**) The t-SNE map labelled with and colored by cluster ID. An 'x' marks the position of a cluster representative. (**right**) Corresponding cluster bundles of *offset spine shapes*.

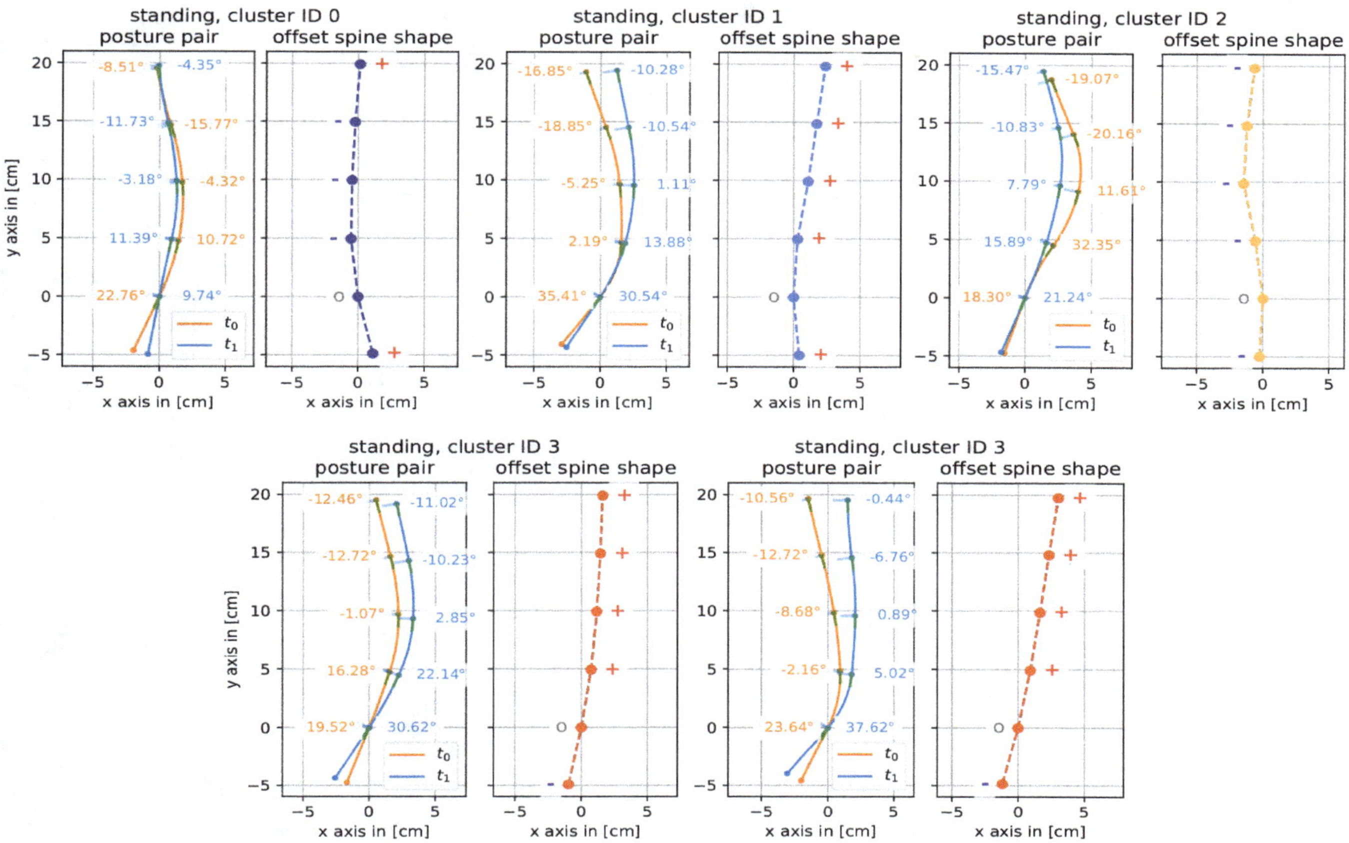

Figure A2. Results for clustering posture pairs of *sitting*: Cluster representative sample posture pairs and offset spine shapes for each cluster. Each sample's position within its cluster is marked by an 'x' in the colored t-SNE map.

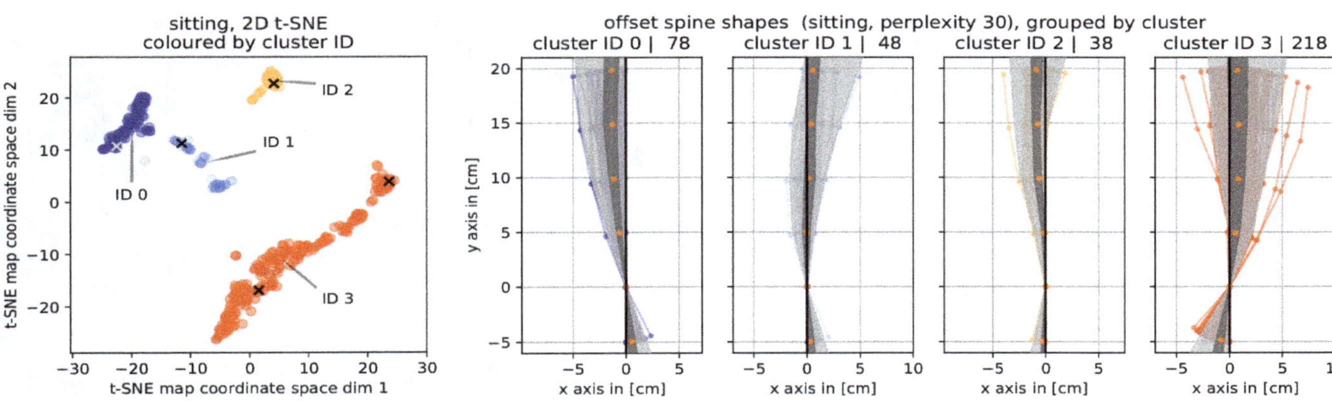

Figure A3. Results for clustering posture pairs of *sitting*. (**left**) The t-SNE map colored by cluster ID. An 'x' marks the position of a cluster representative. (**right**) Corresponding cluster bundles of *offset spine shapes*.

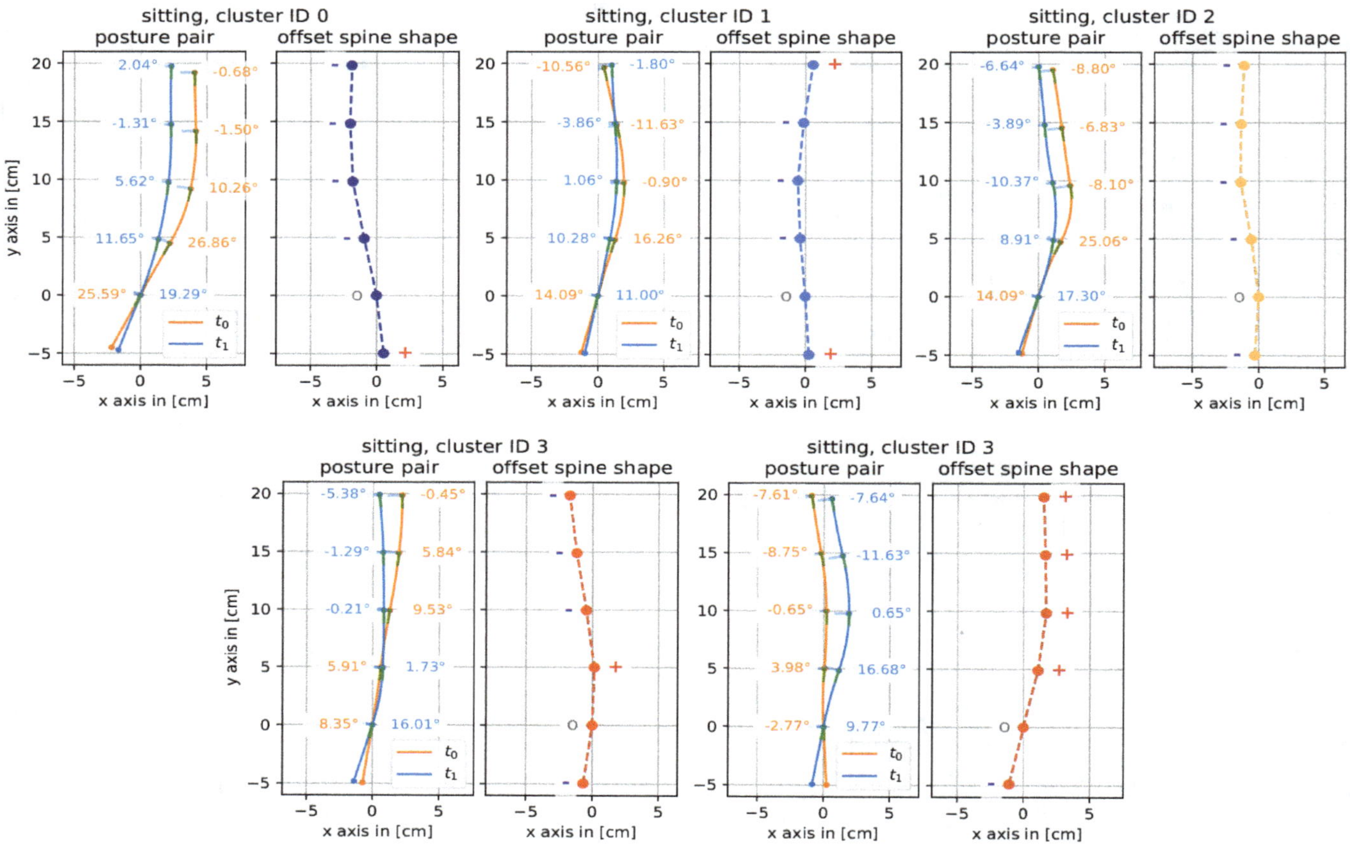

Figure A4. Results for clustering posture pairs of *sitting*: Cluster representative sample posture pairs and offset spine shapes for each cluster. Each sample's position within its cluster is marked by an 'x' in the colored t-SNE map.

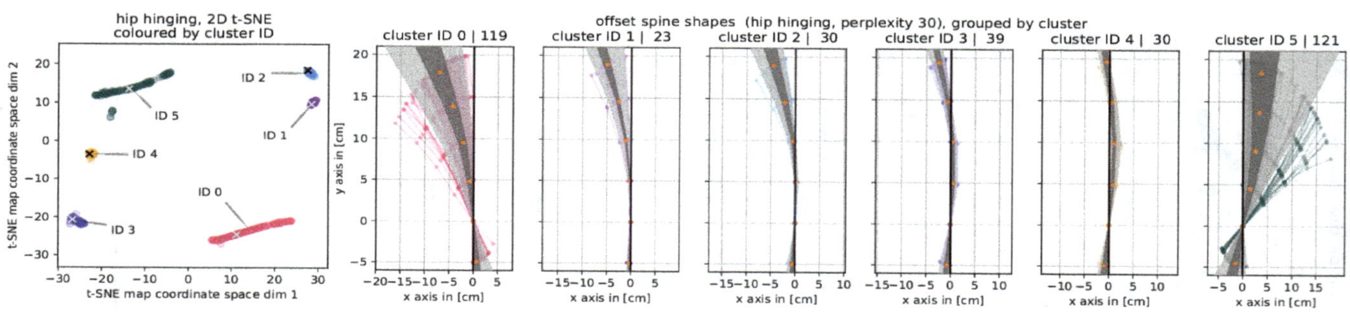

Figure A5. Results for clustering posture pairs of *hip hinging*. (**left**) The t-SNE map colored by cluster ID. An 'x' marks the position of a cluster representative. (**right**) Corresponding cluster bundles of *offset spine shapes*.

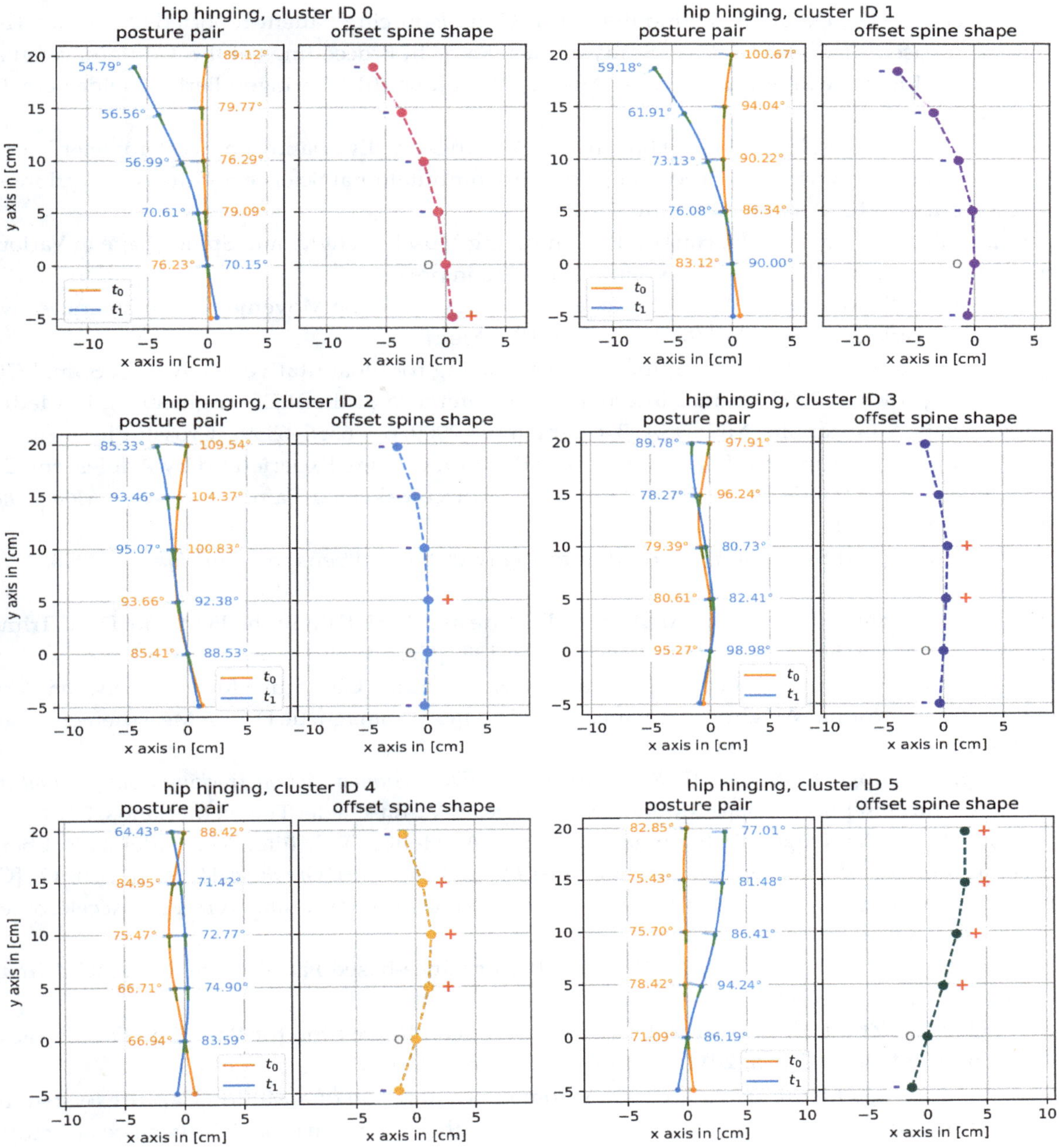

Figure A6. Results for clustering posture pairs of *hip hinging*. Cluster representative sample posture pairs and offset spine shapes for each cluster. Each sample's position within its cluster is marked by an 'x' in the colored t-SNE map. The two posture snapshots are additionally rotated about the origin such that the topmost sensor of the unguided t_0 snapshot lies on the y-axis.

References

1. Manchikanti, L.; Singh, V.; Falco, F.J.E.; Benyamin, R.M.; Hirsch, J.A. Epidemiology of Low Back Pain in Adults. *Neuromodul. Technol. Neural Interface* **2014**, *17*, 3–10. [CrossRef] [PubMed]
2. Hoy, D.; March, L.; Brooks, P.; Blyth, F.; Woolf, A.; Bain, C.; Williams, G.; Smith, E.; Vos, T.; Barendregt, J.; et al. The Global Burden of Low Back Pain: Estimates From the Global Burden of Disease 2010 Study. *Ann. Rheum. Dis.* **2014**, *73*, 968–974. [CrossRef] [PubMed]
3. Nelson, R.J. The Rape of the Spine. *Spine J.* **2015**, *15*, S11–S12. [CrossRef] [PubMed]
4. Rubin, D.I. Epidemiology and Risk Factors for Spine Pain. *Neurol. Clin.* **2007**, *25*, 353–371. [CrossRef] [PubMed]
5. Gaskin, D.J.; Richard, P. The Economic Costs of Pain in the United States. *J. Pain* **2012**, *13*, 715–724. [CrossRef] [PubMed]

6. Peleg, M.; Leung, T.I.; Desai, M.; Dumontier, M. Is Crowdsourcing Patient-reported Outcomes The Future of Evidence-based Medicine? A Case Study of Back Pain. In Proceedings of the Conference on Artificial Intelligence in Medicine in Europe, Vienna, Austria, 21–24 June 2017; Springer: Berlin/Heidelberg, Germany, pp. 245–255.
7. Stollenwerk, K.; Müllers, J.; Müller, J.; Hinkenjann, A.; Krüger, B. Evaluating an Accelerometer-based System for Spine Shape Monitoring. In Proceedings of the Computational Science and Its Applications—ICCSA 2018, Melbourne, VIC, Australia, 2–5 July 2018.
8. Peper, E.; Krüger, B.; Gokhale, E.; Harvey, R. Comparing Muscle Activity and Spine Shape in Various Sitting Styles. In *Biofeedback*; Allen Press: Lawrence, KS, USA, in press.
9. Papi, E.; Koh, W.S.; McGregor, A.H. Wearable Technology for Spine Movement Assessment: A Systematic Review. *J. Biomech.* **2017**, *64*, 186–197. [CrossRef] [PubMed]
10. Hay, O.; Hershkovitz, I.; Rivlin, E. Spine Curve Modeling for Quantitative Analysis of Spinal Curvature. In Proceedings of the 2009 Annual International Conference of the IEEE Engineering in Medicine and Biology Society, Minneapolis, MN, USA, 3–6 September 2009; pp. 6356–6359. [CrossRef]
11. Brink, Y.; Louw, Q.; Grimmer, K. The Amount of Postural Change Experienced by Adolescent Computer Users Developing Seated-related Upper Quadrant Musculoskeletal Pain. *J. Bodyw. Mov. Ther.* **2018**, *22*, 608–617. [CrossRef]
12. Wong, W.Y.; Wong, M.S. Trunk Posture Monitoring with Inertial Sensors. *Eur. Spine J.* **2008**, *17*, 743–753. [CrossRef]
13. Franklin, M.E.; Conner-Kerr, T. An Analysis of Posture and Back Pain in the First and Third Trimesters of Pregnancy. *J. Orthop. Sport. Phys. Ther.* **1998**, *28*, 133–138. [CrossRef]
14. González-Sánchez, M.; Luo, J.; Lee, R.; Cuesta-Vargas, A.I. Spine Curvature Analysis between Participants with Obesity and Normal Weight Participants: A Biplanar Electromagnetic Device Measurement. *Biomed. Res. Int.* **2014**, *2014*, 935151. [CrossRef]
15. Roetenberg, D.; Luinge, H.; Slycke, P. *Xsens MVN: Full 6DOF Human Motion Tracking Using Miniature Inertial Sensors*; Technical Report 1; Xsens Motion Technologies B.V.: Enschede, The Netherlands, 2013.
16. Tautges, J.; Zinke, A.; Krüger, B.; Baumann, J.; Weber, A.; Helten, T.; Müller, M.; Seidel, H.P.; Eberhardt, B. Motion Reconstruction using Sparse Accelerometer Data. *ACM Trans. Graph.* **2011**, *30*, 18:1–18:12. [CrossRef]
17. Riaz, Q.; Guanhong, T.; Krüger, B.; Weber, A. Motion Reconstruction Using Very Few Accelerometers and Ground Contacts. *Graph. Model.* **2015**. [CrossRef]
18. Weise, T.; Bouaziz, S.; Li, H.; Pauly, M. Realtime Performance-based Facial Animation. *ACM Trans. Graph.* **2011**, *30*, 77:1–77:10. [CrossRef]
19. Cao, C.; Hou, Q.; Zhou, K. Displaced Dynamic Expression Regression for Real-time Facial Tracking and Animation. *ACM Trans. Graph.* **2014**, *33*, 43:1–43:10. [CrossRef]
20. Hoffmann, J.; Brüggemann, B.; Krüger, B. Automatic Calibration of a Motion Capture System based on Inertial Sensors for Tele-Manipulation. In Proceedings of the 7th International Conference on Informatics in Control, Automation and Robotics (ICINCO), Funchal, Portugal, 15–18 June 2010.
21. Ma, C.Z.H.; Ling, Y.T.; Shea, Q.T.K.; Wang, L.K.; Wang, X.Y.; Zheng, Y.P. Towards Wearable Comprehensive Capture and Analysis of Skeletal Muscle Activity during Human Locomotion. *Sensors* **2019**, *19*, 195. [CrossRef]
22. Zhao, W.; Chai, J.; Xu, Y.Q. Combining Marker-based Mocap and RGB-D Camera for Acquiring High-fidelity Hand Motion Data. In Proceedings of the ACM SIGGRAPH/Eurographics Symposium on Computer Animation, Lausanne, Switzerland, 29–31 July 2012; pp. 33–42.
23. Stollenwerk, K.; Vögele, A.; Krüger, B.; Hinkenjann, A.; Klein, R. Automatic Temporal Segmentation of Articulated Hand Motion. In Proceedings of the Computational Science and Its Applications—ICCSA 2016: 16th International Conference, Beijing, China, 4–7 July 2016; Part II; Springer International Publishing: Berlin/Heidelberg, Germany, 2016; pp. 433–449. [CrossRef]
24. Drerup, B.; Hierholzer, E. Automatic Localization of Anatomical Landmarks on the Back Surface and Construction of a Body-fixed coordinate System. *J. Biomech.* **1987**, *20*, 961–970. [CrossRef]
25. Betsch, M.; Wild, M.; Johnstone, B.; Jungbluth, P.; Hakimi, M.; Kühlmann, B.; Rapp, W. Evaluation of a Novel Spine and Surface Topography System for Dynamic Spinal Curvature Analysis during Gait. *PLoS ONE* **2013**, *8*, e70581. [CrossRef]

26. Poredoš, P.; Čelan, D.; Možina, J.; Jezeršek, M. Determination of the Human Spine Curve Based on Laser Triangulation. *BMC Med. Imaging* **2015**, *15*, 2. [CrossRef]
27. Williams, J.M.; Haq, I.; Lee, R.Y. Dynamic Measurement of Lumbar Curvature Using Fibre-optic Sensors. *Med. Eng. Phys.* **2010**, *32*, 1043–1049. [CrossRef]
28. Consmüller, T.; Rohlmann, A.; Weinland, D.; Druschel, C.; Duda, G.N.; Taylor, W.R. Comparative Evaluation of a Novel Measurement Tool to Assess Lumbar Spine Posture and Range of Motion. *Eur. Spine J.* **2012**, *21*, 2170–2180. [CrossRef]
29. Cajamarca, G.; Rodríguez, I.; Herskovic, V.; Campos, M.; Riofrío, J.C. StraightenUp+: Monitoring of Posture during Daily Activities for Older Persons Using Wearable Sensors. *Sensors* **2018**, *18*, 3409. [CrossRef] [PubMed]
30. Voinea, G.D.; Butnariu, S.; Mogan, G. Measurement and Geometric Modelling of Human Spine Posture for Medical Rehabilitation Purposes Using a Wearable Monitoring System Based on Inertial Sensors. *Sensors* **2017**, *17*, 3. [CrossRef] [PubMed]
31. Gray, H.; Williams, P.L.; Bannister, L.H. Chapter 6: Skeletal System–Vertebral Column, Ribs, Thorax, Skull. In *Gray's Anatomy*, 38th ed.; Churchill Livingstone: New York, NY, USA, 1995.
32. Wilcoxon, F. Individual Comparisons of Grouped Data by Ranking Methods. *J. Econ. Entomol.* **1946**, *39*, 269–270. [CrossRef] [PubMed]
33. Hotelling, H. Analysis of a Complex of Statistical Variables into Principal Components. *J. Educ. Psychol.* **1933**, *24*, 417–441. [CrossRef]
34. Van der Maaten, L.; Hinton, G. Visualizing Data Using t-SNE. *J. Mach. Learn. Res.* **2008**, *9*, 2579–2605.
35. Kullback, S.; Leibler, R.A. On Information and Sufficiency. *Ann. Math. Stat.* **1951**, *22*, 79–86. [CrossRef]
36. Shapiro, S.S.; Wilk, M.B. An Analysis of Variance Test for Normality (Complete Samples). *Biometrika* **1965**, *52*, 591–611. [CrossRef]
37. Stephens, M.A. EDF Statistics for Goodness of Fit and Some Comparisons. *J. Am. Stat. Assoc.* **1974**, *69*, 730–737. [CrossRef]
38. Wilk, M.B.; Gnanadesikan, R. Probability Plotting Methods for the Analysis of Data. *Biometrika* **1968**, *55*, 1–17. [CrossRef]
39. Wilcoxon, F. Individual Comparisons by Ranking Methods. *Biom. Bull.* **1945**, *1*, 80–83. [CrossRef]
40. Pedregosa, F.; Varoquaux, G.; Gramfort, A.; Michel, V.; Thirion, B.; Grisel, O.; Blondel, M.; Prettenhofer, P.; Weiss, R.; Dubourg, V.; et al. Scikit-learn: Machine Learning in Python. *J. Mach. Learn. Res.* **2011**, *12*, 2825–2830.
41. Van der Maaten, L.; Hinton, G. Visualizing Non-metric Similarities in Multiple Maps. *Mach. Learn.* **2012**, *87*, 33–55. [CrossRef]
42. Wong, W.Y.; Wong, M.S. Detecting Spinal Posture Change in Sitting Positions with Tri-axial Accelerometers. *Gait Posture* **2008**, *27*, 168–171. [CrossRef]
43. Nachemson, A.L.; Schultz, A.B.; Berkson, M.H. Mechanical Properties of Human Lumbar Spine Motion Segments: Influences of Age, Sex, Disc Level, and Degeneration. *Spine* **1979**, *4*, 1–8. [CrossRef]
44. Youdas, J.W.; Garrett, T.R.; EganMayo, K.S.; Therneau, T.M. Lumbar Lordosis and Pelvic Inclination in Adults with Chronic Low Back Pain. *Phys. Ther.* **2000**. [CrossRef]

Permissions

All chapters in this book were first published by MDPI; hereby published with permission under the Creative Commons Attribution License or equivalent. Every chapter published in this book has been scrutinized by our experts. Their significance has been extensively debated. The topics covered herein carry significant findings which will fuel the growth of the discipline. They may even be implemented as practical applications or may be referred to as a beginning point for another development.

The contributors of this book come from diverse backgrounds, making this book a truly international effort. This book will bring forth new frontiers with its revolutionizing research information and detailed analysis of the nascent developments around the world.

We would like to thank all the contributing authors for lending their expertise to make the book truly unique. They have played a crucial role in the development of this book. Without their invaluable contributions this book wouldn't have been possible. They have made vital efforts to compile up to date information on the varied aspects of this subject to make this book a valuable addition to the collection of many professionals and students.

This book was conceptualized with the vision of imparting up-to-date information and advanced data in this field. To ensure the same, a matchless editorial board was set up. Every individual on the board went through rigorous rounds of assessment to prove their worth. After which they invested a large part of their time researching and compiling the most relevant data for our readers.

The editorial board has been involved in producing this book since its inception. They have spent rigorous hours researching and exploring the diverse topics which have resulted in the successful publishing of this book. They have passed on their knowledge of decades through this book. To expedite this challenging task, the publisher supported the team at every step. A small team of assistant editors was also appointed to further simplify the editing procedure and attain best results for the readers.

Apart from the editorial board, the designing team has also invested a significant amount of their time in understanding the subject and creating the most relevant covers. They scrutinized every image to scout for the most suitable representation of the subject and create an appropriate cover for the book.

The publishing team has been an ardent support to the editorial, designing and production team. Their endless efforts to recruit the best for this project, has resulted in the accomplishment of this book. They are a veteran in the field of academics and their pool of knowledge is as vast as their experience in printing. Their expertise and guidance has proved useful at every step. Their uncompromising quality standards have made this book an exceptional effort. Their encouragement from time to time has been an inspiration for everyone.

The publisher and the editorial board hope that this book will prove to be a valuable piece of knowledge for researchers, students, practitioners and scholars across the globe.

List of Contributors

Xiaochen Zhang, Hui Zhang and Fei Hu
Department of Industrial Design, Guangdong University of Technology, Guangzhou 510006, China

Linyue Zhang
School of Communication and Design, Sun Yat-Sen University, Guangzhou 510275, China

Yi Zhu
Department of Industrial Design, Guangdong University of Technology, Guangzhou 510006, China
School of Industrial Design, Georgia Institute of Technology, Atlanta, GA 30332, USA

Ke Lu
School of Engineering Sciences in Chemistry, Biotechnology and Health, KTH Royal Institute of Technology, Hälsovägen 11C, 141 57 Huddinge, Sweden

Liyun Yang, Farhad Abtahi and Mikael Forsman
School of Engineering Sciences in Chemistry, Biotechnology and Health, KTH Royal Institute of Technology, Hälsovägen 11C, 141 57 Huddinge, Sweden
Institute of Environmental Medicine, Karolinska Institutet, Solnavägen 1, 171 77 Solna, Sweden

Kaj Lindecrantz
Institute of Environmental Medicine, Karolinska Institutet, Solnavägen 1, 171 77 Solna, Sweden
Swedish School of Textiles, University of Borås, Allégatan 1, 501 90 Borås, Sweden

Fernando Seoane
Department of Clinical Science, Intervention and Technology, Karolinska Institutet, Hälsovägen 7, 141 57 Huddinge, Sweden
Swedish School of Textiles, University of Borås, Allégatan 1, 501 90 Borås, Sweden
Department of Biomedical Engineering, Karolinska University Hospital, 1, 171 76 Solna, Sweden

Shuai Yu
School of Mechanical Science and Engineering, Huazhong University of Science and Technology, 1037 Luoyu Road, Wuhan 430074, China

Sheng Liu
School of Mechanical Science and Engineering, Huazhong University of Science and Technology, 1037 Luoyu Road, Wuhan 430074, China
Key Lab for Hydropower Transients of Ministry of Education, School of Power and Mechanical Engineering, Wuhan University, 8 East Lake South Road, Wuhan 430072, China
Institute of Technological Sciences, Wuhan University, 8 East Lake South Road, Wuhan 430072, China

Andreas Ejupi and Carlo Menon
Menrva Research Group, Schools of Mechatronic Systems & Engineering Science at Simon Fraser University (SFU), Burnaby, BC V5A 1S6, Canada

Ambra Cesareo, Ylenia Previtali and Andrea Aliverti
Dipartimento di Elettronica, Informazione e Bioingegneria, Politecnico di Milano, 20133 Milan, Italy

Emilia Biffi
Scientific Institute, IRCCS E. Medea, Bioengineering Lab, 23842 Bosisio Parini, Lecco, Italy

Woo Hyung Lee
Department of Biomedical Engineering, Seoul National University College of Medicine, Seoul 03080, Korea

Hyung Seok Nam
Department of Biomedical Engineering, Seoul National University College of Medicine, Seoul 03080, Korea
Department of Rehabilitation Medicine, Seoul National University Hospital, Seoul 03080, Korea

Han Gil Seo
Department of Rehabilitation Medicine, Seoul National University Hospital, Seoul 03080, Korea

Yoon Jae Kim
Interdisciplinary Program for Bioengineering, Seoul National University Graduate School, Seoul 08826, Korea

Moon Suk Bang
Department of Rehabilitation Medicine, Seoul National University Hospital, Seoul 03080, Korea
Department of Rehabilitation Medicine, Seoul National University College of Medicine, Seoul 03080, Korea

Sungwan Kim
Department of Biomedical Engineering, Seoul National University College of Medicine, Seoul 03080, Korea
Institute of Medical and Biological Engineering, Seoul National University, Seoul 03080, Korea

Wei Zhang, Anisoara Paraschiv-Ionescu and Kamiar Aminian
Laboratory of Movement Analysis and Measurement, Ecole Polytechnique Federale de Lausanne, 1015 Lausanne, Switzerland

A. Stefanie Mikolaizak
Robert Bosch Foundation for Medical Research, 70376 Stuttgart, Germany

Michael Schwenk
Robert Bosch Foundation for Medical Research, 70376 Stuttgart, Germany
Network Aging Research, Heidelberg University, 69115 Heidelberg, Germany

Sabato Mellone
Department of Electrical, Electronic and Information Engineering, University of Bologna, 40136 Bologna, Italy

Beatrix Vereijken, Jorunn Helbostad and Kristin Taraldsen
Department of Neuromedicine and Movement Science, Norwegian University of Science and Technology, 7491 Trondheim, Norway

Mirjam Pijnappels and Nini H. Jonkman
Department of Human Movement Sciences, Vrije Universiteit Amsterdam, Amsterdam Movement Sciences, 1081BT Amsterdam, The Netherlands

Elisabeth Boulton
School of Health Sciences, Faculty of Medicine, Biology and Health, University of Manchester, and Manchester Academic Health Science Centre, Manchester M13 9PL, UK

Andrea B. Maier
Department of Human Movement Sciences, Vrije Universiteit Amsterdam, Amsterdam Movement Sciences, 1081BT Amsterdam, The Netherlands
Department of Medicine and Aged Care, @ AgeMelbourne, Royal Melbourne Hospital, University of Melbourne, Melbourne 3050, Australia

Jochen Klenk
Robert Bosch Foundation for Medical Research, 70376 Stuttgart, Germany
Institute of Epidemiology and Medical Biometry, Ulm University, 89081 Ulm, Germany

Chien-Chin Hsu
Department of Emergency Medicine, Chi Mei Medical Center, Tainan 710, Taiwan
Department of Biotechnology, Southern Taiwan University of Science and Technology, Tainan 71005, Taiwan

Bor-Shing Lin
Department of Computer Science and Information Engineering, National Taipei University, New Taipei 23741, Taiwan

Ke-Yi He and Bor-Shyh Lin
Institute of Imaging and Biomedical Photonics, National Chiao Tung University, Tainan 711, Taiwan

Ying Kuen Cheung
Department of Biostatistics, Mailman School of Public Health, Columbia University, New York, NY 10032, USA

Pei-Yun Sabrina Hsueh
IBM Watson Research Center, Yorktown Heights, NY 10598, USA

Ipek Ensari and Keith M. Diaz
Center for Behavioral Cardiovascular Health, Department of Medicine, Columbia University Medical Center, New York, NY 10032, USA

Joshua Z. Willey
Department of Neurology, Columbia University Medical Center, New York, NY 10032, USA

Alexis Fortin-Côté and Philip Jackson
Center for Interdisciplinary Research in Rehabilitation and Social Integration, Quebec City, QC G1M 2S8, Canada
School of Psychology, Université Laval, Quebec City, QC G1V 0A6, Canada

Jean-Sébastien Roy and Laurent Bouyer
Center for Interdisciplinary Research in Rehabilitation and Social Integration, Quebec City, QC G1M 2S8, Canada
Department of Rehabilitation, Université Laval, Quebec City, QC G1V 0A6, Canada

Alexandre Campeau-Lecours
Center for Interdisciplinary Research in Rehabilitation and Social Integration, Quebec City, QC G1M 2S8, Canada
Department of Mechanical Engineering, Université Laval, Quebec City, QC G1V 0A6, Canada

Robert W. Broadley, Jochen Klenk, Sibylle B. Thies, Laurence P. J. Kenney and Malcolm H. Granat
School of Health Sciences, University of Salford, Salford, M6 6PU, UK
Department of Clinical Gerontology, Robert-Bosch-Hospital, 70376 Stuttgart, Germany
Institute of Epidemiology and Medical Biometry, Ulm University, 89081 Ulm, Germany

Stefanie Passler, Niklas Müller and Veit Senner
Technical University of Munich, Department of Mechanical Engineering, Professorship of Sport Equipment and Materials, Boltzmannstraße 15, D-85747 Garching, Germany

David A. Clifton
Institute of Biomedical Engineering, Department of Engineering Science, University of Oxford, Oxford OX2 6DP, UK

Davide Morelli
Institute of Biomedical Engineering, Department of Engineering Science, University of Oxford, Oxford OX2 6DP, UK
Biobeats Group LTD, 3 Fitzhardinge Street, London W1H 6EF, UK

Massimo Cairo
Biobeats Group LTD, 3 Fitzhardinge Street, London W1H 6EF, UK

Alessio Rossi
Computer Science Department, University of Pisa, Largo Bruno Pontecorvo 3, 56127 Pisa, Italy

Samanta Rosati, Gabriella Balestra and Marco Knaflitz
Department of Electronics and Telecommunications, Politecnico di Torino, 10129 Torino, Italy

Katharina Stollenwerk and André Hinkenjann
Hochschule Bonn-Rhein Sieg, Institute of Visual Computing, 53757 Sankt Augustin, Germany

Jonas Müller and Björn Krüger
Gokhale Method Institute, Stanford, CA 94305, USA

Index